EATING DISORDER

3 BOOKS IN 1

Emotional Eating, Intuitive Eating And Mindful Eating. An Ultimate Guide To Healthy Eating And Living.

TABLE OF CONTENT

INTRODUCTION

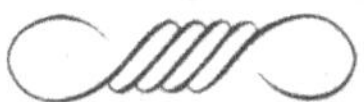

If you could trade out each diet like a frequent flyer program, the vast majority of us would have earned a free trip to the moon and back. The $60 billion per year weight loss industry could finance such a trip for a long time even unto future generations. Amusingly, we appear to have more regard for our expensive automobiles than for ourselves. If you took your vehicle to an auto repairman for normal check-ups, and after time and cash spent, the vehicle continued with its faults, you wouldn't be hard on yourself, right? However, regardless of the way that 90 to 95 percent of all weight loss routines and diets perform below expectations —you will always blame yourself, not the diet! Is it accurate to say it isn't unexpected that, with a high disappointment rate for various weight loss and diet routines—we don't blame the dieting process?

At first, when we wandered into the world of private practice, we didn't have any acquaintance with one another. However, independently, every one of us had strikingly comparative encounters that made us re-examine how we work. This prompted an extensive change in the way we practice and years after; that fact was the driving force for this book.

In spite of the fact that we rehearsed independently of one another, unconsciously, every one of us began by making a promise to maintain a strategic distance from the trap of working with weight control. We would not like to deal with an issue that was just set up to fail in the long run. Be that as it may, while we attempted to stay away from weight reduction programs, doctors continued referring their patients to us. Normally, their blood pressure or cholesterol was high. Whatever their clinical issues were, weight reduction was believed to be the fastest route of treatment. Since we needed to support these patients, we set out on the weight reduction program with a promise to do it better than we had in the past; the major aim was that our patients would succeed. They would be among that 5 to 10 percent success ratio.

We created simple but healthy meal plans based on our patients' preferences, ways of life, and explicit needs. These plans depended on the broadly accepted "exchange system" regularly utilized for diabetic meal plans and weight control. We disclosed to them this was not a diet routine, for even in those days, we realized weight control plans didn't work. We acknowledged that these meal plans were not low-calorie diets since patients could pick chicken, turkey, fish, or lean meat. They could have a bagel, a biscuit, or toast. If they truly needed a treat, they could have one (not five!). They could top off with "free snacks and food" aplenty, so they never needed to feel hungry.

We explained to them that, if they had a craving for a specific food, they could feel free to eat it without feeling guilty. In any case, we likewise advised delicately, yet firmly, that adhering to their customized meal plans would assist them with accomplishing their goals. As the weeks passed, our customers were anxious to please us and strictly followed their meal plans. We weighed them every week; eventually, they met their weight loss target. Regrettably, sometime later, we began getting calls from a good number of these same individuals explaining to us why they desperately needed our services again.

Some way or another, the weight had returned. Their calls were apologetic and persuasive. For reasons unknown, they couldn't stay on track any longer. Perhaps they required somebody to monitor them. Perhaps they needed more restraint. Possibly they simply weren't great at this type of thing, and unquestionably, they felt remorseful and discouraged. Regardless of the "disappointment," our patients put all the blames on themselves. All things considered, they confided in us—we were the "incredible nutritionists" who had helped them shed pounds. Consequently, they had done something wrong, not us. As time went on, it turned out to be evident that something was exceptionally amiss with this weight loss approach.

The entirety of our well-meaning goals was just fortifying some extremely negative, self-destroying ideas that our patients had about themselves—that they didn't have discretion, they couldn't do it accordingly, they were awful or wrong. This prompted blame, blame, and more blames on themselves. At this point, we had both arrived at a defining moment in the manner we counseled. How would we be able to continue showing individuals things that appeared to be logically and nutritionally stable, yet activated such passionate upheaval?

However, then again, how might we disregard an aspect of treatment that could have such a significant impact on a patient's future wellbeing? As we battled with these issues, we started to investigate a portion of the well-known literature that recommended a 180-degree rotation from dieting. It proposed a method for eating that took into consideration all kinds of food choices, without respect for nutritional values. Our underlying responses were exceptionally skeptical, if not absolutely dismissing.

We responded with self-righteous resentment. How would we be able to, as nutritionists (registered dietitians), trained to take a look at the associations among nutrition and wellbeing, endorse a method for eating that appeared to dismiss the very establishment of our philosophy and knowledge? The battle line was drawn. The healthy meal plans were not helping individuals keep up lasting weight control, yet the "toss out nutrition approach" was a hazardous alternative.

The recommendation to overlook food and dismiss how the body feels because of eating "anything you desire" limits the regard for one's body, which is the gift of life. In the long run, we settled the contention by creating the **INTUITIVE EATING PROCESS.**

This book is a link between the developing anti-diet movement and the health community. While the anti-dieting movement counters dieting and hails accepting your body the way it is (fortunately), it frequently neglects to address health dangers. How would you reconcile junk diet issues and still eat healthy meals, while you are not dieting? We will reveal to you how in this book.

If you are like the vast majority of our customers, you are tired of dieting but then alarmed by eating too much. A good number of our clients are uncomfortable in their bodies—however, they don't have a clue how to change for the better.

Intuitive Eating gives another method for eating that is ultimately stress-free and sound for your mind and body. It is a process that releases the shackles of abstaining from excessive food intake (which can prompt hardship, resistance, and rebound weight gain). It implies returning to your underlying foundations—confiding in your body and its signals. Intuitive Eating won't just change your association with food; it might completely change you. We trust that Intuitive Eating will make a huge difference in your life—it has for our customers. Indeed, when our customers discovered that we were writing this book, they were ready to share some particular defining moments with you:

• "Make certain to reveal to them that, if they have a craving, it can end up being an incredible encounter, since they'll find out a lot about their contemplations and emotions because of such cravings."

• "Disclose to them that taking an opportunity to check whether they're hungry doesn't imply they can't eat if they find they're not hungry. It's only an opportunity to ensure they're not eating on autopilot. If they need to eat in any case, they can!"

• "When I go to a session, I feel as though I'm heading off to see the priest for confession. That originates from every one of the occasions I used to go to the dietician, and I would need to disclose to him how I had trespassed after he had weighed me. This isn't originating from you but the internal Food Police."

"I feel like I'm out of jail. I'm free and not pondering about food all the time any longer."

"At times, I blow up, in light of the fact that good food has lost its magic on my taste buds. Nothing tastes as good as it did when it was forbidden. I continued searching for the old rush that food used to give me until I understood that my excitement in life wasn't going to originate from my eating any longer."

"With consent comes a decision. Furthermore, settling on decisions dependent on what I need and not on what another person is letting me know, feels so empowering."

"Subsequent to quitting any pretense of binging, I wound up feeling truly low a portion of the time and even angry on different occasions. I understood that the food was concealing my awful sentiments. Be that as it may, it was likewise concealing my positive sentiments. I'd preferably feel better and terrible rather than not feeling at all!"

"When I perceived the amount I was utilizing dieting and eating to adapt to life, I understood that I needed to change a portion of the stress in my life if I, at any point, needed to relinquish food as a way of dealing with stress."

"In some cases, I have hungry days, and on other days, I feel full. It's so pleasant to eat all the more some of the time and not feel remorseful that I'm conflicting with some dieting plan."

"I get so elated when I see food I used to limit. Presently, I believe—it's free, it's there, and it's mine!"

"I'm so happy you're writing this book; it will enable me to clarify what I'm doing. All I know is that it works!"

"When I'm in the diet mood, I can't consider the genuine issues in my life."

"This is simply the best I've taken care of myself in my life."

MINDFUL EATING VERSUS INTUITIVE EATING—IS THERE A DIFFERENCE?

We very frequently utilize the expression "Mindful eating" since it has gotten generally utilized and practiced by many. The Center for Mindful Eating states that mindful eating incorporates:

- • Allowing yourself to be mindful of the positive opportunities that are accessible through food preparation and utilization, by regarding your very own inner wisdom.

- • Choosing to eat meals that are both satisfying to you and nourishing to your body, by utilizing every one of your senses to explore, enjoy, and taste.

- • Acknowledging reactions to varieties of food (preferences, neutral, or aversions), without judgment.

- • Learning to know about physical hunger and satiety signs to control your choice to start eating and to quit eating. While Intuitive Eating incorporates the standards of careful eating, it likewise envelops a more extensive way of thinking, tending to the issues of intellectual distortions and emotional eating. It incorporates considering fulfillment to be a focal point in eating, physical action/development for feeling better, dismissing the counting calories mindset, utilizing sustenance data without judgment, and regarding your body, paying little respect to how you feel about its shape. Intuitive Eating is a dynamic process that involves coordinating a broader philosophy of mind, body, and nourishment. Let us show you strategic steps on how to be successful with Intuitive Eating.

CHAPTER ONE
WHAT KIND OF EATER ARE YOU?

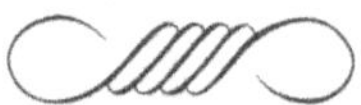

Maybe you are still abstaining from excessive food intake and don't know it! There are numerous kinds of eating styles that are unconscious types of dieting. A good number of our patients have said they were not on a diet—however, after looking into what and how they eat, they were all the while unconsciously dieting! Here's an example: Ted came on the grounds that he needed to lose weight and become fit. He said that, in his fifty years of living, he had been on just four serious diet plans.

When scrutinizing the book titles in the workplace (impulsive overeating books, emotional eating books, dietary disorder books, etc.), he expressed, "You work with a lot of real dieting disorders … well, I'm not one of those." Ted obviously didn't consider himself to be a dieter, only a cautious eater. However, it worked out that he was an oblivious dieter. In spite of the fact that Ted was not effectively dieting, he was under-eating to a level where he was almost passed out in the evening. The explanation—he had consistently been unhappy with his weight!

In the mornings, he would go for a serious bicycle ride for 60 minutes, get back home, and have a little breakfast. Lunch was generally a serving of mixed greens with frosted tea (while this sounds solid, it's excessively low in starches). By mealtime, his body would scream for carbs and good food. Ted was in an extreme calorie shortage, yet in addition, he refused to take enough carbohydrates. Nighttime transformed into a food fest! Ted thought he had a "food volume" disorder with a solid sweet tooth. In all actuality, he had an unconscious diet mindset that naturally set off his late-night eating and sweet tooth cravings.

Alicia likewise was not a conscious dieter. She came in, not to get in shape, but since she needed to build her energy level. During the earlier session, it became evident that she had complicated issues with food. So she was queried as to whether she had been dieting a great deal. She looked shocked. "How did you know that I've been on zillions of diets?"

While Alicia claimed to approve of her present weight, she was still at war with eating right; she didn't trust herself with making appropriate food choices. For reasons unknown, Alicia had been abstaining from excessive food intake since she was a child. In spite of the fact that she was not officially abstaining from excessive food intake, she held (and extended) a lot of food rules that almost deadened her capacity to eat normally. We see this constantly, the headache from dieting: keeping away from specific foods no matter what, feeling crazy the minute a "forbidden" food is eaten, feeling regretful when deliberate food rules are broken, (for example, "Thou shalt not eat after 6 P.M., etc.) unconscious dieting generally happens as meticulous dietary patterns. There can be a barely recognizable difference between eating for dieting and healthy eating. Notice how even the frozen diets, for example, Lean Cuisine and Weight Watchers, are putting their emphasis on wellbeing instead of a diet.

For whatever length of time that you are occupied with some type of dieting, you won't be free from food and stress. Regardless of whether you are a conscious or an oblivious dieter, the effects are comparative— the diet backfires impact. This is described by periods of cautious eating, "blowing-it," and paying retribution with all the more slimming down or extra-cautious eating. In this chapter, we will investigate the dieting/eating styles to help see where you are present. Afterward, you will meet the Intuitive Eater, and the Intuitive Eating style, the answer for living healthy without diets.

THE EATING PERSONALITIES

To assist you with explaining your eating style (or dieting), we have recognized the accompanying key classifications of eaters that show trademark eating designs: the Careful Eater, the Professional Dieter, and the Unconscious Eater. These eating characteristics are displayed in any event, when not formally dieting. It's conceivable to have more than one eating characteristic, despite the fact that we see that there tends to be a dominant trait.

Occasions in your life can likewise impact or move your eating character. For instance, one customer, a tax lawyer, was normally a Careful Eater; however, during charge season, he turned into the Chaotic Unconscious Eater. You may wind up, at times, having the eating qualities portrayed under the three core eating characteristics. Observe this, and if your eating personality exists in one of these domains more often than not, it very well may be a disorder. Peruse each eating personality and see which one best mirrors your eating style.

By understanding where you are present, it will get simpler to figure out how to turn into an Intuitive Eater. For instance, you may discover you have been occupied with a type of dieting and not have known about it. Or on the other hand, you may find qualities that unwittingly neutralize you.

THE CAREFUL EATER

Careful eaters are the individuals who will, in general, be cautious about what food they put into their bodies. Ted was a case of a Careful Eater (by day). Superficially, Careful Eaters give off the impression of being "flawless" eaters.

They are exceptionally food conscious. They usually appear health and wellness conscious (honorable attributes respected and reinforced in our general public).

EATING STYLE.

There is a scope of food practices that the Careful Eater shows. At one point, the Careful Eater may worry over every piece of food permitted into the body. Grocery shopping trips are spent examining food labels. Eating out regularly implies cross-examining the waiter— what's in the food, how is the food prepared—and getting affirmations that the food is prepared explicitly to the Careful Eater's admiration (generally not one bit of oil or other fat utilized in cooking).

What's wrong with this mindset? Aren't label reading and emphatic café requesting in the wellbeing interests of certain individuals? Obviously! The difference, be that as it may, is the power of the cautiousness and the capacity to relinquish any blame with respect to your eating decision. Careful Eaters tend to under-eat in small portions and screen the quality of food eaten. The Careful Eater can burn through a large portion of their waking hours arranging the next healthy snack or meal, frequently worried over what to eat.

While the Careful Eater isn't officially on a diet regimen, their brain is—scrutinizing each "undesirable," greasy, or sugary food eaten. The Careful Eater can run the scarce difference between being truly keen on health and wellbeing and eating cautiously for body image. Now and again, the Careful Eater is guided by time or events. For instance, some Careful Eaters are fastidious during the weekdays, so they acquire their "eating right" to "eat lavishly" on the weekends or for an up and coming

party. Be that as it may, ends of the week happen 104 days of the year—
the overeating can backfire with undesirable weight gain. Therefore, it's
not strange for a Careful Eater to think about going on a diet.

THE PROBLEM

There's nothing amiss with being keen on the health and well-being
of your body. The issue happens when diligent eating influences a sound
association with food—and contrarily impacts your body. Cautious
Eaters take after a chronic dieter style. They may not eat fewer carbs,
yet they examine each food for quality and quantity.

THE PROFESSIONAL DIETER

Professional dieters are simpler to recognize; they are always
dieting. They have typically attempted the most recent commercial diet,
diet book, or new weight reduction trick. Now and again, abstaining
from excessive food intake happens through fasting or "cutting back."
Professional Dieters know a great deal about of nourishments, calories,
and "slimming down stunts," yet the explanation they are consistently
starting another diet routine is that the first one never worked. Today,
the Professional Dieter is likewise knowledgeable in checking
sugar/carbohydrate grams.

EATING STYLE

Professional dieters likewise have cautious eating characteristics.
The distinction, in any case, is that chronic dieters control each eating
decision for the sake of getting in shape, not really for health reasons.
When the dieter isn't formally on a diet, the person is generally
pondering on how quickly he/she can get started with the next diet. She
frequently awakens, trusting this will be a decent day—the fresh start.

While Professional Dieters have a ton of dieting information, it
doesn't work well for them. It's not irregular for them to binge or take

part in Last Meal eating the minute a forbidden food is eaten. That is on the grounds that chronic dieters genuinely accept they won't eat such food anytime soon; for tomorrow, they diet; tomorrow they begin once again with a fresh start. Better eat now; it's the last possibility. Of course, the Professional Dieter gets disappointed at the worthlessness of the endless loop. Diet, get in shape, put on weight, irregular binges, and back to dieting.

THE PROBLEM

It's difficult to live along these lines. Slimming down makes it progressively hard to shed pounds, not to mention eat refreshingly. Chronic under-eating typically brings about indulging or occasional binges. For some Professional Dieters, the disappointment of getting in shape turns out to be escalated to the point that they may attempt laxatives, diuretics, and diet pills. What's more, because these "diet aids" don't work, they may attempt outrageous strategies, for example, ceaseless limiting, as anorexia nervosa, or purging, (for example, vomiting after a binge), like bulimia.

While anorexia and bulimia are multi-factorial and established in psychological disorders, a growing body of research has shown that chronic dieting is not uncommon with dieting disorders. One study specifically found that, when weight watchers arrive at the age of fifteen years, they are multiple times as liable to experience the ill effects of a dietary issue as non-dieters.

THE UNCONSCIOUS EATER

The Unconscious Eater is frequently occupied with paired eating— which is eating and doing another action simultaneously, for example, sitting in front of the TV and eating or reading and eating. Due to the nuances and absence of mindfulness, it may be hard for an individual to recognize this eating character. There are numerous subtypes of unconscious eaters. The Chaotic Unconscious Eater frequently carries on with an over-planned life, excessively occupied, such a large number of activities. The disorderly eating style is heedless; anything that's accessible will be snatched—candy machine toll, inexpensive food, it'll all do.

Nutrition and diet are frequently essential to this individual—only not in the crucial point in time of the chaos. Chaotic Eaters are regularly so bustling, putting out flames that they experience issues recognizing natural hunger until it's furiously insatiable. Of course, the unconscious eater goes on long stretches of time without eating. The Unconscious Eater is helpless against the insignificant nearness of food if very hungry or full. Sweet jolts, food lying around at gatherings, food sitting on a kitchen counter—none will, for the most part, be left behind by the unconscious Eater. More often than not, in any case, the Unconscious eater doesn't know that they are eating or the amount they are eating. For instance, the Unconscious Eater may cull up a few confections while in transit to the bathroom without monitoring it.

Social trips that rotate around food, for example, mixed drink parties and occasion buffets, are particularly extreme for the Unconscious Eater. The Unconscious Eater values every dollar used in eating. Their eating drive is frequently impacted by getting as much as they can for the cash.

The Emotional Unconscious Eater utilizes food to adapt to feelings, particularly awkward feelings, for example, stress, outrage, and dejection. While Emotional Eaters see their eating as the issue, it's regularly a side effect of a more profound issue. Eating practices of the Emotional Eater can go from snatching a sweet treat in stressful conditions to chronic compulsive binges of tremendous amounts of food.

Unconscious eating in its different structures is an issue if it brings about constant indulging (which can easily happen when you are eating and not exactly mindful of it). Remember that somewhere close to the first and last nibble of food is the place the slip by of consciousness happens. As in, "Gracious, everything is gone!" For instance, have you at any point purchased a huge box of sweets at the motion pictures and started to eat it just to find your fingers all of a sudden scratching the base of the unfilled box? That is a basic type of unconscious eating.

Yet, unconscious eating can likewise exist at a serious level, to some degree, a modified condition of eating. For this situation, the individual doesn't know about what is being eaten, why he began eating, or even how the nourishment tastes. This is daydreaming with nourishment.

In the end, the eating styles of the Careful Eater, the Professional Dieter, and the Unconscious Eater become an inadequate method for eating, in any event, when superficially, they show up OK. The answer to the frustrated eater: Try harder with another eating routine! From the start, the new diet appears to be elating and hopeful; however, inevitably, the natural weight gain returns. Abstaining from excessive food intake gets progressively troublesome, and in any event, when you continue your gauge eating character, it might feel more awkward than before.

This is on the grounds that, with each diet, the internal food rules get more grounded. These foods frequently propagate sentiments of blame about eating in any event, when you are not officially abstaining from excessive food intake (dieting). Likewise, the organic impacts of dieting make it progressively hard to have an ordinary association with food.

The Intuitive Eater character, be that as it may, is the special exception. It is the one eating style that doesn't work against your health and can assist you with chronic dieting and weight fluctuations.

INTRODUCING THE INTUITIVE EATER

Intuitive Eaters walk to their inward craving sign and eat whatever they pick without feeling guilt or any moral dilemma. The Intuitive Eater is an unaffected eater. However, it is hard to be an unaffected eater in the present health-conscious society when you think about the types of food, and weight loss messages from ads, media, food professionals, and health experts.

Whenever we portrayed the basic eating characteristics of the Intuitive Eater to our customers, it's astonishing how regularly we'll hear the reaction, "That is how my husband eats." or "That is how my girlfriend eats." When we ask how that individual's weight and relationship to food are, the reaction is "zero issues!"

Consider babies. They are the natural Intuitive Eaters—basically free from cultural messages about food and self-perception. Babies have intrinsic knowledge of food, if you don't meddle with it. They don't eat dependent on abstaining from excessive food intake rules or health, yet various studies have shown that, if you let a little child eat spontaneously, he will eat what he needs when given free access to quality meals. (This is presumably the hardest thing for a concerned parent to do—to let go and believe that children have an inborn capacity to eat!).

A milestone study, led by Leann Birch, Ph.D., published in the New England Journal of Medicine affirmed that preschool-age kids have a natural capacity to direct their eating as per their body's requirement for development. This remains constant; with every meal, the little children's eating seems, by all accounts, to be a parent's bad dream. Researchers have found out that, at a given meal, caloric intake was an exceptionally factor; however, it balanced out after some time. However, numerous guardians expect that their little youngsters can't manage their food consumption. Therefore, parents frequently embrace coercive systems trying to guarantee that the youngster eats healthy nutrition suitable for a growing child. In any case, past research by Birch and her partners demonstrates that such control strategies are counterproductive.

Besides, Birch notes that "guardians' endeavors to control their youngster's eating were accounted for more regularly by obese grown-ups than by grown-ups of normal weight." Similarly, Duke University analyst, Philip Costanzo, Ph.D., found that abundant weight in school-age kids was exceptionally connected with how much guardians attempted to limit their kids' eating. Indeed, even benevolent guardians meddle with Intuitive Eating. When a parent attempts to overrule a kid's regular eating signs, the tissue deteriorates, instead of getting better. A parent who provides food for a child at whatever point a craving signal is heard and who quits encouraging when the child shows that he's had enough can assume a powerful role in the initial development of Intuitive Eating.

Actually, notable work by specialist and dietitian Ellyn Satter has demonstrated that, if you get the parents of overweight children to back off and give them a chance to eat without parental pressure, the children will, in the end, eat less than necessary. Why? The child starts to hear and comprehend his own inward signals of craving and satiety. The youngster additionally realizes that the individual will need to access food. As indicated by Satter, "Kids denied nourishment trying to be thinly gotten distracted with food, apprehensive they won't get enough to eat and are inclined to binge when they find the opportunity." We have seen this as valid for grown-up dieters too. Only for grown-ups, the Intuitive Eating process has been covered for quite a while, regularly a long time.

Rather than having a parent slacken the pressure, this relaxing of weight needs to originate from inside and against society's fantasy of dieting and distorted body worship. Luckily, we all have the characteristic Intuitive Eating capacity; it's simply been suppressed, particularly by regular dieting. This book is dedicated to telling you the best way to stir the Intuitive Eater within you!

HOW YOUR INTUITIVE EATER GETS BURIED

As babies get somewhat older, the mixed messages start to sneak in—from the early impacts of the Saturday morning commercial to the good-natured parent who cajoles his youngster to "Clean your plate." The coercion doesn't stop when you are a kid. There are a few external powers that impact our eating, which can additionally bury Intuitive Eating.

You have just observed the harm that chronic dieting plays, including but not limited to:

Increased binge-eating

Decreased metabolic rate

Increased distraction with food

Increased sentiments of deprivation

Increased feeling of disappointment

Decreased feeling of self-discipline

This alone serves to erode your trust with food and urges you to depend on outside sources to direct your eating patterns (a meal plan, a diet, the hour of the day, food rules, etc.). The more you go to outside sources to "judge" if your eating is under wraps, the further away you are from becoming an Intuitive Eater. Intuitive Eating depends on your inner prompts and signals.

EAT HEALTHY-OR-DIE MESSAGES.

Messages about eating healthily are all over, from philanthropic health organizations to food companies touting the medical advantages of their particular item. The innate message? What you eat can improve your wellbeing. On the other hand, take one wrong move (nibble), and you're one bit nearer to the grave. Is this an exaggeration? No. For instance, a 1994 official statement released by the Harvard School of Public Health expressed that eating trans-unsaturated fats (found in margarine) may cause thirty thousand deaths every year in the U.S. from coronary illness. That sort of message can easily leave you feeling remorseful for eating "an inappropriate" food and feeling confounded about what you ought to eat.

Magazines and papers have additionally significantly expanded their inclusion of nutrition and wellbeing. One food editorial manager, Joe Crea, of a significant metropolitan paper, the Orange County Register (California), noticed that in a six-year timeframe (1987–1993), his accounts on nutrition increased fivefold. Of about 800 nutrition stories, 200 were on health-related issues. While there is no uncertainty that what you eat can affect your wellbeing, the exponential media inclusion has filled in as a course to building nutrition distrustfulness in the buyer, particularly the dieter.

Joe Crea agrees, "You open the paper, see a wonderful lead story about cheesecake, and at the same time, another piece on how indulging in it will make you fat. It places the confusion in strife." Are we saying you ought to overlook the virtues of healthy eating? Of course not. Nonetheless, when you have a "weight loss" mindset, the torrent of "good dieting" messages can make you feel guiltier about the food you decide to eat.

Obesity and Health announced a study on 2,075 grown-ups in Florida that uncovered that 45 percent of grown-ups felt regretful in the wake of eating foods they like. Women might be particularly guilt-ridden. An American Dietetic Association survey demonstrated that ladies feel guiltier than men about the nourishment they eat (44 percent versus 28 percent). Could this be on the grounds that ladies diet more often than men? Or then again, maybe ladies are normally the objective of health messages and food advertisements (think about the number of ladies' magazines).

Ladies are the key leaders for the family's health and nutrition planning and are typically the watchmen of food and nutrition issues; also, they fill in as a practical objective. We have discovered that setting up nourishment or good dieting as an underlying need in the Intuitive Eating process is counterproductive. To start, we disregard nutrition, since it meddles with relearning how to turn into an Intuitive Eater. Nutrition heresy? No. It's conceivable to regard and respect quality food choices. It can't be the principal need when you've been dieting for your entire life. Or then again take a look at it along these lines; if you have concentrated all your thoughts on dieting, has it made any significant difference? The most nutritious eating plan (absolute) can be embraced as another type of dieting. The rest of this book will tell you bit by bit the best way to turn into an Intuitive Eater.

CHAPTER TWO
AROUSING THE INTUITIVE EATER: STAGES

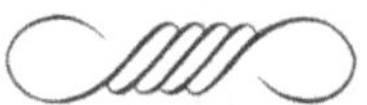

The journey to Intuitive Eating resembles taking a cross-country trip. Before you even lash on your climbing boots, you need to realize what's in for your store during your adventure. While a guide is useful, it doesn't portray what you'll have to know to be sufficiently prepared, for example, trail conditions, atmosphere, uncommon touring spots, what sort of clothes to wear, etc. The motivation behind this section is to enable you to comprehend what's in store during your voyage to Intuitive Eating.

Regardless of whether it's climbing or relearning a more fulfilling eating style, you will experience numerous phases en route. The measure of time that you have to remain in a specific stage is variable and profoundly individualized. For instance, crossing new hiking trails relies upon how physically fit you are, the manner by which you manage dread of new trails, how much time you need to climb, and the accessibility of climbing trails. Essentially, your adventure back to Intuitive Eating relies upon to what extent you've been dieting, how emphatically entrenched your diet thinking is, to what extent you've been utilizing nourishment to adapt to life, so that you are so ready to confide in yourself and you are so ready to make weight reduction an optional objective and figure out how to turn into an Intuitive Eater, which is the essential objective.

Here and there, you'll move to and fro among the stages. If you acknowledge this is a normal part of the process, it will assist you to keep going without feeling that you are breaking faith or not gaining ground.

Think about this situation: You are on a hiking trail and experience a byway that is difficult to interpret with your trail map. Do you go to right or left? You contemplate for some time and choose to go left. While strolling, you spot something you've never observed, a splendid green caterpillar shimmying up a purple blossom. A couple of steps ahead, you find an unusual bird. In any case, a couple of steps past these wonders of nature is a major rock flagging that you picked an inappropriate way. You pivot, return to the fork, and take the other way. Was this alternate route an exercise in futility? No. Thus, on the way to Intuitive Eating, you will take many turns and examinations with new musings and practices.

Intuitive Eating is altogether different from dieting. Dieters generally get disappointed when they don't pursue the dieting precisely as recommended. We have seen numerous chronic dieters simply go astray at one meal, be critical for that error, and "blow" the dieting for that day or weekend or significantly more! Remember that the journey to Intuitive Eating is a process complete with high points and low points, in contrast to dieting, when the regular desire is straight progress (losing a specific measure of weight in a particular time span).

The way to Intuitive Eating resembles "investing in a long-term mutual fund." After some time, there will be a return on the interest, regardless of the day by day fluctuations of the securities exchange. Such should be normal and anticipated. How amusing that we have been instructed in economic matters, the everyday changes in the securities exchange are typical, and there is rarely a speedy get-rich fix, yet in the weight reduction business, "get slim quick" is regularly observed as the main objective for success.

Remember Webster's meaning of process: "a continued improvement involving numerous changes," and "a specific strategy for accomplishing something, by and large including various operations or activities." As with any process, it's essential to remain centered in the present and develop from the numerous encounters you will experience. Assuming, nonetheless, you focus on the final product (which for a great many people is the number of calories or pounds lost), it can make you feel discouraged and overwhelmed and wind up disrupting the process. Rather, if you recognize little changes en route and value the learning process (which can be stressful), it will assist you with remaining on the Intuitive Eating way and pushing ahead. When you really become an Intuitive Eater, your body will come back to its regular weight ' level and stay there. For some individuals, that implies shedding pounds.

To see whether you are a good candidate for weight reduction, ask yourself these questions:

Have you routinely eaten past your agreeable fullness level?

Do you routinely indulge when you're preparing for your next diet (knowing there will be a lot of meals you won't be permitted to eat)?

Do you indulge as a method for dealing with stress in troublesome occasions or to top off time when you're exhausted?

Have you likewise been impervious to work out?

Do you possibly practice when you diet?

Do you skip suppers or stand by to eat until you're eagerly very hungry, possibly to find that you indulge when you at long last eat?

Do you feel regretful, either when you binge or when you eat an "a wrong meal," which brings about all the more indulging?

If you answered "yes" to a few or all of these inquiries, then, all things considered, you will come back to your natural healthy weight after this process. When you've quit any pretense of slimming down perpetually, you'll end up eating far less nourishment and needing to exercise consistently. You'll see that your body feels so much better when your stomach isn't overloaded, when your muscles are conditioned, and your heart is fit.

If you focus on how you feel, instead of weight reduction, you'll find, unexpectedly, that you can't resist the urge to get in shape; rather, you will keep concentrating on weight reduction as the objective. You'll get tied up in the old eating routine mindset, thinking and searching for that perfect weight reduction resembling a carrot dangling on that stick before you—you're always dieting without being successful. Throughout the years, we have seen that our patients experience a five-step movement in figuring out how to become Intuitive Eaters.

The next section will assist you with getting a thought of what's in store on your personal journey to intuitive eating.

STAGE ONE: READINESS—HITTING DIET BOTTOM

This is the point where many people start. You are painfully mindful that each endeavor to get in shape has ended in disappointment. You are burnt out on valuing every day, depending on whether the scale is up or down a pound or two (or if you've overeaten the day preceding). You think about food constantly. You talk about the unhealthy and restrictive food talk—"If only I didn't need to watch my weight, I could eat that," or "1 had two snacks—I was quite awful at my weight game today."

Your weight could can be categorized as one of three examples: It's higher than any time in recent times; you are stuck at a level, and the pounds won't shed; or while not significantly overweight, you pick up and lose five or ten pounds much of the time. You have put some distance between biological appetite and satiety signals. You have overlooked what you truly prefer to eat and rather eat what you figure you "should" eat. Your association with food has built up a negative tone, and you fear eating the meals you love since it might be difficult to stop.

When you surrender to the temptation of the "forbidden foods," it's not surprising to binge since you already feel regretful.

However, you earnestly promise you will never eat them again. It's not uncommon to find that you eat to comfort, occupy, or even numb yourself from your emotions. If that is the situation, you will detect that a mind-blowing quality of life has been truncated by obsessive thoughts about nourishment and by thoughtless eating. You already developed a negative opinion about your body image—you don't care for the manner in which you look and feel in your body, and your sense of pride is diminished. You have gained from your own experience that slimming down doesn't work—you have wound up in a sorry situation and feel stuck, baffled, and disheartened.

This stage continues until you conclude that you are troubled eating and living along these lines—and you are prepared to take care of business. Your first considerations may veer toward finding another eating routine to take care of your issues. Be that as it may, very quickly, you understand that you can't do that until the end of time. If this is the place you find yourself, at that point, you are prepared for the procedure that will take you back to eating naturally.

STAGE TWO: EXPLORATION—CONSCIOUS LEARNING AND PURSUIT OF PLEASURE

This is a phase of discovery and exploration. You will experience a period of hyper consciousness to help reacquaint yourself with your Intuitive sign: hunger, taste inclinations, and satiety. This stage is a lot like figuring out how to drive a vehicle. For the new driver, simply getting the vehicle out of the carport requires a lot of conscious deductions, complete with a psychological checklist:

Put the key in the start, ensure the gear is in park or neutral, turn on the ignition, check the rearview mirror, remove the hand brake, etc. This hyper consciousness is important to secure the entirety of the means required just to get that vehicle in first gear! In a similar sense, you will focus in on the details of eating that have advanced without such focused reasoning (this is important to discover the Intuitive Eater in you). It might appear to be cumbersome and awkward, even over the top.

In any case, hyper consciousness is unique in relation to over the top reasoning. Fanatical believing is inescapable and is described by stress. It fills your psyche during the day and shields you from considering anything else. Hyperconsciousness is more explicit. It zooms in when you have an idea about food, however, leaves when the eating experience is finished. Also, much the same as the means required to drive a vehicle become autopilot for the experienced driver, Intuitive Eating will, in the long run, be experienced without this underlying awkwardness. You may feel that you are in a hyperconscious state for a significant part of the time during this stage. This may feel awkward from the outset and maybe even weird. Keep in mind, a lot of your past eating was either, for the most part, oblivious or diet-coordinated.

In this stage, you'll start to make peace with food by giving yourself unrestricted permission to eat. This part may feel alarming, and you may decide to move gradually (within your comfort zone). You will figure out how to dispose of guilt-induced eating and start to find the significance of the fulfillment factor with food.

The more fulfilled you are when eating, the less you will consider nourishment when you are not hungry—you will never again be lurking in the shadows. You will try different things with nourishments that you have not eaten for quite a while. This incorporates dealing with your actual nourishment of different preferences. You may even find that you don't care for the flavor of a portion of the foods you've been longing for! (Remember that long periods of counting calories or eating what you "should," just serve to separate you from your inside eating drive and genuine nourishment inclinations).

You will figure out how to respect your appetite and understand your body signals that show the numerous degrees of craving. You will figure out how to isolate these natural signs from the enthusiastic sign that may likewise trigger eating. In this stage, you may find that you are eating larger amounts of nourishments than your body needs. It will be hard to regard your completion at this stage since you need time to explore different avenues regarding the amount it takes to fulfill a denied sense of taste. It likewise requires some investment for you to create trust with nourishment again and realize that it's genuinely alright to eat.

How might you respect fullness if you are not totally sure it's alright to eat a specific nourishment or if you dread it won't be there tomorrow? During this stage, weight gain normally stops or is constrained to only a few pounds. If you have been utilizing food emotionally, you may find that you start to feel your emotions and may encounter distress, trouble, or even sorrow now and again. The greater part of your eating might be in foods that are heavier in fat and sugar than you've been familiar with—despite the fact that you may have been eating huge amounts of these foods unintentionally or with guilt. The manner in which you eat during this stage won't be the example that you will set up or need for a lifetime. You will see that your wholesome parity is unbalanced, and you may not feel physically in control during this time.

This is all normal and anticipated. You should release yourself through this phase for whatever length of time that you need. Keep in mind; you are compensating for a considerable length of time of hardship, negative self-talk, and blame. You are modifying positive nourishment encounters, similar to a strand of pearls. Every nourishment experience, similar to each pearl, may appear to be irrelevant, yet on the whole, they have any kind of effect.

STAGE THREE: CRYSTALLIZATION

In this stage, you will encounter the first arousals of the Intuitive Eating style that has consistently been a part of you, yet was covered under the thought of dieting. When you enter this stage, a significant part of the investigation work from the past stage starts to solidify and feels like big conduct change. Your considerations about foods are never again excessive. You barely need to keep up the hyper consciousness about eating that was initially required. Therefore, your eating choices don't require a lot of coordinated ideas. Rather, you find that your meal decisions and reactions to biological signals are primarily intuitive.

You have a more prominent feeling of trust—both in your entitlement to pick what you truly want to eat and in the way your biological signals are reliable. You are more comfortable with your food decisions and will begin to enjoy true fulfillment at your mealtimes. Now, you respect your craving more often, and it's simpler to observe what you want to eat when you are hungry. You keep making peace with nourishment. What feels new in this stage is that it's simpler to stop amidst your meal to intentionally measure how much of your stomach is filling up.

You will be able to understand when you are full and regard the presence of that signal, despite the fact that you may find that you regularly eat past the fullness mark. The same principle applies when an archer focuses on another objective; it regularly requires shooting numerous arrows before figuring out how to hit the bull's eye. You may be picking heavier foods more often than not, yet you will find that you don't require as much to fulfill you.

If you've been an emotional eater, you'll become proficient at isolating biological hunger signals from emotional hunger. In view of this clarity, as a rule, you will encounter your feelings and discover approaches to comfort and occupy yourself without the utilization of food. Some weight reduction may happen during this stage, particularly if you have a lot of weight to lose. If not, you'll see that you're keeping up your weight instead of dealing with weight issues here and there. However, more significant than weight reduction, at this stage, is the feeling of prosperity and strengthening that starts to happen. You won't feel powerless and miserable any longer. You will start to regard your body and comprehend that it is at this place because of the dieting attitude, as opposed to the absence of self-discipline.

STAGE FOUR: THE INTUITIVE EATER AWAKENS

When you arrive at this stage, all the work you have been doing comes full circle in an agreeable, free-flowing eating style. You reliably pick what you truly need to eat when you are eager. Since you realize that you can have more nourishment, based on your personal preference, at whatever point you are hungry, it's anything but difficult to quit eating when you feel full. You will start to find that you pick lighter and more beneficial nourishments, not on the grounds that you figure you should but since you feel better physically when you eat along these lines. The dire need to demonstrate to yourself that you can have heavier nourishments will have decreased. You genuinely know and trust that these once illegal foods will consistently be there, and if you truly need to eat them, you can—so they lose their charming quality.

Chocolate begins to take on a similar emotional undertone as a peach. You won't have to test yourself any longer, and your deprivation troubles will be no more. When you do pick heavier foods, you will get extraordinary delight and feel happy with littler amount than any time in recent memory and without guilt.

If adapting to your emotions has been hard for you, you will be less reluctant to encounter them and become progressively capable of sitting with them. Finding solid choices to divert and comfort yourself when fundamental will get normal for you. Your self-talk will be certain and non-judgmental. Your peace agreement with nourishment is immovably settled, and you will have discharged any contention or left-over blame about nourishment decisions that you have conveyed. You will have quit being furious with your body and making disrespectful remarks about it. You will regard it and acknowledge that there is a wide range of sizes and shapes on the planet. Now, weight reduction will turn out to be progressively obvious, and your body will be en route to moving toward its common weight.

STAGE FIVE: THE FINAL STAGE—TREASURE THE PLEASURE

Now, your Intuitive Eater has been recovered. You will confide in your body's Intuitive capacities—it will be anything but difficult to respect your appetite and regard your completion. At last, you will feel no blame about your nourishment decisions or amounts. Since you like your relationship to nourishment and fortune the delight that eating presently gives you, you will dispose of uninspiring eating circumstances and unappealing food sources. You will need to encounter eating in the most ideal of conditions and not pollute it with emotional stress. You will feel an inward conviction to quit any pretense of utilizing nourishment to adapt to enthusiastic circumstances if that has been your habit. You will find that you would much rather manage your sentiments or occupy yourself from them with something besides nourishment when feelings become excessively overpowering.

Since your eating style has become a wellspring of joy instead of a source of worry, you will see nutrition and exercise in a new way. The weight of the exercise activity will be lifted, and practicing will start to look alluring to you. Exercise will never again be utilized as the main impetus to consume more calories; rather, you become resolved to practice as an approach to feel much improved, physically and rationally.

Similarly, quality nutrition will never again be another system for making you feel terrible about the manner in which you eat; rather, it turns into a way to feel as physically great and sound as you can. When you arrive at the last stage, your weight will normally diminish (if you had weight to lose) to a spot that is comfortable and fitting for your stature. If your weight was normal, you would find that you can keep up it with no exertion and will be freed of the emotional good and bad times that go with the restriction/binging cycles. Finally, you will feel engaged and shielded from external powers revealing to you what and the amount to eat and how your body should look. You will feel free of the weight of counting calories. Furthermore, you will become an Intuitive Eater in every respect!

YOU CAN DO IT!

These stages and the progressions that happen with your eating and thoughts may appear to be unimaginable. Or on the other hand, they may appear to be excessively scary to follow through. For instance, the idea of giving yourself unending permission to eat may appear to be startling—and you may expect that you will never quit eating and will put on more weight. The rest of this book clarifies in extraordinary detail how to actualize every guideline, why it is required, and the basis behind it. You will likewise discover how other chronic dieters became Intuitive Eaters and how it transformed them. When you are done reading this book, you will realize that you also can turn into an Intuitive Eater and stop the madness associated with dieting.

CHAPTER THREE
REJECT THE DIET MENTALITY

Toss out the diet books and magazine articles that offer you the false teachings for getting thinner rapidly, effectively, and for all time. Reject the falsehoods that have driven you to feel as though you were a disappointment each time a new a diet quit working for you and you regained the entirety of the lost weight. If you permit even one little hope to believe that another and better diet may be hiding around the corner, it will keep you from allowing yourself to rediscover Intuitive Eating.

If you're like most customers we see, the possibility of not dieting can be terrifying, in any event, when you realize that you can't force down one more diet plan or drink. It's entirely expected to feel panicky about relinquishing dieting, particularly when everyone around you is on a diet. It has been the main instrument you have known to get more fit, though briefly.

Winding up in a real diet, the predicament is a paralyzing feeling—one where you are doomed if you diet and accursed if you don't. A good number of our customers feel stuck between these two clashing feelings of fear: "If I keep dieting, I'll ruin my digestion and put on weight," and "If I quit dieting, I'll put on more weight." Other normal apprehensions that we hear are:

FEAR: If I quit dieting, I won't quit eating.

REALITY: Dieting regularly triggers indulging.

Obviously, it's difficult to quit eating when you've been under-eating and restricting good nutrition; it's an ordinary reaction to starvation. But once your body learns, and believes, that you won't starve it any longer through dieting, the extreme drive for eating will diminish.

FEAR: I don't have a clue about how to eat when I'm not dieting.

REALITY: When you quit dieting and become an Intuitive Eater, you will eat in light of an inward flag, which will manage your eating. This resembles figuring out how to swim just because. The feeling of being surrounded by water can be unnerving to the beginner swimmer, particularly when completely submerged.

Likewise, being encompassed by food can be startling to the interminable dieter, who is figuring out how to eat once more. Yet, you won't figure out how to swim by simply remaining at the edge of the pool (even while accepting that figuring out how to swim is something worth being thankful for). First, you start by considering going all in and figuring out how to take in the water. In the end, you will place your head in the water when you are prepared—and you get increasingly agreeable.

FEAR: I will be out of control.

REALITY: You will feel in charge through Intuitive Eating, as opposed to depending on external factors and authority figures that you will undoubtedly resist. You will figure out how to tune in to and respect your inward signs, both physical and passionate—an incredible capacity.

THE DIET VOID

For some individuals, dieting has been an approach to adapt to life, from time to practicing a similarity to control. Think about the occasions throughout your life in which you started a diet. How regularly did your dieting harmonize with difficult transitions or moments? It's not bizarre to start a diet during the accompanying life transitions: going from childhood to adolescence, leaving home, wedding, beginning a new job or encountering marital troubles. While counting calories may have been useless, it offered fervor and expectation—the invigoration of brisk weight reduction and the energy of watching the scale inch downwards, the expectation that this diet will be it. It's like setting off to a beautician for another cut, with the desire that it will alter the way you look and feel about yourself and perhaps transform you. However, when you bid farewell to the rush and fervor of dieting, you'll likewise be relinquishing the bogus expectation and dissatisfactions from dieting.

There is a social component to dieting that you may miss, diet holding. When you choose to quit any pretense of abstaining from excessive food intake, you may be shocked how frequently new diets and dieting are the themes of discussion at parties, with companions, at work—and now you won't play that game. It may feel like an unquestionable requirement, like the motion picture everybody is discussing, just you haven't seen it and have no designs to see it. You may feel somewhat left out, isolated. Keep in mind, as long as there is cash to be made, there will consistently be another program or diet for a fast weight reduction fix.

PSEUDO-DIETING

A considerable lot of our customers state, "I've quit all forms of dieting"; however, they experience difficulty shaking off the diet attitude. They might be physical off a diet. However, the dieting contemplations remain. The issue is those dieting thoughts, as a rule, convert into a diet like practice, which becomes pseudo-dieting or oblivious abstaining from excessive food intake. So, these customers will, in any case, endure the symptoms of dieting, yet it's a lot harder to spot (and afterward they truly feel wild with their eating).

Pseudo-dieting practices are not typically obvious to the individual occupied with them. Remember that eating is universal, which makes it difficult to be objective. It very well may be hard to discover the loopholes in your eating mindset/conduct if you don't have the foggiest idea of what you are searching for. To the shock of our customers, they frequently don't find that they have been pseudo-dieting until together we audit their eating history. Here are a few instances of pseudo-dieting :

Meticulously checking sugar grams is the advanced adaptation of counting calories. While being aware of what you eat has its merits, the demonstration of checking starch grams to control weight is actually the same as counting calories. A considerable lot of our constant calorie counters are geniuses at rationing their starch grams for the afternoon— and they are trapped.

Eating just "safe" foods. This typically implies staying with fat-free as well as low-calorie meals, beyond calculating fat grams. For instance, one customer would not eat any food that recorded more than one gram of fat on the food label, paying little attention to what her complete fat and calorie admission for the day was. Keep in mind, notwithstanding, that one meal, one snack, or one day won't represent the truth of your health status or your weight.

Eating just at specific times of the day, regardless of whether you are hungry, is a normal habit from dieting, particularly not eating after a specific time of night, for example, after 6:00 P.M.

Reality: Our bodies don't punch clocks; we don't, all of a sudden, reduce our requirement for energy. This can particularly be an issue for a dieter who practices after work, returns home late—around 7:30 P.M.— and chooses it's past the point where it is possible to eat for fear that the fat meter is in high gear! While it is sensible not to have any desire to want to hit the bed on a full stomach, to deny a hungry body any food or energy requirements is preposterous. Paying penance for eating "bad" foods, for example, treats, cheesecake, or frozen yogurt. The punishment can include skipping the next meal, eating less, vowing to be "great" tomorrow, or doing additional exercise.

Cutting back on food, particularly when feeling fat or for a unique occasion, for example, a wedding or class get-together. While cutting back sounds guiltless enough, it's stunning how frequently this gets carried on as oblivious under-eating. Keep in mind, under-eating as a rule triggers indulging.

Pacifying hunger by drinking espresso or diet pop. This is a typical slimming down stunt to mollify food cravings without eating or calories.

Limiting carbohydrates: We are struck by the number of customers who claim they are aware of the significance of devouring this fuel, yet eat a lacking measure of starches, for example, bread, pasta, and rice, since they are afraid they will put on weight.

Putting on a "false food face" out in the open, eating just what is "legitimate" before other individuals. One customer, Alice, ate an agreeable meal with companions. When the treat plate came around, she truly needed a bit of pie, yet battled the desire since she needed to give an impression of being a sound, chronic dieter. Be that as it may, on her way home, the desire for the pie expands into a wild hankering. Alice stopped at the store, purchased an entire pie, and ate one-fourth of it, which was more than she would have eaten had she respected her actual food inclination before that moment!

Competing with another person who is dieting —feeling committed to being similarly serious-minded (if not more). Since dieting is seen as a temperate characteristic in our general public, it isn't surprising that you would get sucked into seeming upright. This can easily happen when companions, family, or a noteworthy other is abstaining from excessive food intake.

Second-guessing or passing judgment on what you have the right to eat depends on what you've eaten before in the day, as opposed to hunger signals. One customer, Sally, ate two huge bowls of puffed rice grain for breakfast, subsequent to running for 60 minutes. She felt that was an excessive amount of nourishment and, later in the midmorning, didn't enable herself to eat, in spite of the fact that she was hungry. Sally figured, "How might I be hungry just two hours after I had a major breakfast?" The truth for Sally was that, while her volume of food toward the beginning of the day was bigger than her standard, it was as yet insufficient for the measure of activity she had done. Her body was attempting to advise her, "I need more fuel," yet Sally felt remorseful for being hungry. She additionally felt regretful for having a major breakfast, until she understood that, in reality, she had under-eaten. Because a feast or bite doesn't fit the "standard" size from your dieting days, it doesn't mean you are indulging!

Becoming a veggie-lover just to get thinner. A vegetarian's way of life can be a sound method for eating and living, yet if it is understood with a diet attitude, it turns out to be only another diet. For instance, Karen started eating meatless to get more fit. Yet, a month into her veggie lover eating, she started desiring meat. At no other time had she encountered meat desires! Karen acknowledged she never truly planned to turn into a veggie lover. She wasn't keen on vegetarian eating for wellbeing or moral issues, just as a vehicle to get more fit; thus, her dieting exploded.

THE DIETER'S DILEMMA

Whether you are occupied with genuine dieting or pseudo-dieting, any type of dieting will undoubtedly prompt issues. The Dieter's Dilemma is activated with the craving to be slim, which prompts abstaining from excessive food intake. That is the point at which the quandary unfurls. Dieting builds yearnings and inclinations for nourishment. The dieter surrenders to the cravings, and in the long run, regains any shed pounds. At that point, he has returned to where he began, at the first weight—or higher. What's more, by and by, the dieter wants to be thin; thus, another diet starts. The Dieter's Dilemma is propagated and deteriorates with each turn of the cycle. The dieter gets heavier and gets a handle on a greater amount of control with eating. How would you break the pointless Dieter's Dilemma? In spite of the fact that the anti-dieting development is developing in prominence, there is constantly another dieting or program around the corner. You should essentially settle on the choice to quit any form of dieting.

THE MOST EFFECTIVE METHOD TO REJECT THE DIET MENTALITY

To relinquish the dieting legend and the slimming down mentality, our minds require another frame. In his best-seller book, The 7 Habits of Highly Effective People, writer Stephen Covey advanced the idea of how we see and understand the world around us. A paradigm is a model or reference by which we see and comprehend the world. In the realm of weight management, slimming down is the social paradigm by which we endeavor to control our weight.

A change in outlook is a break from the norm of cultures with old perspectives, with old ideal models. We should change our mindset to "I refuse to diet"; at exactly that point would we be able to construct a sound association with food and our bodies. While Covey's work is known in the business network, he hits upon an issue that sounds accurate for ceaseless dieters. He accepts that individuals are regularly attracted to cure the issue regardless of the long-term implications of this "handy solution." He feels that this methodology really worsens the issue instead of understanding it. He identified the physical body like a prized resource that frequently is destroyed, while one is on the race for fast outcomes and transient advantages. Here are the means of starting your change in perspective and dismissing the diet mentality.

STEP I: RECOGNIZE AND ACKNOWLEDGE THE DAMAGE THAT DIETING CAUSES

There is a significant number of research on the health issues caused by dieting. Recognize that the damage is genuine, and that continued dieting will just worsen your issues. A portion of the key symptoms can be put in two classes, emotional and biological. As you read, take personal stock and inquire from yourself which of the issues you are encountering. Knowing that dieting is the issue will assist you with getting through the wrong cultural myth that diets work. Keep in mind, if dieting is the issue, how might it be a piece of the grand solution?

HARM FROM DIETING: BIOLOGICAL AND HEALTH

In every century, starvation has existed. Unfortunately, this is genuine even today. Survival of the fittest in the past meant survival of the fastest—just those with satisfactory energy stores (fat) could endure starvation. Therefore, our bodies are as yet prepared in this cutting edge age to battle starvation at the cell level. To the extent the body is concerned, dieting is a type of starvation, despite the fact that it's intentional. Constant slimming down has been shown to:

Teach the body to hold increasing fat when you start eating once more. Low-calorie diets are the catalysts that make and store fat in the body. This is a type of organic remuneration to enable the body to store more vitality, or fat, in the wake of dieting. Slow weight reduction with each progressive endeavor to abstain from food. This has been demonstrated to be valid in both rodent and human studies.

Decrease digestion - Dieting triggers the body to turn out to be progressively effective at using calories by bringing down the body's requirement for vitality

Increase binges and cravings - People and rodents have been shown to indulge after chronic food restriction. Food restriction animates the mind to dispatch a course of desire to eat more. After significant weight reduction, research shows that rodents lean toward eating progressively fat, while individuals have been shown to incline toward nourishments both high in fat and sugar.

Increase danger of premature death and coronary illness - A thirty-two year investigation of in excess of 3,000 people in the Framingham Heart Study has demonstrated that paying little respect to beginning weight, individuals whose weight more than once goes here and there—known as weight cycling or dieting —have a higher demise rate and double the typical danger of dying from coronary illness. These outcomes were free of cardiovascular hazard factors and remained constant whether an individual was slim or stout. The harm from dieting might be equivalent to the dangers of remaining obese. Likewise, the results of the Harvard Alumni Health Study show that individuals who lose and gain at least eleven pounds within ten years, don't live as long as individuals who keep up a steady weight.

Satiety prompts atrophy - Weight watchers, for the most part, quit eating because of self-imposed limits as opposed to internal signals of fullness. This, joined with skipping meals, can condition you to eat suppers of an increasingly bigger size.

May cause body shape to change - Dieters who ceaselessly regain the shed pounds will, in general, regain weight around the stomach. This sort of fat stockpiling increases the danger of coronary illness. Other recorded reactions include cerebral pains, menstrual inconsistencies, weariness, dry skin, and male pattern baldness.

HARM FROM DIETING:

Psychological and Emotional Psychological specialists detailed the accompanying unfriendly impacts at the Landmark 1992 National Institutes of Health, Weight Loss and Control Conference:

Dieting is connected to dietary problems.

Dieting may cause pressure or make the dieter more helpless against its effects.

Independent of body weight, dieting is connected with sentiments of disappointment, lower confidence, and social uneasiness.

The calorie counter is regularly powerless against loss of control of overeating while damaging "the guidelines" of the diet, regardless of whether there was a genuine or perceived offense of the dieting! The insignificant view of eating prohibited nourishment, paying little mind to genuine calorie content, is sufficient to trigger indulging. In a different report, therapists David Garner and Susan Wooley present a convincing defense against the significant expense of bogus expectation from dieting.

They infer that:

Dieting progressively disintegrates certainty and self-trust.

Many large people accept they couldn't have become stout except if they had some principal character shortage. Gainer and Wooley contend that, while numerous stout people may encounter gorging and sadness, these mental and social manifestations are the aftereffect of abstaining from excessive food intake. Be that as it may, these overweight people effectively decipher these side effects as additional proof of a basic issue. However, corpulent individuals don't have over the top mental unsettling influences contrasted with typical weight individuals.

STEP 2: BEWARE OF DIET-MINDSET TRAITS AND THINKING

The diet mindset surfaces in subtle forms when you choose to dismiss dieting. It's essential to perceive basic attributes of the dieting mindset; it will fill you in regarding whether you are as yet playing the dieting game. Disregard self-control, being respectful and failing.

DISREGARD WILLPOWER

While no specialist would anticipate that a patient should "will" circulatory strain to typical levels, doctors every now and again anticipate that their overweight patients should "will" their weight reduction by confining their nourishment, as per Susan Z. Yanovski, M.D. This is likewise an overall frame of mind among our customers and numerous Americans—all you need is resolution and a little discretion.

In a 1993 Gallup survey, the most widely recognized impediment to getting more fit referred to by ladies was self-control. For instance, Marilyn is a successful legal advisor who moved to the highest point of the corporate ladder. She credits hard work, determination, and self-control as being liable for her prosperity. However, when she attempted to utilize these model standards in her dieting endeavors, she was terrible at it. Whatever achievement she had accomplished in her professional life was dulled by her feeling of disappointment with eating.

For what reason was Marilyn ready to be so taught in one part of her life, however, not in the other? "Discipline" is gotten from the word "disciple." According to Stephen Covey's work, if you are a follower of your very own profound qualities that have a superseding reason for existing, almost certainly, you'll have the will to complete them.

Marilyn accepted profoundly that composing demanding agreements and keeping flawless records were imperatives to building certainty with her customers and her law office. However, some way or another, hearing that bread wasn't right on one diet and anything with sugar wasn't right on another didn't cause a similar sort of profound conviction.

Attempt as she may, she couldn't generally accept that chocolate chip treats were that underhanded! Self-discipline can be characterized as an endeavor to counter characteristic wants and supplant them with prescriptive principles. The longing for desserts is regular, ordinary, and very lovely! Any diet that lets you know, you can't have desserts is conflicting with your common want. The dieting turns into a lot of inflexible guidelines, and these sorts of rules can trigger resistance. Self-control doesn't have a place in Intuitive Eating. As Marilyn turned into an Intuitive Eater, she found that tuning in to her own sign fortified her characteristic impulses, as opposed to battling them. She had nobody else's proscriptive principles to pursue or to oppose. Marilyn has quit taking on the apparition determination conflict, and she has lost all the weight with which she had been battling.

DISREGARD BEING OBEDIENT

A benevolent recommendation by a companion, for example, "You ought to have the seared chicken "or "You shouldn't eat those fries" can set off an inward nourishment resistance. In this kind of nourishment battle, your solitary weapon to battle back turns into a twofold request of fries. Our customers call this overlook your eating. In material science, opposition consistently happens as a response to compelling. We see this rule in real life in the public arena—revolts frequently eject when the power turns out to be excessively incredible.

Additionally, the straightforward demonstration of being determined what to do (regardless of whether it's something you need to do) can trigger a defiant chain response. Much the same as "horrible two-year-olds or young people who revolt to demonstrate they are free, dieters can start defiant eating in the light of the demonstration of dieting, with its arrangement of unbending rules directing what to eat. As it's not astonishing to get notification from our customers that disrupting the guidelines of a diet makes them feel simply like they did when they were rebellious teenagers. In any case, cheer up, disobedience is an ordinary demonstration of self-safeguarding—securing your space or individual limits.

Think about an individual limit as a tall block fence encompassing you, with just one door. No one but you can open that door if you choose. Accordingly, nobody is permitted inside, except if you welcome the individual in. Inside your fence live private emotions, considerations, and organic signals. Individuals who accept they realize what you need and instruct you are picking the lock to your door or attacking your limits. Nobody might comprehend what's inside except if you let him know by welcoming him in. What slims down or eat less advocate can know when you are hungry or what amount of nourishment it will take to fulfill you?

In what capacity can anybody know what surface and taste sensations will satisfy your sense of taste? In the realm of abstaining from excessive food intake, individual limits are crossed at numerous levels. For instance, you are determined what to eat, the amount to eat, and when to eat it. These choices should all be close to home decisions, with deference to singular independence and body signals. While nourishment direction may originate from somewhere else, you ought to at last be liable for the when, what, and the amount of eating. When a nutritionist or diet attacks your limits, it's not unexpected to feel weak. The more you pursue the nourishment limitations, the more prominent the attack on your self-governance. Here is the place the oddity lies. When abstaining from excessive food intake, you will probably revolt by eating more—to reestablish your independence and secure your limits. In any case, the demonstration of revolting can make you feel as wild.

Rather, you have an inward nourishment battle on your hands. In any case, when the nourishment insubordination is released, its force fortifies sentiments of the absence of control and the conviction that you don't have self-control. At last, you start to suffocate in an ocean of self-uncertainty and disgrace. What starts as mentally sound conduct finishes in calamity. At last, weight reduction is undermined because of individual limit security. With Intuitive Eating, there is no compelling reason to revolt, since you become the one in control! Limits are additionally attacked when somebody makes remarks about your weight or how you should look. Once more, you will undoubtedly revolt by indulging. It's a method for saying, "You reserve no option to disclose to me what to gauge."

DISREGARD FAILURE.

A lot of our dieting clients walk into our offices feeling as though they are disappointments. Regardless of whether they are government officials, prominent big names, or straight-A students, they all discuss their food encounters disgracefully, and they question whether they'll ever have the option to feel successful in the area of eating. The dieting can trigger feelings of progress or disappointment. You can't come up short at Intuitive Eating—it's a learning process at each point along the way. What used to be thought of as a difficult will rather be viewed as a growth experience. You'll get directly in the groove again when you see this as improvement, not disappointment.

STAGE 3: GET RID OF THE DIETER'S TOOLS

The dieter depends on external forces to control his eating, adhering to a controlled food plan, eating because it is the ideal time or eating a predetermined (and estimated) amount of food, regardless of whether they are hungry. The dieter additionally approves progress by external forces, essentially using the scale, asking, "What number of pounds have I lost? Is my weight up or down?" It's an ideal opportunity to toss out your dieting tools and books. Dispose of the meal plans and the bathroom scales. If all it took was a decent "reasonable" calorie-restricted meal plan to become fit, we would be a country of thin individuals—free meal plans are accessible from magazines, papers, and even some nourishment organizations.

THE SCALE AS FALSE IDOL

"If it's not too much trouble given the number a chance to be ... " This unrealistic number of prayers isn't happening in the gambling clubs of Las Vegas, yet in private homes all through the nation. In any case, much the same as the desperate gambler trusting that his fortunate number will come in, so is it worthless for the dieter to pay tribute to the "scale god." In one scope of the scale roulette, expectations and desperation make a daily dramatization that will, at last, shape what state of mind you'll be in for the afternoon. Incidentally, "good" and "bad" scale numbers can both trigger indulging—regardless of whether it's a salutary eating festivity or an encouragement party. The scale ritual undermines the body and mind endeavors; it can in one minute debase days, weeks, and even a very long time of dieting progress.

WHEN A POUND IS NOT A POUND

Numerous components can impact an individual's weight, which doesn't mirror the individual's ratio of muscle to fat. For instance, two cups of water gauge one pound. If you will, in general, hold water or swell, the scale can undoubtedly raise a couple of pounds without an adjustment in what you have eaten. However, for the dieter, the outcomes of water weight can appear to be extreme. For instance, we have had numerous patients feel terrible about eating an additional pastry throughout the end of the week and gauge themselves on the next Monday. The scale shoots up five pounds—and they accept they increased five pounds of fat.

Since lots of dieters are fast with the calorie calculator cruncher, we ask, "Did you eat an extra 17,500 calories throughout the end of the week?" Obviously not, would be their answer. However, to make five pounds of fat requires a caloric overabundance of 17,500 calories more than average eating (one pound of fat is identical to 3,500 calories). So how would you clarify the weight gain?

WATER WEIGHT

Whenever the scale all of a sudden ascents or falls, it is normally a result of a liquid component in the body. Eating high-sodium foods can likewise incite water maintenance (not fat retention) in salt-touchy people. However, how effectively interminable dieters accept they accomplished something incorrectly; they should have without any assistance eaten five pounds worth of nourishment! No! No! No! Likewise, shedding two pounds quickly from an hour of heart stimulating exercise is anything but a two-pound fat loss. Or maybe, it's generally water loss from sweat.

Happy dieters who imagine that they have shed ten pounds in seven days might be in for an undesirable shock. While the facts may confirm that the scale demonstrated ten pounds less than they weighed days back, the real question is, what sort of weight did they lose? To shed ten pounds of fat in a week requires an energy loss of 35,000 calories or a deficiency of 5,000 calories every day! The normal lady just eats around 1,500 to 1,600 calories for each day.

The sad truth is that this individual is losing a ton of water weight, for the most part, to the detriment of their muscles because of the process of muscle-wasting. Muscle is made up of the most part of water (around 70 percent). When a hungry body isn't given enough calories, the body rips apart itself for an energy source. The prime order of the body is that it must have vitality at any cost—it's a piece of the endurance system. The protein in muscles is changed over to important vitality for the body. When a muscle cell is crushed, water is discharged, and in the long run, discharged—there's your valuable weight reduction.

The lost muscle adds to reducing your digestion. Muscles are metabolically dynamic tissue—for the most part, the more muscle we have, the higher our metabolic rate.

That is one reason men consume a bigger number of calories than ladies—they have more bulk. Muscle additionally occupies less room than fat.

While this is positively valuable, a chronic dieter regularly gets baffled by the rising or constant scale number. The scale doesn't reflect body creation—simply like gauging a bit of steak at the butcher doesn't reveal to you how to fit the meat is. Saying something regarding the scale just serves to keep you concentrated on your weight; it doesn't help with getting back to reality with Intuitive Eating. Consistent weight checks can leave you baffled and hinder your progress. The best option—quit weighing yourself!

INTUITIVE EATING TOOLS

The instruments of the Intuitive Eater are inward signals, not outside powers revealing to you what, when, and the amount to eat. Yet, to acquire and comprehend these internal signals, you need another arrangement of intensity power tools—or rather, strengthening tools, which will be talked about in the following sections of this book.

CHAPTER FOUR
HONOR YOUR HUNGER

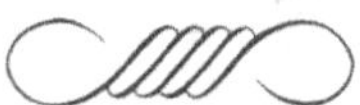

Keep your body sustained biologically with sufficient nutrients as well as carbohydrates, or you can trigger a basic drive to overeat. When you arrive at the point of excessive appetite, all aims of moderate, conscious eating are fleeting and irrelevant. Figuring out how to respect this first biological sign makes way for revamping trust with yourself and with food. A dieting body is a destitute body. Crazy comparison? No. While a dieting body may not resemble a starving individual in Ethiopia or Somalia, the "manifestations" from slimming down display a striking likeness to the starvation state.

The body doesn't have a clue that there is a McDonald's everywhere as you set out on a diet. To the extent the body is concerned, it is living in a starvation state and needs to adjust. Our requirement for nutrients (energy) is so basic and base that, if we are not getting enough vitality, our bodies normally repay with incredible biological and mental systems. The intensity of food restriction was distinctly exhibited in a landmark starvation study directed by Dr. Ancel Keys during World War II, intended to help famine sufferers.

The subjects of the examination were thirty-two solid men who were chosen since they had predominant "psychobiological stamina"—prevalent mental and physical wellbeing. During the initial three months of the examination, the men ate however they wanted, 3,492 calories every day. The following half-year was the semi-starvation timeframe. The men were required to lose 19 to 28 percent of their weight contingent upon their body creation. Calories were sliced almost down the middle to a norm of 1,570 every day. The impacts of semi-starvation were surprising, and strikingly reflect the side effects of chronic dieting :

Metabolic rates diminished by 40 percent.

The men were fixated on nourishment. They had uplifted nourishment longings and discussed nourishment and gathering plans.

The eating style changed—wavering from covetous swallowing to slowing down the eating experience. A few men played with their nourishment and tarried over a feast for two hours.

The scientists noticed that "Few men neglected to hold fast to their eating regimens and revealed scenes of bulimia." One man was accounted for to have endured a total loss of "self-discipline" and ate a few treats, a sack of popcorn, and two bananas. Another subject, "outrageously defied the dietary guidelines" and ate a few sundaes and malted grains and even took penny treat.

Some men practiced intentionally to acquire expanded nourishment proportions.

Personalities changed, and as a rule, there was the beginning of lack of care, touchiness, irritability, and wretchedness. During the refeeding time frame, when the men were permitted to eat freely, hunger got voracious. The men thought that it was hard to quit eating. The end of the week meant adding 8,000 to 10,000 calories. It took most of the men five months to standardize their eating. It's essential to recollect that during the time of these exemplary studies, there were no Arnold

Schwarzeneggers or wellness and nourishment divas. Sustenance inquiries were in its earliest stages.

However, these men encountered a base fixation on food that was not media-driven or society-driven; rather, it was activated by a natural endurance system.

Such conduct had never been seen in these men before their nourishment hardship experience! Despite the fact that this is an exemplary starvation study, the caloric level is illustrative of a cutting edge weight reduction diet for men of 1,500 calories. These men were eating. Envision if a similar report was held under the present weights to be flimsy. We have had a few customers peruse the exemplary Keys study, and they are struck by the comparability of their own encounters to those of the semi-starved men.

MECHANISM THAT TRIGGERS EATING

Regardless of whether you are a chronic dieter, amazing organic components are activated when your body doesn't get the vitality from food that it needs. It's no accident that food is incorporated as one of the basic human needs in Maslow's Hierarchy of Needs—a model that positions human needs, proposing that specific fundamental needs should be met before you can proceed to satisfy increasingly complex ones. Food and vitality are so basic to the endurance of the human species that, if we don't eat enough, we set off a natural circuit that turns on our eating drive both physically and mentally.

The craving drive is genuinely a mind-body association. Eating is critical to such an extent that the nerve cells of hunger are situated in the nerve center of appetite located in the hypothalamus of the brain. A variety of biological signals trigger eating. What numerous individuals accept to be an issue of self-discipline is rather a natural drive. The power and force of the organic eating drive ought not to be thought little of. The neurochemicals from the mind coordinate our eating behavior with our body's natural need. Through an unpredictable arrangement of a compound and neural criticism, the mind screens the vitality needs of all our body frameworks, minute to minute. Furthermore, it makes decided compound orders concerning what we ought to eat. Fasting is especially dangerous to hunger control. It basically turns on the hormone switches that initiate us to eat.

Numerous studies have demonstrated that bringing down body weight by nourishment limitation and dieting has neither rhyme nor reason metabolically or to our mind science. Truth be told, it's counterproductive. The hormones that control craving likewise influence dispositions and perspective, our physical vitality, and our sexual experiences. Most professionals concur that there are both complex biological and mental components that impact our eating. In this section, we will concentrate on the essential natural systems that turn on our longing to eat, particularly if we have denied our bodies of good food or dieting. There is increased digestion in starved people as studies have demonstrated that the body gets naturally prepared for the moment of eating, similar to a sprinter squatted in prepared for a race, the minute the beginning gun is activated.

Salivation increases with the increase of food deprivation, in any event, when there is no nourishment present or proposal of eating! This has been shown in research both on dieters and normal (non-dieting) people.

Increased digestive hormones have been found in dieters both before and after eating.

THE CARBOHYDRATE CRAVER:

Neuropeptide Y (NPY) is a hormone produced by the cerebrum that triggers our drive to eat carbohydrates, the body's essential and favored wellspring of vitality. While the majority of what we think about NPY originates from research on rodents, there is a great deal of proof that shows that this mind synthetic can profoundly affect human eating conduct too by expanding both the size and term of starch-rich meals. Food deprivation or under-eating drives NPY without hesitation, making the body look for more carbohydrates. When the following meal or eating opportunity moves around, it can easily transform into a high-starch gorge—not on the grounds that you need determination or are crazy; it's your science (rather, NPY) shouting, "Feed me." NPY is fired up after any forced time of food deprivation, including a medium-term fast from dinner to breakfast. NPY's levels are normally the most noteworthy in the first part of the day as a result of the momentary food deprivation from a medium-term fast.

The raised NPY levels are a part of the natural reason for eating early in the day! During an overnight fast, your body's stores of sugars in the liver are depleted and need topping off. You truly wake up on void in the first part of the day. Be that as it may, if you skip breakfast, you are probably going to pay for it with an increase in NPY level, which can lead to mid-evening time pigging out. The mind likewise makes more NPY when sugars are being used as fuel and in the midst of stress.

Eating carbohydrates reduce NPY through its impact on serotonin, another hormone in the brain. As we eat more starches, it builds the generation of serotonin, which stops the creation of NPY and puts an end to the desire for sugars. The more you deny your actual appetite and battle your characteristic science, the more grounded and increasingly serious food yearnings and cravings become. Fasting or limiting particularly fires up the NPY and drives the body to look for more sugars. So when the following eating opportunity happens, it can easily become a high-sugar gorge. For what reason is there such a compound drive for starches? How about we take a look at the basic job starches play in the body—it will assist you with understanding the base yearning drive.

THE IMPORTANCE OF CARBOHYDRATES

Carbohydrates are the highest quality level of food energy available to the body. Cells work best when they get a specific unit of sugars, such as glucose, and even little deficiencies can cause issues. The mind, sensory system, and red blood cells depend solely on glucose for fuel. Due to the significance of glucose, the degrees of it in the blood are firmly managed by two hormones, insulin, and glucagon. There is an exceptionally restricted measure of sugar put away in the liver, as glycogen, that causes supply more glucose to the blood when levels get excessively low. However, this valuable fuel keeps going just three to six hours (except around evening time, when liver glycogen endures longer because the requirement for vitality is lower). How does this fuel hold get exchanged?

Eating starch-rich foods. If the diet is deficient in sugars, the body needs to go to innovative energizing systems to supply indispensable vitality to the body. Protein predominantly from muscle will get dismantled and changed over to vitality, principally as glucose. It resembles taking wood from the system structure in your home to use as fuel in your chimney.

The wood will consume and give important fuel; however, it does as such at a significant expense. You start to lose the respectability of your structure! If you believe that eating a high-protein diet will keep this from happening, it's not really. When you eat a deficient measure of vitality or starches, the protein will likewise be redirected to be utilized as vitality. In this way, this "high-protein diet" is no protection. Instead, the protein is utilized as a costly wellspring of fuel, as opposed to its expected use in the body. It resembles having a structure provider give loads of wood to modify your home.

If you are always utilizing that heap of wood to make campfires rather than to fix your home, you are still left with a frail structure. So, protein is expected to keep up and construct muscles, hormones, compounds, and cells in the body. When starches and vitality are inadequate, protein is moved from its essential job to give fuel. A considerable lot of our customers accept that, when we need more vitality, our bodies will, at last, start consuming fat. It doesn't work that way. Keep in mind, the cerebrum and different pieces of the body need starches solely for fuel.

Just a tiny part (5 percent) of the put-away fat can be changed over to a starch fuel. Then again, the body has a lot of compounds to change protein to glucose. One reason individuals get more fit so rapidly on low-starch or fasting, eating fewer carbs is that they are eating up their very own protein tissues as fuel. Since protein contains just half the same number of calories per pound as fat, it vanishes twice as quick. With each pound of body protein, three or four pounds of related water are lost. If your body were to keep expending itself in light of current circumstances, demise would happen in around ten days.

All things considered, the liver, heart muscle, and lung tissue—every fundamental piece—is being singed as fuel. In any event, when the heart muscle is weakening, regardless, it needs to keep up a similar measure of work, with less power and at a slower pulse. Generally, the torn apart heart muscle needs to work more enthusiastically with a littler, flawed motor; siphoning execution isn't diminished about the measure of heart tissue lost. In the long run, the body can change over put away fat to a type of usable vitality for the cerebrum and sensory system called ketones. This process is known as ketosis.

Ketosis is an adjustment to delayed fasting or starch hardship. Be that as it may, just about a portion of the synapses can utilize these mixes for vitality. In this way, when fat is being utilized under these hardship conditions, the body's slender tissue (protein) keeps being lost at a fast rate to supply glucose to sensory system cells that can't utilize ketones as fuel. The main concern? Sufficient sugars and vitality are significant! The Powerhouse Cell Theory Hunger signals are not influenced by low starches alone.

As indicated by cell analysts Nicolaidis and Even, the craving signal is produced by the general vitality need. When cell control is low, it will create a sign that actuates hunger. While cells get their vitality principally from starch, protein and fat are calculated into the cell control condition, which could trigger yearning. For instance, regardless of whether one of your family unit apparatuses runs on unadulterated power, it could likewise get its vitality from batteries or a gas controlled generator. They all give vitality yet have various expenses and efficiencies. All supplements that give vitality (sugars, protein, and fat) in the long run get changed over to one widespread vitality division utilized by the cells, ATP. ATP is the synthetic vitality that powers the cells and, along these lines, our bodies. Nicolaidis and Even suggest that the appetite signal is activated by the general ATP need of the cell. To summarize—we need vitality. Vitality originates from nourishment.

STEP BY STEP INSTRUCTIONS TO HONOR BIOLOGICAL HUNGER

It's too difficult to think about hearing your appetite if you are never tuning into it. The initial step regarding your natural appetite is to start to tune into it. The ensemble of craving has numerous sounds that are shifted for various individuals. Similarly, as an ensemble director can recognize the voices of each instrument in an orchestra, you will, in the end, have the option to enter into explicit substantial sensations and what they mean. In the first place, you might have the option to perceive a clear greedy appetite; however, experience issues perceiving delicate food cravings. Likewise, to the non-trained melodic ear, noisy cymbals may be anything but difficult to distinguish, yet it will require some serious energy and tuning in to get on the subtler voices of the bassoon or oboe. - Each time you eat, ask yourself: "Am I hungry? What's my craving level?" If the sentiment of yearning is difficult to distinguish, ask yourself: "When was the last time I felt hungry? How did my stomach feel? How did my mouth feel?" Any mix of the accompanying can be experienced as yearning sensations or indications (running from delicate to insatiable):

Mild murmuring in the stomach

Growling within the stomach

Light-headedness

Difficulty concentrating

Uncomfortable stomach torment

Irritability

Feeling faint

Headache

The rhythmic movement of your appetite probably won't coordinate other people's—that is alright, it's personal. Take care not to get excessively hungry or greedy. If this is hard for you to check, a general rule is to go no longer than five waking hours without eating. This depends on the science of filling up your starch tank in the liver, which runs out each three to six hours.

We have seen that customers who go longer than five hours without eating will, in general, indulge at the following eating opportunity. To connect with the subtleties of yearning, it checks the heat of craving at ordinary interims. Check in with your body, and ask, what's my appetite level? It's useful to do this each time you eat and between eating events. Keep in mind, despite the fact that this may appear hyperconscious, it's an engaged advance to get you reacquainted with your body and its science. We have utilized an assortment of apparatuses to enable our customers to check in with their appetite; however, one is especially useful and is somewhat less demanding.

Monitor your craving level each time you eat, prior, and then afterward, utilizing the Hunger Discovery Scale. What example do you see developing? Is there a specific time during which you eat? Is there any connection between the amount you eat and the time allotment between eating? You may find that your eating style inclines toward snacking. Try not to be frightened.

If you eat modest quantities of nourishment, for example, a tidbit or little meal, you may find that you are very hungry all the more frequently, for example, each three to four hours. In addition to the fact that this is ordinary, it might have favorable metabolic circumstances. Snacking research (in which individuals are given various tidbits or smaller than usual suppers) has demonstrated that the arrival of insulin is lower in individuals bolstered snacking counts calories contrasted with bigger conventional meals of indistinguishable calories. Insulin is a fat building hormone.

The more insulin released, the simpler it is for the body to accumulate fat. Once in a while, our customers get stressed when they suddenly feel more hungry than expected—as though something isn't right. In any case, after looking into it further, they generally locate that two or three days earlier, they had a bizarrely light day of eating—not counting calories, however, just not a great deal of nourishment. The body plays catch-up. The vast majority of our customers experience issues recalling what they ate one day ago, not to mention two days prior. Research on kids has shown that they compensate for their wholesome needs in normal time from two or three days to seven days.

For what reason should grown-ups be any different? Actually, new research is starting to show the equivalent is valid for grown-ups. The body may do a portion of its vitality calibrating over a time of days, as opposed to from hour to hour. We discover this is particularly valid if, despite everything, you tend to eat diet kinds of nourishment, for example, rice cakes or serving of mixed greens. You may feel full, yet the absence of vitality makes up for lost time with you. The body needs to redress.

Different Voices of "Craving": A typical mix-up with our more up to date customers is that they at first grasp the respect your yearning idea as a dieting mantra, "Thou will eat just when hungry." The issue here is that this unbending translation can leave you feeling as though you have disrupted a guideline or fizzled if you eat for some other explanation than hunger. When you have a feeling that you have defied a norm, you can get maneuvered directly over into the diet mindset. Recognize that typical eaters don't generally eat just from unadulterated yearning, yet they keep up their weight.

Taste Hunger. Now and then, individuals may eat basically in light of the fact that it sounds great or on the grounds that the event calls for it. We call this taste hunger. Ordinary eaters can acknowledge this— they don't see it as a major diet infringement. In each culture, nourishment assumes a significant job in rituals of entries and celebratory occasions. OK, chide a lady of the hour or lucky man for eating a bit of wedding cake when she or he was not very hungry? However, it's not uncommon for weight watchers to feel awful about any apparent nourishment offense and afterward feel like they should quit. Furthermore, that is when gorging regularly happens.

Practical "Craving"— Planning Ahead. While it's critical to eat dependent on your organic appetite, it's likewise imperative to be viable and not unbending. For example, suppose you are going to a play with companions from 7:00 to 10:00 P.M. Furthermore, your chance to eat is at 6:00 P.M. You may not be hungry at that point, yet you absolutely will be later. Do you stay there at the café and not eat and let hunger move indirectly in the center of the play, just to come full circle in greedy yearning by the last demonstration? No. Eating a light meal or bite heretofore is a reasonable arrangement.

Emotional Hunger. When you are really ready to recognize and accept your biological appetite, it gets simpler to explain why you need to eat. It isn't surprising for some of our customers to eat due to emotional yearning—to extinguish awkward feelings (for example, dejection, weariness, and outrage). Unexpectedly, a considerable lot of our customers are regularly flabbergasted that what they thought to be emotional eating was, in numerous cases, primal hunger eating. Be that as it may, the out-of-control feeling of overeating is almost indistinguishable, regardless of whether it was activated biologically or emotionally.

CHAPTER FIVE
FEEL YOUR FULLNESS

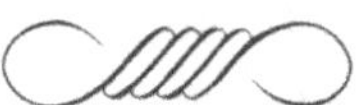

Tune in to the body signals that disclose to you that you are filled. Watch out for the signs that show you're comfortably full and can't eat anymore. Take a pause in the midst of eating and ask yourself how the food tastes and what your present completion level is. The greater part of chronic dieters we have worked with has a place with the spotless-plate club. What's more, the vast majority of them state that they've done whatever it takes not to eat everything. It might appear that an obvious step to weight reduction is to regard your fullness, instead of to routinely "clean your plate."

However, leaving food can be hard to accomplish, particularly for chronic dieters. Dieting imparts a license to eat just at mealtime—when it is "legitimate." Ironically, this feeling of privilege strengthens a clean-your-plate attitude. This is especially valid for our customers who have used over-the-counter fluid weight control plans, for example, Slim-Fast. (Fluid diet programs commonly have you drink a "refreshment supper" for breakfast and lunch, and afterward "enable you to have a reasonable supper" of "genuine" nourishment).

Naturally, the greater part of our patients, for all intents and purposes, licked their plates clean when allowed the chance to eat their one genuine meal. It isn't so much that they indulged; rather, they ate the entirety of their exact and "entitled" divides. Other diet plans utilizing normal nourishment commonly offer little divides at meals. This, as well, urges you to eat while you can. Who might leave any piece of nourishment when amounts are pitiful? For instance, even frozen diet suppers float at around 300 calories (and regularly less), which ordinarily leaves you not exactly fulfilled. Truth be told, there is another pattern of frozen diet dishes offering considerably fewer calories—more like 200 calories for each. This sort of eating scarcely cultivates connecting with your internal eating signals, particularly the signal of satiety. Rather, you eat everything.

Maybe you've hurled your diet plans out years prior, however now cautiously count fat grams. You may discover, in any case, that you clean-your-plate with regards to eating without fat nourishments. We've had a few customers eat a whole bundle of fat-free chocolate cake (or other sans fat treats) with cheerful surrender on account of the qualification factor. They would justify, "There's no fat, so I can eat as much as I need." Unfortunately, without fat, it isn't really sans calorie. Be that as it may, the calories wouldn't be an issue if individuals were regarding their completion level. Obviously, different variables can easily condition you to finish each piece on your plate, including:

Having been educated to complete everything on your plate by well-meaning parents.

Respecting economics and the value of nourishment—thou will not squander. Keep in mind, nonetheless, that whichever way the food can be squandered; on account of incessantly eating more than you need, it turns into an issue of increase in waist size.

Having an instilled habit of eating to finish. Out of sheer habit, you finish a whole plate of food, or an entire burger, or an entire sack of chips, paying little heed to how very hungry or full you are. This is a dependence on outer prompts. You quit eating when the nourishment is gone, paying little heed to the size of the underlying part.

Beginning a meal (or snack) in an excessively covetous state. In this state, gobbling power is fired up, and it's simple to sidestep typical satiety signals. Regardless of whether you don't clean your plate, it's still conceivable that you might be indulging or bypassing your agreeable satiety level. With our customers who don't clean their plates, we have frequently found that, while there may be nourishment left on the plate, it took an awkward degree of totality to get them to quit eating. The issue is the failure to perceive comfortable satiety or to regard fullness.

THE KEY TO RESPECTING FULLNESS

Regarding fullness, or the capacity to quit eating since you have had enough to eat naturally, is based on giving yourself unqualified permission to eat. By what means can you or any dieter hope to leave food on your plate if you accept that you won't have the option to eat that specific food or meal once more? Except if you genuinely give yourself permission to eat again when you are hungry, or to approach that specific nourishment, regarding totality essentially turns into a one-sided counting calories practice without roots. It won't grab hold.

The Intuitive Eater figures out how to quit eating when the individual has had only enough to fill the stomach easily without being overfull. It's simpler to quit eating now and abandon nourishment when you realize you can eat it again later.

RECOGNIZING COMFORTABLE SATIETY

We are amazed at how regularly our customers don't have the foggiest idea of what comfortable satiety level feels like. Goodness! However, they can, for the most part, portray incredible detail of how indulging or being overstuffed feels. Information on what agreeable satiety feels like is frequently elusive, particularly to the chronic dieter. However, if you don't have the foggiest idea what agreeable satiety feels like, how might you expect to accomplish it? It resembles attempting to take shots at an objective while never observing it or knowing where it dwells. While fullness is the objective, it could easily be missed if you don't have the foggiest idea where to search for it, particularly when you have been adapted to clean your plate. Additionally, if you start eating when you are not hungry, it's difficult to tell when to stop. How would you envision agreeable satiety feels? Here are some regular portrayals offered by our customers:

An unpretentious sentiment of stomach fullness

Feeling fulfilled and content

Nothingness—neither hungry nor full

The sensation is exceptionally personal, and keeping in mind that we can depict it perpetually, it's similar to attempting to tell somebody what snow feels like. We can give you an idea or picture—however, it's something that should be experienced at the individual level, with the goal that you know how it feels in your body.

HOW TO RESPECT YOUR FULLNESS

When you routinely clean your plate, your eating style effectively goes on autopilot—you eat until completion until the food is no more. To break this example of eating, we have thought that it was useful to be acutely mindful or hyperconscious of your eating. This implies being conscious or aware of your eating experience. While you may positively know that you are occupied with the habit of eating, we find that somewhere close to the first bite and subsequent bites, there is a huge degree of knowing when you are full. Regularly, the food isn't being tasted! In like manner, it's very simple to sidestep agreeable satiety.

Here are a few models:

I didn't know how many treats I would eat at the motion pictures until all of a sudden, my hands were scratching at the sight of the unfilled box.

I wouldn't consider parting a meal when eating out until my manager inquired as to whether I would part a course at her preferred eatery. Hesitantly, I concurred. Shockingly, I was altogether happy with a large portion of a dish, realizing that had I requested the full segment, I would have eaten everything out of sheer propensity.

Once I open a pack of any food, I intend to eat everything. God helping me, I'd leave a couple of goodies. I know I'm not tasting the food more often than not.

CONSCIOUS EATING

The underlying advance away from the visually impaired autopilot eating mode is conscious eating. It's where you impartially watch your eating as though under a magnifying instrument. (Your Food Anthropologist voice will be useful here.) We have broken this phase into a progression of steps that starts with taking a scaled-down break from eating. This will assist you with regrouping and evaluate where you are in your eating. It resembles the break that competitors and mentors take during a game to help improve their play or methodology. This is what to do.

Pause the meal or snack for a while. Remember that this break isn't a promise to quit eating. Or maybe, it's a promise to being under tight restraints with your body and taste buds. (If you felt that, by stopping, you were committed to leaving food on your plate, you'd be hesitant to experience this progression. Truth be told, huge numbers of our customers who seemed uninterested in this progression later owned up that they were anxious about the possibility that they would need to prevent eating from thereon.)

During this break, play out these checks:

TASTE CHECK:

We find that this check is normally pleasurable, which is the reason we like it. Ask yourself how the food tastes. Is it deserving of your taste buds? Or on the other hand, would you say you are proceeding to eat in light of the fact that the food is there?

SATIETY CHECK:

Ask yourself what your appetite or fullness level is. Is it accurate to say that you are as yet hungry, do you feel unsatisfied, or is your appetite leaving and would you say you are starting to feel fulfilled? To start, this may appear to be an all-in or all-out process. Be tolerant and recall you are becoming acquainted with yourself from the back to front. Similarly, as you would not hope to become more acquainted with an individual more than one feast, how might you hope to comprehend your satiety level in one meal or bite? It will require some investment. Nonetheless, the more in order you are with your yearning level, and the more you respect your appetite, the simpler this progression will be.

Make sure to be available to any answer. There can be extensive vacillation in your totality levels relying on the last time you ate and what you ate. If you find you're as yet hungry, at that point, continue eating.

When you wrap up (whatever the sum), ask yourself where your totality level is currently. Did you arrive at agreeable satiety? Did you outperform it? By what amount? Utilize the Fullness Discovery scale to assist you with connecting.

Discovering your totality level will assist you in recognizing your Last-Bite Threshold. This is the endpoint. You realize that the chomp of food in your mouth is your last—finis! It might require some investment to get to this point. The more you have been detached from your body's feeling of totality, the more it will take to characterize this point. If you respect your appetite (Principle Two), it is a lot simpler to know totality. Assuming you don't eat from organic hunger, how might you hope to prevent natural completion (or to try to recognize what it feels like)? It will be ideal if you show restraint toward yourself. • Don't feel committed to leaving food on your plate. If you find that you have a degree of obstruction for this action, it might be from past dieting experience. You might be feeling committed to leaving food on your plate— - which is a remainder of the diet mindset. Keep in mind; there is no pledge to leave food on your plate. The dedication, rather, is to become more acquainted with your satiety level and your taste buds. It's impeccably typical, in any event, when you find your particular satiety level, to indulge. That is alright. We have discovered that numerous customers keep on picking more food—they are as yet testing the "unequivocal authorization" to eat.

Sooner or later, when the originality wears off, you will find that it's very simple to leave food on your plate. It requires a level of awareness—checking in with yourself. Be that as it may, if more often than not, you can perceive your completion and regard it, it will have a significant effect in your capacity to keep up a characteristic weight.

INSTRUCTIONS TO INCREASE CONSCIOUSNESS

It's extremely hard to accomplish two conscious things immediately. While you unquestionably may shuffle a zillion exercises, your brain centers basically on one. That is the reason, for instance, such huge numbers of individuals lock their keys in their vehicle. Their brains are centered elsewhere, for example, getting into the workplace on schedule or emptying some food supplies. We find that to capitalize on eating, it should be a conscious action, at whatever point conceivable. • Eat Without Distraction. Esteem and appreciate the eating experience whenever the situation allows. For instance, Adelle, a fast-paced, hard-determined legal counselor, constantly utilized her time and would typically eat while accomplishing something different. Adelle would understand briefs while having lunch at work and would feast with a magazine at home. She stepped forward when she chose to have a go at eating without interruption when at home (she was excessively occupied at work to try to consider "simply eating" lunch). Adelle found that, if she ate a meal or bite at home without participating in perusing, she would, for the most part, eat less. Amazingly, she discovered that she ate less, not on the grounds that she was attempting to eat littler sums, but since she could identify her completion level a lot sooner. She was excited that "easily" she was eating less food, feeling fulfilled without hardship, and not abstaining from excessive food intake. Adelle was happy to eat along these lines at home, yet didn't see it as reasonable for work—and this was advancement!

Reinforce Your Conscious Decision to Stop. A considerable lot of our customers have discovered that, when they choose to quit eating, since they've arrived at the edge, it's useful to plan something to make it a conscious demonstration, for example, delicately pushing the plate forward an inch or putting their utensils or napkin on their plate. This just helps them to remember their choice. Else, it might be very simple to guiltlessly snack on the rest of the food, despite the fact that you had no goal of doing as such. (If you experience difficulty with squandering food, take a stab at taking care of your scraps for tomorrow's lunch or meal or offering them to a vagrant.) • Defend Yourself from Obligatory Eating. This typically implies working on saying, "No, thank you!" I never understood the criticalness of this demonstration until I went to an extremely exquisite mixed drink party in which there appeared to be one server for every visitor! The minute my hand was unfilled of food or drink, a very anxious server was there to offer more food or refreshment. I discovered it was simpler to state "yes," particularly if I was in a discussion. It took considerably more vitality to state "no." The equivalent is valid if you go to any capacity wherein there are benevolent "food pushers" from the thoughtful host to the offensive family member. A unique note of alert to those of you who appreciate wine by the jug at a decent café: A great server will frequently keep your glass full. Except if you are aware of that, you may drink more than you mean. Keep in mind; you are responsible for the amount you eat or drink.

THE FULLNESS FACTORS

"I just ate two hours prior—I regarded my craving and regarded my totality, so how might I be hungry again unexpectedly early?" While the ebb and tide of satiety signs may appear to be bewildering, it's ordinary to have various degrees of yearning and completion, particularly when you start tuning in to your body's eating prompts. There are, likewise, a few factors that influence totality. These components are both natural and educated. When you have a general comprehension of a portion of these satiety factors, it makes it simpler to confide in your body and feel your totality. The capacity to perceive agreeable satiety or completion can eventually decide how a lot of food will be expended in a supper. What's more, the measure of food eaten in a meal is impacted by these fullness factors:

The measure of time since you ate. The more regularly you eat, the less hungry you will be. This has been seen as valid in snacking research. These are pondering in which individuals are given a few tidbits or little suppers for the duration of the day.

The kind of food you eat. The macronutrients, protein, sugars, and fat impact is resulting in food admission by their commitment to the aggregate sum of food vitality in the stomach. Other food factors, for example, fiber, will likewise influence the fullness factor as a result of its mass and water retention properties. Protein specifically appears to have a suppressive/impact on consumption past its commitment to add up to calories, as indicated by a few investigations. • The measure of food staying in the stomach at the hour of eating. If your stomach is vacant, you will eat more than if some food is present (from an earlier bite or feast).

Initial yearning level. If you start a meal or snack in a starving state, you are bound to gorge and abrogate satiety signals.

Social impact. Eating with other individuals can impact the amount you eat. Studies have indicated:

— The more individuals assembled at a feast, the more individuals will, in general, eat.

Eating with others increases the length of the meal.

— Eating more on weekends is ordinarily due to being around individuals.

— Dieters, be that as it may, have been shown to eat less when they realize somebody is "watching" them. The equivalent is valid for non-dieters when they feast with a "model" eater. In one examination, when the model eater ceased from eating, so too did the non-dieter.

There is a habit of disregarding or being diverted from biological signals in social settings. We have discovered that the way into the social issue is to keep making eating a conscious action with deliberate food decisions. Obviously, there are numerous variables that impact how full you feel from eating. With such huge numbers of factors that impact on your eating, it ought to be nothing unexpected that the measure of food you want to eat can and will change. A major key is to remain tuned in and to eat intentionally.

BE CAREFUL WITH AIR FOOD

Just pushing some food in your mouth like a pacifier to ease cravings for food may reverse the desired effect, and the comforting effect may not last long. This is particularly valid for "air food"— food that tops off the stomach yet offers little sustenance. Air food incorporates such low-calorie foods as air-popped popcorn, rice cakes, puffed rice oat, without fat saltines, celery sticks, and sans calorie refreshments. There's nothing intrinsically amiss with these foods. In any case, if you eat them hoping to get full, it will frequently take large amounts—and you may wind up waiting for something increasingly considerable to "top off the meal." That's the place having a decent snack or meal, which incorporates a heavier sugar, some protein, or fat, is particularly useful, if you're searching for a touch of "backbone," or something to keep you from eating. If you realize you will go out for a breathtaking meal or to a gathering and need only a touch of something to offer some relief from your craving; lighter foods may fill your need.

Foods with Staying Power Snacks or meals with a little fiber, complex starches, some protein, or even a little fat will help increment satiety. Amusingly, huge numbers of our ceaseless weight watchers avoid the very foods that could assist them with feeling increasingly fulfilled at suppers—complex starches. Here are some basic unacceptable food decisions and recommendations for how you can balance them to be all the more fulfilling. (There's nothing naturally amiss with these light foods; they just may not give backbone).

IMAGINE A SCENARIO IN WHICH YOU CAN'T STOP EATING.

If you find after time that you are eating despite the fact that you are not very hungry, there's a decent possibility that you may be utilizing food as a method for dealing with stress. This isn't generally as clear and emotional as certain magazines recommend.

IMAGINE A SCENARIO IN WHICH YOU FEEL THERE'S SOMETHING MISSING.

If you've found what it feels like to feel easily full, but then feel that something is missing, it could be the fulfillment factor. This is so significant we've committed an entire rule to it—and talk about it in the next chapter.

CHAPTER SIX
DISCOVER THE SATISFACTION FACTOR

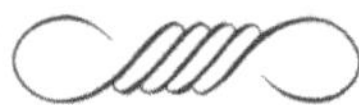

The Japanese have the wisdom to advance joy as one of their objectives for healthy living. In our anger to be slight and solid, we frequently disregard one of the most fundamental blessings of presence—the joy and fulfillment that can be found in the eating experience. When you eat what you truly need, in a situation that is welcoming, the delight you determine will be incredible power in helping you feel fulfilled and content. By giving this experience to yourself, you will find that it takes considerably less food to choose you've had "enough."

How often have you eaten a rice cake when you truly needed potato chips? What's more, what number of rice cakes, carrots, and apples have you eaten endeavoring to get a similar fulfillment you would have found with a bunch of chips? If you feel genuinely happy with your eating experience, you will find that you eat far less food. On the other hand, if you are unsatisfied, you will probably eat more and be sneaking around, paying little heed to your satiety level. For instance, one customer, Fran, needed a bit of cornbread with lunch, yet she demandingly avoided eating it.

Fran contemplated having cornbread with supper, however again halted herself. That night, she ate six Weight Watchers pastries and understood that what she was truly looking for was cornbread—no measure of diet sweets would fulfill her cornbread hankering. Amusingly, the calories from the dieting sweets far surpassed the calories from a solitary bit of cornbread. When Fran was eating the dieting pastries, she was pursuing her apparition food—attempting to fill the void made by denying the fulfillment factor from the food she initially needed.

THE WISDOM OF PLEASURE

Americans have gotten so centered on the speculative chemistry of foods—regardless of whether as an aide to getting more fit or looking for wellbeing—that we have dismissed a significant job that eating plays in our lives—arrangement of delight. The Japanese promote joy as one of their objectives of good dieting. "Make all exercises relating to food and eating pleasurable ones," is one of their Dietary Guidelines for Health Promotion. How unexpected this exhortation is for Americans, particularly dieters, who have come to consider food to be the foe and the eating experience as the battleground between "enticing" food sources and the resolve to maintain a strategic distance from them.

Most calorie counters with whom we work have dismissed that it is so critical to have a delightful, not to mention pleasurable, eating experience. For a few, any encounter that bears a resemblance to delight triggers sentiments of blame and bad behavior. It's not very amazing since we live in a rather judgmental society. Dieting plays directly into this ethic—do penances, settle for less. However, if you settle for food that is substandard, it will frequently leave you needing food, eating, and possibly overeating.

DON'T BE AFRAID TO ENJOY YOUR FOOD

Like many people, our customers are at first apprehensive that, if they let the joy of eating into their lives, they may keep looking for food in an excessive way. However, giving yourself a chance to appreciate food will really bring about self-limiting, as opposed to crazy eating. Keep in mind; hardship is a key factor that prompts kickback eating. Fulfilled Now—Dieting for a significant number of our customers, creates a feeling of fulfillment in a feast that really diminishes their longing for foods sometime in the not too distant future. We have had our customers analyze having a luxurious meal versus a meal with simply "picking" or rummaging. When they set aside the effort to set up a meal that draws in their feeling of smell, taste, locate, etc., they perpetually report a sentiment of fulfillment and a diminished requirement for more food later at night.

The individuals, who get back home and lie on the couch with a box of fries and a soft drink, wind up getting up for one more snack. They feel that they haven't generally eaten and never appear to be fulfilled. Before the finish of the night, they feel overfull and baffled. Kelly is a bustling individual who regularly ignores her very own needs. At times, she'll be so occupied with work and her kid that she doesn't stop to set up a feast for herself. When she sets aside the effort to make sense of what she truly needs to eat and winds up eating precisely what she needs for lunch or supper, she finds that she has no longing for dessert. When she diets throughout the day and never feels fulfilled, her treat cravings around evening time are alarming. When you permit yourself joy and fulfillment from each conceivable eating experience, your absolute amount of food will diminish.

HOW TO REGAIN YOUR PLEASURE IN EATING

Because of dieting, and the dread of surrendering it, dieters have lost their pleasure in eating, and they don't have a clue how to get it back. Here are the means we use with our customers to assist them with accomplishing joy and fulfillment in their eating.

Stage 1: ASK YOURSELF WHAT YOU REALLY WANT TO EAT

Fulfillment is inferred when you set aside the effort to make sense of what you truly need to eat, give yourself the full consent to eat it, and afterward eat in an unwinding, comfortable environment. The issue for most dieters with whom we've worked is that they have made sense of such huge numbers of "stunts" to abstain from eating that they never again realize what they like to eat! When you're going to start another diet, have you at any point asked yourself what you want to eat? That idea, once in a while, enters a dieter's brain. All things considered, the fundamental reason of dieting is to determine what to eat—for what reason would you start to scrutinize your very own needs!

Stage 2: DISCOVER THE PLEASURES OF THE PALATE

Our customers are focused on each part of the food aside from the present time and place. They mourn the past and stress over the future (what will I eat, in what manner will I work off these calories); however, once in a while, they focus on the genuine encounter of eating. In this way, they are not tasting—not encountering or appreciating food. It's as though the skill of eating should be relearned without inclination.

THE SENSUAL QUALITIES OF FOODS

To find what foods you truly like and how to build fulfillment in your eating, investigate the wonderful characteristics of foods. For many people, this implies a conscious time of experimentation. Take your taste buds and sense of taste for a moonlight trip. Before you eat, consider:

• **Taste.**

Put a specific food in your mouth to see which of your taste sensations gets excited. Roll the food around on your tongue to check whether it's sweet, salty, sour, or unpleasant. Is that taste lovely, indifferent, or possibly hostile? Attempt this test on different occasions during the day to check whether certain preferences are increasingly pleasurable on various occasions. A few people are attracted to the sweet taste at breakfast and need waffles or hotcakes. Something hot, for example, eggs with salsa, may be a mood killer in the first part of the day. Others can't eat something sweet until some other time toward the evening.

• Texture.

As you roll the food around on your tongue and start to bite on it, experience the different kinds of textures that food can give. How does crunchy feel to you? Is it rough to need to break into a crunchy food, or is it a delightful encounter? What response do you have to a food that is smooth or rich? Does it help you to remember baby food, and is that engaging or irritating? A few foods are chewy and require a ton of work by your teeth and tongue. How is that for you? At times, you may very well need the progression of fluid through your mouth and down your throat. Certain food surfaces may be engaging at various times of the day or even on multiple days.

• Aroma.

The fragrance of food will have a greater impact on your craving for it than does its taste or surface. Welcome the different fragrances that foods can transmit. Stroll by the pastry shop and smell the yeasty bread leaving the stove or breathe in the espresso fumes as the espresso is trickling through the channel. If the smell of food isn't engaging, you presumably won't get your ideal fulfillment from it. If it smells incredible to you as it is cooking or served to you, it will most likely build your fulfillment.

• Appearance.

Food craftsmen who plan business food sets or menus for eateries realize that food sources that look engaging are charming and make an individual need to attempt them. Investigate the food you're going to eat. Is it appealing to your eye? Is it crisp looking? Is its shading intriguing to you? Envision a plate with a poached chicken bosom, a bubbled potato, and cauliflower—not very exciting. You'll most likely get less fulfillment from that feast than one that is all the more energizing to look at.

• Temperature.

A hot bowl of soup may very well be the request for the day if it's cold and stormy outside. But yogurt isn't typically attractive when you're shuddering under an umbrella. Ask yourself what the most engaging temperature of your foods is. Do you like your hot foods bubbling hot or calm? Do you like your drinks with loads of ice or practically nothing? Or is room temperature fine and dandy for you?

• Volume or Filling-Capacity.

A few foods are light and breezy, while others are substantial and filling. The filling limit of your food decisions can have any kind of effect in how much food you have to fulfill you or how you feel after you're done eating. A few days, you may just be fulfilled by a plate of pasta that fills your stomach, while at different times, a lighter serving of mixed greens is all the more engaging. Regardless of whether something tastes and feels incredible on your tongue and in your mouth, if it makes your stomach feel squeamish or too substantial, it will reduce the fantastic experience. Regard Your Individual Taste Buds. Remember that everybody has an alternate involvement in taste and surface sensations. Not all foods will be attractive to you. (If you once became ill on corn, paying little respect to the reason, corn may never appear to be engaging again.) Your inclinations might be deep rooted or may change every now and then. Stay in contact with what is mouthwatering to you so you can pick what is generally fulfilling. Consider What You Really Feel Like Eating. Once you've experienced this hyperconscious experimentation with the tactile characteristics of foods, whenever you feel like a feast or a tidbit, take a couple of seconds to choose what you truly need to eat. If you experience difficulty choosing what to eat or need a little help, ask yourself:

What do I want to eat?

What food smell may speak to me?

How will the food look?

How will the food taste and feel in my mouth?

Do I need something sweet, salty, harsh, or even somewhat severe?

Do I need something crunchy, smooth, rich, delicate, uneven, liquid, and so on?

Do I need something hot, cold, or moderate?

Do I need something light, breezy, overwhelming, filling, or in the middle?

How will my stomach feeling when I'm done eating?

If you have general information on your taste inclinations, it will lead you to the correct spot on the menu or in the market. Checking in with yourself before a meal will give you the points of interest existing apart from everything else. A further basic key to discovering fulfillment in your eating is to take a break after you've had a couple of bites of your food. Are the taste and texture reliable with your craving? Is the food fulfilling enough to eat? If you keep n eating a food since it's there, regardless of the way that it's unappealing, you'll possibly wind up feeling unsatisfied when you're done and end up waiting for something different that will fulfill you.

Stage 3: MAKE YOUR EATING EXPERIENCE MORE ENJOYABLE

Relish Your Food

Europeans appear to have cornered the market on moderate, erotic eating encounters. Organizations frequently shut down briefly to take into account a long lunch, so the meal can be enjoyed and savored. Friends will, in general, assemble to appreciate the discussion and the food. Americans, then again, regularly take part in work area eating (fifteen minutes if they're fortunate) while going over notes for a gathering. Who do you think has the most fulfilling meal experience? Maybe you don't have the opportunity to value the engaging quality of the various hues and states of the food. You can scarcely take in their smells or feel their surfaces on your tongue and teeth—not to mention appreciate their taste. To assist you with appreciating your food and getting more fulfillment from your meals:

Make time to love your food. Give yourself a particular time for a meal. Indeed, even fifteen minutes is superior to nothing.

Sit down at the table or your work area. Remaining at the fridge or strolling around diminishes consideration and fulfillment.

Take a few full breaths before you start to eat. Profound breathing quiets and focuses you, so you can be centered on eating gradually.

Pay thoughtfulness regarding eating as gradually as possible. Keep in mind that your taste buds are on your tongue, not in your stomach. Eating your food removes your opportunity to taste it truly.

Taste each bite of food that you put in your mouth. Experience the distinctive taste and surface sensations the food can give.

Put your fork down once in a while all through the feast. This will back you off.

Food won't taste as great or be as fulfilling after you've arrived at the last bite.

EAT WHEN GENTLY HUNGRY RATHER THAN WHEN FAMISHED

If you plunk down for a feast when you're very hungry to such an extent that you could eat dairy animals, you won't have the option to differentiate between a tasty steak and the bovine itself! In case you're famished, your biological requirement for energy takes over your capacity to eat gradually and taste what's before you.

Moreover, if you start to eat when you aren't generally hungry, it very well may be hard to choose whether what you're eating is truly what you need and whether it's wonderful. When you're not very hungry, food isn't as convincing. If you discover this is valid for you, this might be an indication that you're not prepared to eat at this time. Hold up a short time, until your appetite is, to some degree, increasingly self-evident, and you'll see that you'll have a simpler time connecting with what you truly need to eat.

EAT IN A PLEASANT ENVIRONMENT (WHEN POSSIBLE)

Most individuals find that they get the best fulfillment from their suppers by eating them in a satisfying setting. Cafés invest a lot of energy and cash making a domain that is engaging and will step individuals back over and over. The style of an eatery can be as significant as the flavor of the food. At home, something very similar goes. If you put everything out on your table in a satisfying way (a placemat or tablecloth, pretty china, etc.), your food pleasure will increase. In any case, eating while standing or driving can lessen fulfillment. If you eat in the vehicle, you are diverted by the traffic and by adjusting food on your lap.

Probably the surest approach to diminish your fulfillment in eating is to attempt to eat when you're having a contention with a relative or companion. You'll most likely wind up eating quicker and may even utilize your biting as an approach to show your resentment. You certainly won't have your attention on the food and might eat everything before you without seeing it—not a wonderful encounter! Give Variety. Eating an assortment of foods isn't just healthfully insightful, but it will give you a more extensive and more fulfilling eating experience. Huge numbers of our customers invest wholeheartedly in keeping void fridges and fruitless pantries.

They accept that, if certain foods aren't anywhere near, they'll be less enticed to indulge. Actually, an absence of engaging food decisions makes a feeling of hardship and advances an imaginative food searching experience that never appears to create a delightful outcome. Give yourself the luxury of keeping a variety of foods around, from soups to pastas to treats or products of the soil. No one can really tell what you may want to eat. Discovering fulfillment in your eating will be a purposeless endeavor if what you need isn't there.

Stage 4: DON'T SETTLE

You are not under any duress to finish your food because you took a bite of it. However, how frequently have you tasted what seemed, by all accounts, to be a divine sweet, just to find it was average—but then you continued eating? Perhaps the greatest resource of being an Intuitive Eater is the capacity to hurl aside food that isn't just as you would prefer.

This can be effectively done when you are genuinely tasting and encountering food, joined with the information you can eat anything you desire once more. Generally, embrace the saying: "If you don't love it, don't eat it, and if you love it, appreciate it." Order something different, discover something different in the fridge, or eat the pieces of the meal that you like and leave the rest.

Stage 5: CHECK IN: DOES IT STILL TASTE GOOD?

Have you at any point eaten an entire box of treats or an entire container of Haagan Daaz? Assuming this is the case, you can likely validate the way that the main couple of treats or spoonfuls of frozen yogurt tasted far superior to those at end. Indeed, even the taste fulfillment of a huge apple wanes when you get down deeply. In investigations of hedonics to food prompts (hedonics is the part of psychology that deals with managing pleasurable and unpleasurable feelings), specialists locate that proceeded with introduction to a similar food brings about a lessening of want for that food. We additionally observe that in our customers. Attempt your very own hedonic experiment. Rate the joy you get from the initial bite of a food from one to ten—one being the least pleasurable and ten being the most. At that point, stop part of the way through eating the food and check your taste buds.

At long last, rate the food when you're down to the last nibble. You're probably going to find that the numbers lessen alongside the food. Routinely check-in with yourself to check whether the food tastes tantamount to how it did when you began. If it doesn't, think about halting, as your fulfillment level is lessening by the bite. Hold up until you're hungry again. Food will taste better, and you'll be increasingly fulfilled. What's more, recollect, nobody is going to remove that food from your eating collection. You can have it for a mind-blowing remainder. So why burn through your time and your food on a not exactly fulfilling experience!

IT DOESN'T HAVE TO BE PERFECT

We've examined how setting aside the effort to make sense of what you truly need to eat and how eating in a good environment can lead you to progressively pleasurable, fulfilling eating encounters. In any case, imagine a scenario where this isn't constantly conceivable. There will be times when you don't have the alternative of getting precisely what you need. You may be served a meal at a companion's or relative's home that wants to sit quietly for it. Many a customer has lamented meals made by a relative or an old companion who may heat up the vegetables until unrecognizable or cook the chicken until it's the surface of an old shoe. On those occasions, recall the guideline of deduction in dim instead of in high contrast.

Intuitive Eating isn't a process that looks for flawlessness, yet one that offers rules to a comfortable association with food. Keep in mind, the majority of your eating encounters will be more fulfilling and pleasurable than you've encountered in long stretches of diets. It's just a single feast—you will endure. It's the manner by which you bounce again into dealing with yourself thereafter that has the effect. Now and then, respecting your appetite is all the better. Also, for a considerable lot of our patients, that by itself is a noteworthy advancement. In any case, if endurance eating involves the majority of your encounters with food, your fulfillment factor will, in all likelihood, be low.

RECLAIM YOUR RIGHT TO PLEASURABLE, SATISFYING EATING

If dieting has been a noteworthy part of your life for a long time, you may need to endeavor to recover your entitlement to make the most of your food. You may have been so customized to eat what you were told, particularly foods that have little taste delight, that you barely realize where to start to discover fulfillment. Realizing what you like to eat and accepting that you reserve the option to appreciate food are key factors in a lifetime of weight control without slimming down. If it requires some investment to achieve the entirety of this, show restraint. All things considered, it's taken you numerous years to lose your capacity to appreciate eating.

CHAPTER SEVEN
COPE WITH YOUR EMOTIONS WITHOUT USING FOOD

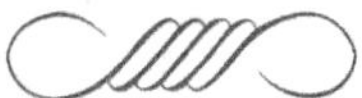

Discover approaches to comfort, support, divert, and resolve your issues without utilizing food. Nervousness, depression, weariness, and outrage are feelings we all encounter all through life.

Everyone has their own trigger, and everyone has its own deal-breaker. Food won't fix any of these emotions. It might comfort for the present moment, divert from the torment, or even numb you into a food headache. Be that as it may, food won't take care of the issue. If anything, eating for an emotional craving will just exacerbate how you feel over the long haul. You'll eventually need to manage the wellspring of the feeling, just as the distress of indulging. Eating doesn't happen in a void. Despite your weight, food, as a rule, has passionate affiliations. If you have any uncertainty, look at food advertisements. They push our eating catches—not through our stomachs but through the enthusiastic association. They infer that in sixty seconds or less you can:

Capture the romance with an intimate mug of espresso.

Make somebody happy.

Reward yourself with a rich pastry.

Eating can be one of the most genuinely loaded encounters that we have in our lives. The passionate mood to eating is set from the principal day that the baby is offered the bosom of its mother to control his crying. It's at that point strengthened each time a treat is offered to alleviate a scratched knee, or frozen yogurt is eaten to commend a Little League triumph. Almost every culture and religion utilizes food as a significant emblematic custom, from the American Thanksgiving blowout to the Jewish Passover Seder. Dieting itself can trigger feelings that lead to utilizing food to adapt to these emotions—chalk up another endless loop brought about by dieting.

THE CONTINUUM OF EMOTIONAL EATING

Food can be utilized to adapt to sentiments in a lot of ways. Utilizing food thusly isn't a segment of organic yearning but of enthusiastic craving. Enthusiastic eating is activated by sentiments, for example, weariness or outrage, not by hunger. These emotions can trigger anything from a benevolent snack to a crazy gorge. Understand that this way of dealing with stress lies on a continuum of power that starts toward one side with mellow, practically all inclusive tangible eating to the furthest edge with desensitizing, regularly anesthetizing eating. The accompanying graph shows this range: tangible satisfaction • comfort • interruption • sedation • discipline.

SENSORY GRATIFICATION

The mildest and most normal inclination that food can call forward is joy. The importance of getting joy from eating is to Discover the Satisfaction Factor. This idea isn't just basic to Intuitive Eating but is an ordinary, normal piece of living. Try not to think little of the significance of satisfying your sense of taste. As we clarified before, by allowing yourself to appreciate and value eating, you will really diminish the measure of food you have to feel fulfilled when naturally hungry. For instance, permitting yourself little tastes of the exceptional foods accessible at Thanksgiving will generally counterbalance gorging.

SOLACE

Simply the idea of specific foods can bring out emotions from an agreeable time or spot. For instance, do you ever long for chicken soup when you are debilitated or macaroni and cheddar on inauspicious days—since that is what your mother fixed on these events? Those are instances of comfort foods. It's entirely expected to have a collection of comfort foods. If you need to twist up with a cover before a chimney and taste hot cocoa with your meal, that is fine. Eating comfort foods once in a while can be a piece of a sound association with food, if you do it while keeping in contact with your satiety levels and without blame. Assuming, in any case, food is the sole thing that helps you deal with yourself when you are feeling tragic, forlorn, or awkward, it can turn into a damaging adapting component.

DISTRACTION

If you go somewhat further on the continuum of emotional eating, food can be utilized to divert you from sentiments you decide not to encounter. Utilizing food to adapt along these lines can get irksome, as it very well may be a tempting conduct that hinders your capacity to recognize your Intuitive sign. It additionally can restrain you from finding the wellspring of the sentiments and dealing with your actual needs.

Regardless of whether you're the young person who sits before the TV with a pack of chips to occupy you from the sentiments of weariness in getting your work done, or you're an official who experiences an entire bowl of peanuts around your work area to divert you from the tension of a laborious gathering, this sort of eating should be stood up to. There is nothing amiss with periodically needing to divert yourself from sentiments. Encountering your sentiments twenty-four hours daily can be monotonous and overpowering. However, food isn't a proper distraction for that brief period.

Sedation •

An increasingly genuine type of utilizing food to adapt is eating to numb or anesthetizing. One customer calls this type of eating a "food coma." Another proposes that this sort of eating brings about a "food hangover." In either case, eating to calm yourself can be as sincerely risky as utilizing medications or liquor for this reason. It shields you from encountering any inclination for broadened timeframes. It becomes difficult to detect your Intuitive sign of yearning and satiety, and it denies you of the wonderful experience that food can bring to your life. Most customers who use food along these lines talk about feeling crazy, withdrawn from life, and for the most part sleepy. They additionally experience difficulty perceiving essential vibes of craving and completion. Connie is a young lady who had an oppressive adolescence.

She figured out how to utilize food at an early age as a desensitizing tool. She keeps quieting herself through the tension, dread, and bitterness of her present life. Connie's weight can increase five pounds every week when she is normally going into her "food trance like states." But significantly more startling than her weight gain is the finished separation from life that she encounters each time. She disengages herself from her companions, phones in sick to work, and feels totally miserable about existence itself. Connie is figuring out how to use other adapting devices with the goal that she can improve an amazing nature. When eating to numb and quiet is incidental and present, it will in general have minimal impeding impact. In any case, this sort of eating can grow into an addictive conduct before you even notice it.

DISCIPLINE

Here and there, eating with the end goal of sedation turns out to be so serious that self-blame results and at last triggers rebuffing practices. Customers end up eating huge amounts of food in a furious, intense way. This is the most extreme type of passionate eating and can prompt loss of confidence and self-loathing. Customers who use food to rebuff themselves report no joy in their eating and really start to despise food. Luckily, this kind of eating conduct vanishes when the Nurturer voice can be enticed to give comprehension and sympathy. If there's no wrongdoing submitted, no discipline needs to be offered.

EMOTIONAL TRIGGERS

We've taken a look at general emotional explanations behind eating; presently, how about we look at the particular sentiments included. A craving for specific foods or just a longing to eat can be activated by a variety of emotions and circumstances. A few people use food to adapt when they have no clue that is what they're doing.

They feel that they're binging "on the grounds that it tastes great." If you find that you're doing a considerable amount of eating when you're not naturally very hungry, at that point, there's a decent possibility that you are utilizing food to adapt. You might not have profound situated passionate purposes behind eating; however, simply overcoming life's problems with a portion of its annoying assignments and weariness may trigger you to look for food to make everything simpler.

FATIGUE AND PROCRASTINATION

One of the most widely recognized reasons our customers eat when they're not hungry is weariness. Actually, studies have demonstrated that paying little heed to an individual's weight, fatigue is one of the most widely recognized triggers of emotional eating. One specific study partitioned students into two gatherings. One bunch had the tedious errand of composing similar letters again and again for almost 30 minutes. The other group was occupied with an exciting composing task. Students in each group were given a bowl of wafers to snack on. Guess which gathering ate more. Notwithstanding weight, the "exhausted" bunch ate the most saltines.

In weariness eating, food is utilized as an approach to fill time just as a path to put off doing everyday work. For certain individuals, the idea of the food and the genuine encounter of making it work and eating it breaks the monotony. Here are a few circumstances that produce weariness eating.

Lying around the house on a Sunday evening when you've made no plans for the afternoon.

Having to traverse an evening of contemplating, administrative work, or a writing task.

Watching an exhausting night of TV with nothing else to do except for take food breaks.

Killing time: trusting that a gathering will begin, sitting tight for a telephone call, etc. We likewise observe this kind of eating in our exhausted customers—they believe they should consistently be accomplishing something, being profitable. The minute a small gap opens up in their timetable, they want to fill it—regularly with food. (It's satisfactory to eat, yet not to rest!)

PAY OFF AND REWARD

Have you, at any point, guaranteed yourself that you could have a treat once you wrapped up a research paper or cleaned the house? Provided that this is true, you have encountered remunerate eating. It's not unordinary to utilize food as an inspiration for achieving undesired errands. For instance:

Children are frequently paid with treats, for example, sweet or frozen yogurt if they act well—at the shopping center, for a sitter, etc.

People regularly remunerate themselves for taking a stab at work, at home, or at school with an additional bagel or a biscuit, for instance. Utilizing food as a reward can act naturally propagating, as there will consistently be continuous assignments and difficulties that can be made progressively middle of the road if they're moderated by food blessings.

FERVOR

Food and the eating experience itself can fill in as an approach to add energy when life starts to feel dull. At an unpretentious level, arranging an exceptional meal or reserving a spot at a most loved café can make a feeling of energy. The thought of starting a better diet can trigger sentiments of expectation. This is one reason dieting is so appealing. Our customers discuss how, in any event, mulling over another diet gives them a surge of adrenaline—simply envisioning another body and another life. When the diet fails, the energy is supplanted with despair. Now, the experience of setting off to the store to purchase huge amounts of taboo foods can be one approach to reproduce the fervor. And afterward, the cycle proceeds—diet/gorging, diet/indulging. This is energizing, however, at what cost?

MITIGATING

It's not hard to comprehend the mitigating power that food can give. It very well may be all the more telling to go to the kitchen for treats and milk than to sit on the lounge chair and experience awkward sentiments. This is especially valid if those treats and milk help you to remember a period that was charming, and life felt less confounded. Routinely eating to calm what upsets you can develop into an issue with food. Food can have other emblematic relationships with comfort. Ellen is a sixteen-year-old who has fought with her dad since she was a little youngster. She depicts him as mean and frightful with a severe character. It was not amazing to hear Ellen talk about her fixation on eating a lot of treats each day as an approach to bring "sweetness" into her life. To her, the desserts countered the sharpness of her everyday encounters with her dad.

LOVE

Food can get associated with the sentiment of being cherished. There is unquestionably a sentimental connection with food—chocolate on Valentine's Day is an exemplary model. When dating, there's an implicit standard process that your relationship is raised to a progressively close level when you have encountered a home-prepared feast for two. Customers often recount how their folks' best way to show love was through food. These guardians might not have had the option to show physical consideration or address them in cherishing ways, yet the food was constantly ample.

DISSATISFACTION, ANGER, AND RAGE

If you wind up experiencing a pack of hard and crunchy pretzels when you're not hungry, it's a decent wager that you might be feeling disappointed or irate. The physical demonstration of gnawing and crunching can fill in as an approach to discharge these affections for certain individuals. One customer, Nancy, a legal counselor, found that she had a propensity for curbing her resentment at a portion of her customers by snatching some hard food, regardless of whether it was carrots or wafers, and chomping endlessly.

STRESS

A significant number of our customers state they head for the closest treat under distressing times. However, in many people, biological signals related to stress turn off the longing to eat. The surge of adrenaline during unpleasant occasions gets a course of natural occasions underway to give prompt vitality. Accordingly, glucose is raised, and assimilation is eased back. These two components alone will, in general, stifle hunger and elevate the feeling of satiety when eating. The natural responses are a type of self-conservation—to prepare our bodies for "fight or flight." While this was very valuable for endurance—warding off a man-eating tiger or escaping from peril required prompt vitality—a developing assortment of research proposes that in our advanced society, this system may really add to heftiness. It might be upsetting to ward off heavy traffic or to escape from a cutoff time, yet you needn't bother with the additional glucose that the pressure response gives. Where does it go?

If you don't utilize it (say, for physical movement), excess glucose gets changed to fat. This organic issue is possibly aggravated if you adapt to worry by eating. Studies have likewise demonstrated that individuals who have been dieting are particularly defenseless against indulging during unpleasant occasions. Stress becomes one more motivation to "blow" the diet. Dieting itself can likewise be a wellspring of stress.

Tension of any size, from an up and coming last to holding on to hear if you landed the position, can trigger a critical need to eat to mitigate uneasiness. Now and then summed up tension can be depicted as that awkward inclination you can't put a finger on; our customers state it feels like butterflies in your stomach. With the emphasis on the stomach, so goes the food.

GENTLE DEPRESSION

It's normal for some individuals to go to food when they are somewhat discouraged. In mellow sadness, weight gain is regularly observed, particularly in dieters. In one examination, 62 percent of the weight watchers and 52 percent of non-dieters expressed they ate more when feeling discouraged.

BEING CONNECTED

They need to feel some portion of a gathering or to feel an association with others can be amazing for certain individuals and can even influence how and what they eat. This experience was piercingly portrayed by Mathew, when he was discussing the meal he had eaten one night with certain companions. In spite of the fact that he didn't care for the food served, he ate it in any case. He settled on the decision to feel associated yet disappointed with the food as opposed to feeling extraordinary. How frequently have you eaten to be a part of the group—from heading out to get dessert to sharing a pizza?

SLACKENING THE REINS

Regularly, customers who are exceptionally effective in each part of their lives, with the exception of in their eating, markdown their achievements. They feel as though their food issues demonstrate they are really disappointments throughout everyday life. We have discovered that, by and large, gorging is the main component such an individual has for giving up and letting free the reigns of command over their life.

COPING WITH EMOTIONAL EATING

Regardless of whether your reaction to passionate hunger is gentle enthusiastic eating or crazy gorging, there are four key strides to making food less significant in your life. Ask yourself:

1. Am I naturally hungry? If the appropriate response is yes, your subsequent stage is to respect your appetite and eat! If you are not hungry, answer the accompanying inquiries.

2. What am I feeling? When you wind up going after food when there is no natural appetite, take an opportunity to discover what you are feeling. This isn't such a simple inquiry to reply, particularly if you are not in contact with your emotions. Attempt the accompanying:

Write out your emotions.

Call a companion and discuss your sentiments.

Talk about your emotions into a recording device.

Just sit with your sentiments and experience them if you can.

Talk to a guide or a psychotherapist.

3. What do I need? Lots of individuals eat to satisfy some neglected need, which is identified with the passionate or physical inclination being experienced. If you are a ceaseless dieter, you can be especially helpless. Eating to soothe a neglected need can be blamed so as to eat.

MEETING YOUR NEEDS WITHOUT FOOD

There are different manners by which we figure out how to deal with the unending emotions that life can trigger. A few people adapt from the get-go that it's alright to express their feelings or to request an embrace. Others aren't fortunate enough to be instructed how to deal with themselves in profitable, supporting ways. The primary errand in figuring out how to adapt without utilizing food is to recognize that you are qualified for having your needs met. In any case, essential needs are regularly limited, including:

Getting rest

Getting arousing delight

Expressing emotions

Being heard, understood, and acknowledged

Being mentally and inventively invigorated

Receiving comfort and warmth

LOOK FOR NURTURE

Feeling sustained can enable you to feel solace and warmth, so food loses its main situation in this job. There are numerous courses and roads accessible for supporting yourself and getting sustainment from others.

Rest and unwind.

Take a sauna or a Jacuzzi bath.

Listen to jazz music.

Take time to inhale profoundly.

Learn to contemplate.

Play cards with your friends.

Take a bath in candlelight.

Take a yoga class.

Get a back rub.

Play with your pets.

Develop a system of friends.

Ask companions for embraces.

Buy yourself little shows.

Put new blossoms in your home.

Spend time cultivating.

Get a nail trim, pedicure, facial, hair style, and so forth

Get a teddy bear and embrace it.

MANAGE YOUR FEELINGS

If you get a steady flow of solace and nurturing, you'll be better arranged to confront the feelings that have been so startling. Recognize what is upsetting you—enable your sentiments to come up. This will diminish your need to drive them down with food. Here are a few proposals of how to manage your sentiments.

Write your sentiments in a diary.

Call a companion (or a few).

Talk about your emotions into a recording device.

Release outrage through beating a cushion or a punching pack.

Confront the individual who is setting off your sentiments.

Let yourself cry.

Breathe profoundly.

Sit with your emotions and find how the force will reduce with time.

If you experience difficulty recognizing your sentiments or adapting to them, it might be useful to chat with a specialist, particularly if it is a tenacious issue.

LOCATE A DIFFERENT DISTRACTOR

Numerous individuals use food as their essential interruption from their emotions. It's alright to escape from your sentiments every once in a while; however, you don't need to blame food. Numerous young people reveal to us that they get back home from school each evening and sit before the TV with a pack of chips and a pop. When inquired as to why they do this, they state that they're maintaining a strategic distance from the exhausting sentiments of getting their work done. When it's recommended that they initially have a bite to deal with their organic craving and afterward observe some TV to occupy themselves for some time before settling down to schoolwork, they shout that their folks would never let them.

For whatever length of time that they're eating, they can honestly put off doing schoolwork, however having different distracters isn't permitted! This is likewise valid for some compulsive worker customers. It's socially worthy to require some investment out to eat (a rest); however, to simply sit at the work area, even while qualified for a break, isn't permitted. They dread that it will show up as though they are sitting idle. Others use food to divert themselves from depression, dread, and nervousness. Since it is overpowering to attempt to feel your sentiments twenty-four hours per day, give yourself consent to take a break from them for some time. Take the decisive position of diverting yourself in a genuinely sound manner. Attempt the accompanying:

Read an interesting book.

Rent a film.

Talk on the phone.

Go out to a movie theater.

Take a drive.

Clean out your storage room.

Put on some music and move.

Read a magazine

Go for a walk around the square

Work in the nursery

Listen to a novel on tape.

Do a crossword puzzle.

Work on a jigsaw baffle.

Play with the PC.

Take a rest.

HOW EMOTIONAL OVEREATING HAS HURT AND HELPED

As you analyze your utilization of food as a way of dealing with stress, it's useful to investigate how food has really helped you. The thought that indulging can have advantages may sound insane to you, particularly if you're feeling troubled by this conduct and by your weight. In any case, if there were no upside to binging, you presumably wouldn't proceed with it. Take a bit of paper and separate it down the middle. On one half, make a rundown of "How utilizing food serves me"— refer to every one of the advantages you get from indulging.

HOW USING FOOD SERVES ME

HOW USING FOOD DOES ME A DISSERVICE

It tastes good

It makes me overweight.

It's reliable—it's always there.

My clothes don't fit.

It keeps me from feeling bored.

I'm uncomfortable walking and exercising.

It soothes me.

My cholesterol is high.

It numbs my bad feelings.

I'm numbed to the joys of life.

As you investigate your rundown, you may be amazed to discover that the utilization of food isn't only a negative encounter for you. Actually, it might give you some significant advantages. In any case, if you're feeling awful and remorseful about utilizing food to adapt, it will be difficult for you to perceive that its advantages may even out its weights. By perceiving that there are a few advantages to utilizing food, you'll start to claim your eating experience instead of feeling wild.

WHEN FOOD IS NO LONGER IMPORTANT

Numerous customers have discussed having weird, awkward sentiments when they're never again utilizing food to adapt to their feelings. Simultaneously, they're feeling cheerful and secure in their new Intuitive Eating style and might be losing the weight that has consistently been a battle for them. There are two or three purposes behind the clashing sentiments.

You never again have the "benefits" of utilizing food. While adapting to food can be ruinous, one customer noticed that, on intense days, she realized she could generally return home to her chocolate. Presently, rather, she's "trapped" with encountering her sentiments. You may even need to experience a lamenting period for the loss of food as sofa and partner.

You may likewise see that you're encountering your emotions in a more profound, more grounded way. Since you're never again concealing them with food, they may profoundly affect you. This is a time when a few people conclude that it is useful to get guiding as an approach to process these since a long time ago covered sentiments.

A STRANGE GIFT

You may go for quite a while without utilizing food to adapt, when out of the blue enthusiastic eating gets you off guard. If this happens, it is anything but an indication of disappointment or that you've lost ground; rather, it's a weird blessing. Overeating is basically a sign that worries throughout your life outperform the ways of dealing with stress that you have created. A portion of these anxieties are separation, work change, a transition to another city, the passing of somebody close, marriage, or the introduction of a youngster. These might be new or surprising encounters for you.

Therefore, you haven't had the chance to create adapting aptitudes to manage them. In this way, you return to eating as the natural method to deal with yourself. Indulging can likewise repeat when your way of life gets unequal with such a large number of duties and commitments, with too brief period for joy and unwinding. Subsequently, food is utilized to enjoy, escape, and unwind (but quickly). When you discover this occurrence, it might be a sign for you to rethink your life and discover approaches to place more emphasis on it. If you don't make these vital changes, food stays significant by filling a neglected need.

In both of these circumstances we've depicted, indulging turns into a red banner that tells you that something isn't directly in your life. When you genuinely value this, eating won't feel wild—rather it's an early cautioning framework.

Perceive that you are so fortunate to have this instrument to alarm you that something is out of kilter in your life! (From the start, our customers think this thought is somewhat ludicrous, until they understand the reality behind it in their very own lives.) Those individuals who have never had a passionate eating issue regularly have no unmistakable admonition of abundant worry in their lives. If you can see that your eating issue can have benefits just as awful impacts, you won't slip into an example of reckless practices that become ruinous and hard to switch.

UTILIZING FOOD CONSTRUCTIVELY

When you adapt better approaches for adapting to your feelings, consider how food can keep sustaining you in a productive manner. You reserve an option to feel better—and that implies not feeling stuffed, yet in addition feeling happy with your food decisions, being solid now, and decreasing future wellbeing dangers. Your association with food will turn out to be progressively positive as you relinquish food as a method for dealing with stress and bring it into your life as a nonthreatening, pleasurable encounter. Be that as it may, first you have to figure out how to regard your body and acknowledge how it feels when you work out.

CHAPTER EIGHT
RESPECT YOUR BODY

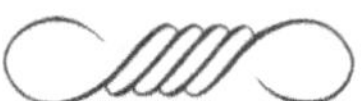

Acknowledge your genetic imprint. Similarly as an individual with a shoe size of eight would not expect sensibly to squeeze into a size six, it is similarly worthless (and awkward) to have a comparative assumption regarding body size. Respect your body so you can rest easy thinking about what your identity is. It's difficult to dismiss the diet attitude if you are ridiculous and excessively condemning of your body shape. Body vigilance brings forth body stress, which stirs up food stress, which energizes the cycle of dieting.

So what do you do, simply overlook it? Crawl into a dark hole, avoid the world, and eat everything in sight? No. Be that as it may, as long as you are at war with your body, it will be hard to find a sense of contentment with yourself and food. With each trashing look in the mirror, the Food Police gain control, and with that comes pledges of only one more diet. Has all the self-hatred on account of your body made a difference? Has harping on your blemished body parts helped you to become less fatty or only aggravated you? Does berating yourself each time you step on the scale make your weight any less?

We presently can't seem to discover one customer who says that concentrating on their body in such negative manners became useful in the end. Studies have demonstrated that, the more you focus on your body, the more awful you feel about yourself. However, the body torment game goes on—Mirror, mirror on the wall, who's the slimmest of them all? It's difficult to get away from the body torment game when the entire nation is playing it. For the sake of wellness, a fit and hard shape has become the body symbol since the nineties. Self-acclaimed fitness experts demand that you can "shape" your body as though it were a chunk of clay, that you can change your hereditary shape with an aerobic huff and puff. We are ardent advocates of being fit and knowing the medical benefits of activity, yet we believe we should call attention to the ridiculous desires being painted.

It is generally acknowledged in the exploration network that you can't spot-reduce (lose fat in only one indicated place). So how might it be that you can shape your body by taking a shot at certain body parts? Indeed, you can fabricate explicit muscles through quality and exercise. What's more, you can lose muscle versus fat through aerobic activity. In any case, you can't select where that fat will be lost. It's conceivable to manufacture muscle underneath fat layers, yet this isn't the idea of body chiseling that most overweight individuals have as a primary concern. Most customers we talk with take body-chiseling classes in order to chisel off the fat. The design world has formed the perfect search for ladies into different renditions of dainty—from the sixties Twiggy figure to the cutting edge starving stray look epitomized by supermodel Kate Moss. Indeed, even the full-bodied design watch ends up being excessively flimsy by therapeutic norms.

BODY IMAGE: A WAIST IS A TERRIBLE THING TO MIND

The majority of our customers are skilled at being excessively basic or despising their bodies. Also, putting an end to body stress and self-hatred is no simple assignment. A large portion of us experience difficulty tolerating a compliment, not to mention tolerating our bodies.

We have discovered that the thought of tolerating your body was an over the top stretch for our customers as a starting point. They expected that, if they acknowledged their present body size, it would mean smugness, surrendering, and getting considerably greater. It's one thing to lose the skirmish of the lump, they'd state, however also absolutely surrendering would mean extreme disappointment.

At any rate, there's respect and pride in proceeding with the battle. Our customers likewise contended that grasping the thought of body acknowledgment felt fraudulent. All things considered, they looked for our assistance on the grounds that they didn't acknowledge their present body—they needed a change. What a mystery. Our experience has given us that, to get to your normal perfect weight, you have to extricate yourself and approach your body with deference. Keep in mind, rehashed lost calories and a wrong frame of mind toward your body have not helped—it's a piece of what got you to where you are at this moment. When you are trapped in the I-detest my-body mentality, it's very simple to continue postponing beneficial things for yourself, holding up until you have a body that is all the more meriting. Be that as it may, that day never comes (particularly when your benchmarks are inaccessible).

So you put off treating yourself better. Numerous parts of your life actually get weighted down. "I'll join the fitness center after I shed ten pounds," "I'll go on a unique get-away after I arrive at my objective weight," "I'll start going out with my companions when I simply get a portion of this weight off"— thus the vacant guarantees go. Also, life gets somewhat emptier during these occasions. Body-image expert and clinician Judith Rodin notes in her book, Body Traps, "You don't have to shed pounds first before you deal with your body image. Indeed, the process really happens very in the invert!" We likewise have discovered that, if you are hungry to make weight reduction an auxiliary objective and regarding your body an essential objective, it will help push you ahead.

We are not saying ignore your body—we are encouraging you rather to respect it. This doesn't imply that you should quit. This doesn't imply that you should ignore your wellbeing. Actually, respecting your body implies dealing with your wellbeing. It is the start of making harmony with your body and your genetics. It is presumably the most difficult thing that you will do. If you put your priorities on making harmony with your food and body, that is turning into an Intuitive Eater, it will enable you to loosen up. Else, it will be a steady back-and-forth. It's entirely expected to feel panicky when pondering about respecting your body.

However, by doing so, it will enable you to experience the Intuitive Eating steps considerably more effectively. Incidentally, we watch a checked distinction between our customers who can regard their bodies and the individuals who are definitely not. The individuals who can arrive at a position of regard for their bodies have more persistence for the Intuitive Eating process. This persistence permits them to investigate further and push ahead faster. The individuals who experience difficulty regarding their bodies regularly wind up in struggle. When they feel nefarious toward their bodies, they battle with a serious want to slim down and "simply get the weight off." Then they sway with irregular sentiments of harmony when working through the Intuitive Eating process. It is those snapshots of harmony that give them trust, in any case, to proceed with Intuitive Eating.

WHY "RESPECT"

We picked the word respect cautiously as a starting point for working through your body issues. It's an intense spot to start for a large portion of our customers. Simply remember these couple of focuses, which will slide you into body-regard: You don't need to like all aspects of your body to regard it. Indeed, you don't need to acknowledge where your body is currently to regard it. Respecting your body implies treating it with poise and meeting its essential needs. A large number of our customers treat their pets with more respect than their very own bodies—they feed them, take for them out for strolls, and are benevolent to them.

At last, if you are somebody who has utilized food as an approach to adapt to your feelings over a lifetime, your present body shape might be illustrative of the manner in which you dealt with yourself when you knew no other way. As opposed to disparaging the consequences of this method for dealing with stress, regard yourself for enduring. Regarding your body is a basic defining moment in turning into an Intuitive Eater. It is difficult. Our way of life has a worked-in inclination against enormous body sizes while setting a premium on appearance. It's imperative to perceive that these inclinations exist, since it might appear as though you are a salmon swimming toward the social standard.

All things considered, it's inside and out in both in blatant and subtle form, from the slight on-screen characters in diet soda promotions to glaring magazine covers, for example, People magazine's January 1994 issue, "Diet Winners and Sinners of the Year. Here's the inside scoop on who got fat, which got fit and how they did it." It removes a conscious exertion to move from this cultural standard. Because looking for a thin body is the cultural standard doesn't make it right.

THE MOST EFFECTIVE METHOD TO RESPECT YOUR BODY

Consider respecting your body in two different ways: first, by making it comfortable, and second, by meeting its fundamental needs. You have the right to be comfortable. You have the right to get your essential needs met. Or on the other hand, the more hopeless you feel, the more desperate you'll be. Think about these fundamental premises of body regard:

My body has the right to be fed.

My body has the right to be treated with pride.

My body has the right to be dressed serenely, and in the way I am accustomed to.

My body has the right to be touched tenderly and with regard.

My body has the right to move easily.

We should investigate how you can offer more regard to your body (and to yourself). It's a simple idea to see, however unmistakably progressively hard to actualize. The accompanying thoughts and apparatuses have helped our customers start another association with their bodies.

GET COMFORTABLE.

How about we get personal here. When was the last time you purchased new underwear? Try not to laugh. Very frequently, we have customers who feel that they don't merit new clothing (not to mention new garments) until they arrive at a specific weight or apparel size. Consider what that implies at a fundamental level. Wearing underwear, a bra, or briefs that are continually squeezing or riding up is exceptionally awkward.

How can you be calm in your body when you have a constant unpleasant token of your size? Indeed, even an old vehicle still needs another arrangement of tires. While at first, you may chuckle at the straightforwardness of changing your clothing, it's significantly affected a considerable lot of our customers. "I had an infant a couple of months back. My maternity clothing was ludicrously huge; however, my regular underwear fit too cozily. They were a consistent reminder that it was too enormous. I felt hopeless until I put resources into clothing that fit. Interestingly, I would not like to spend the cash—even though I had dished out a bounty on a health improvement plan that didn't work. I was astonished at how a straightforward demonstration had such an effect on resting easy thinking about myself."

Cassandra was in her fifties and hadn't purchased new bras in years. (The ones she had been of high caliber and very costly, so they had kept going.) Sadly, the under-wires in her bras were poking and scarring her, yet she didn't feel she had the right to purchase new bras until she shed pounds. However, consistently, she was hopeless. Her initial move toward her body was to buy new bras and pantyhose. Even though she realized it would be some time before she contacted her optimal, yet sensible, weight, she discovered that wearing convolutedly tight underwear would not cause the process to happen any speedier. When she was increasingly loose in her clothing, she had the option to be successfully free about her eating.

The comfort standard goes past underpants. How you dress can be a stage toward a freshly discovered regard for your body. We are not saying you ought to be a captive to the design business but dress in the way in which you are acclimated. If you are accustomed to dressing in a customized suit troupe, for what reason would it be advisable for you to stop because your body isn't the place you need it to be? You ought not need to make do with scraps or frump duds.

There's nothing amiss with dressing in frayed pants and a curiously large shirt if that is the thing that you are utilized to and agreeable in. Assuming you lean toward wearing dress pants and an easygoing jacket and settle for destroyed pants, it might influence how you feel about yourself and your body. It's an issue of being steady. Very regularly, health improvement plans asked you to "dispose of your fat garments", else, they caution, you are giving a greeting for disappointment. By following this proclamation, in any case, you are setting yourself up to feel awkward and more body-phobic.

Instead, dress for your present time and body; be agreeable. Change Your Body-Assessment Tools. We have discovered that the higher the number of our customers who weigh themselves as often as possible experience issues living in their present body—they get too stressed over the numbers. Our recommendation: Stop gauging yourself. Keep in mind; the scale is the apparatus of a ceaseless calorie counter. And be careful with substituting a tight pair of pants as a pseudo-scale or body appraisal apparatus. Clinging to a little bit of attire and giving one it a shot day by day or week after week can similarly undermine how you feel about yourself and your body. Jamie, a youthful record official for an advertising firm, was doing very well with Intuitive Eating. She quit abstaining from excessive food intake, regarded her appetite, regarded her totality, etc. Jamie had likewise disposed of the scale. However, she started to evaluate her advancement by taking a stab at a tight smaller than usual skirt. Each time she gave the dress a shot, she felt awful about herself. It passed on the message, "You haven't gained enough ground. You are still excessively fat." Jamie inevitably disposed of the skirt and her terrible emotions about her body. Indeed, even a thin individual will feel fat in some jeans that are excessively tight.

CHAPTER NINE
EXERCISE—FEEL THE DIFFERENCE
FORGET ACTIVIST EXERCISE.

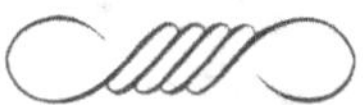

Simply get active and feel the distinction. Move your concentration to how it feels to move your body, as opposed to the calorie-consuming impact of exercise. If you focus on how you feel from working out, for example empowered, it can affect turning up for an energetic morning walk and hitting the snooze alarm. If, when you wake up, your only objective is to lose/weight, it's typically not a propelling component at that moment. If you were to arrange your demeanor toward work out, would it be "just-do-it" or "simply overlook it"? A significant number of our customers fall into the last class.

They are worn out. Turning out frequently went with the negative encounters of insufficient dieting. Our customers detested exercise for two key reasons. They may have begun practicing when they started a diet, or they mishandled their bodies with ridiculous measures of activity, which prompted wounds. In any case, they truly felt regretful for not doing what's needed. If you started an activity program while beginning a diet, your energy (calorie) intake was excessively low. When you need more vitality, practice isn't stimulating, not to mention fun. It turns into an errand, pure drudgery. When you are deprived of eating, it's inevitably hard to work out, mainly if starches are deficient (which is frequently the situation with our incessant calorie counters).

Carbohydrates are the favored fuel of activity.

As should be evident with starch control, running two miles utilizes 50 to 55 grams of carbohydrates. This is the measure of starches found in three cuts of bread. If you usually limit carbohydrate foods (for example, potatoes, bread, and pasta) and afterward include workout, you are troubling the body with a starch shortfall. Keep in mind, for normal, natural capacities, the body must have starches. If you don't sustain your body with enough starches, it will destroy its muscle protein to make indispensable vitality. This has been shown even in research on continuance competitors.

Continuance competitors who didn't get enough sugars for their activity action consumed fanned chain amino acids (a part of a protein) to help make essential vitality to fuel their bodies. Remember that even fit and spurred competitors experience issues working out if they are low on sugars! This impact was represented in an investigation of top school swimmers by practice physiologist David Costill of Ball State University in Indiana. He found that swimmers who didn't eat enough carbohydrates were not able to finish their exercises.

If top athletes experienced difficulty working out because they didn't eat enough, for what reason would you hope to be any different? If you have never delighted in working out, not to mention encountering the "sprinter's high" from working out, there's a decent possibility it was a direct result of dieting or the dieting attitude of constraining foods. When a diet comes up short, practice frequently stops since it was just done as assistance to dieting. You are left with recollections of feeling terrible, which makes you less inclined to need to practice later on. No big surprise, the chronic weight watcher experiences issues with predictable exercise. Who needs to regularly expose his body to something that doesn't feel better?

However, customers frequently reprimand themselves for not having enough resolve or not having the outstanding "take care of business" mantra of activity.

This resembles feeling remorseful for not having enough resolution to "will" a vehicle to work on a vacant tank of gas. However, to harvest the numerous positive outcomes from practice, there should be a predictable exertion. A large number of our customers have been worn out both rationally and physically from "crash working out." Like crash slims down, crash practicing doesn't keep going long. This regularly happens when somebody is resolved to get fit rapidly. They start with a lot of movement in a brief span and end up either sore, or despising exercise, or both. Others feel scared by not having a fit enough body to go to the rec center or work out. It's a one-two terrorizing punch.

To begin with, they don't feel hungry enough by the various hard bodies. Second, they get a glaring unsure update from floor-length mirrors put on each vacant divider. There are different reasons ceaseless dieters don't want to begin or proceed to work out:

Bad encounters growing up, including being compelled to run laps or do the workout as a discipline, being prodded for being clumsy, not getting picked for groups.

Rebelling against guardians, life partners, and other people who pushed working out, similar to a "decent" diet: "You ought to go run," "You ought to go to the rec center," etc.

BREAKING THROUGH EXERCISE BARRIERS

As opposed to demanding that our clients quickly set out on an exercise routine, we hold up until they are prepared. Deferring action for half a month, even a couple of months, won't have a major effect on a profound rooted responsibility. In this way, don't stress if you don't feel like tying on your shoes and running a couple of laps, particularly if you have inclined toward being an activity abuser. There are a few keys to getting through the hindrances that keep you from working out.

CONCENTRATE ON HOW IT FEELS

We have discovered that one key to steady exercise is to concentrate on how it feels, instead of playing the numbers round of checking calories burned. Rather than simply sticking around for your chance or gritting your teeth when working out, investigate how it affects you for the day (counting during exercise and following). How would you feel in regards to:

Stress level—Are you ready to deal with pressure better? It is safe to say that you are less tense? Is it simpler to accept circumstances, move with the punches?

Energy level—Do you feel progressively alert? Somewhat more spunky?

A general sense of wellbeing—Do you have an improved outlook on life?

Sense of strengthening—Do you feel more in charge? Do you say, "I can do it," and hold onto the day?

Sleep—Do you rest all the more soundly and wake up refreshed? If you are in a time of inertia, it's particularly critical to take note of these emotions. They will fill in as your benchmark. Look at the contrast between when you did and didn't work out. Note how you felt. When you can truly feel the distinction between practicing reliably and being dormant, the positive sentiments can be a persuading factor for proceeding. For what reason would you quit accomplishing something that feels better? Instead, if you practice with the dieting attitude, you become accustomed to halting and beginning, much the same as each new dieting endeavor. It has been demonstrated that 70 percent of the individuals who start an activity program quit during the first year. Keep in mind; practice is considerably more than a calorie-eating machine.

DISASSOCIATE FROM WEIGHT LOSS EXERCISE

Are we stating that exercise doesn't influence weight reduction? No. It's all around acknowledged that physical movement is the one steady component related to long-term weight upkeep. Exercise assumes a critical job in digestion and protecting slender bulk. However, practice solo records for just a piece of weight reduction. So if your solitary spotlight is on weight reduction, it won't spur you to exercise for long. It will only serve like a period card being punched by an exhausted sequential construction system worker.

Furthermore, when the result isn't brisk enough, it could be debilitating. Utilizing weight reduction as an ultimate purpose behind physical action could likewise drive you to practice misuse. And still, after all that, regardless, you may not be content with your body.

CONCENTRATE ON EXERCISE AS A WAY OF TAKING CARE OF YOURSELF

Regardless of whether you are heavy or thin in stature, youthful or old, everybody profits by being active. It makes you feel better and averts medical issues sometime down the road. Explicit benefits include:

Increased bone quality

Increased pressure resilience

Decreased pulse

Reduced danger of constant sicknesses, including coronary illness, diabetes, osteoporosis, hypertension, and a few malignant growths

Increased level of good cholesterol (HDL); diminished complete cholesterol level

Increased heart and lung quality

Improved digestion—keeps up fit weight and fires up vitality creation in the cells

TRY NOT TO GET CAUGHT IN EXERCISE MIND GAMES

If you've had a diet attitude for several years, there's a decent possibility that parts of it have penetrated do-not-practice-traps. The "It's-Not-Worth-It" Trap. We know numerous individuals who wouldn't walk except if they could get in 60 minutes—anything under that "doesn't check." Therefore, a fifteen-minute walk break during lunch doesn't count. Instead, they don't do anything. We usually observe customers rebate their exercise since they didn't arrive at their recommended quantity. It "didn't count" since they just practiced multiple times in seven days, as opposed to five.

GETTING STARTED ON A LIFELONG COMMITMENT

Kids are generally dynamic—squirming, running, and bouncing. In any case, as we get more seasoned, our physical action decreases regardless of quick-paced living. In contrast to youngsters, we have to search for approaches to build our regular activity intentionally. Start by asking how you can be increasingly dynamic in your everyday living. For instance, consider leaving your vehicle down the square to work in a ten-minute stroll to work. When you factor in the arrival walk, you've quite recently fabricated twenty minutes of strolling into your day.

Include a ten-minute walk break during lunch, and you've met the base level for physical wellness and its medical advantages. Do this five times each week, and you've strolled 130 hours or around 400 to 500 miles in a single year!

Keep in mind; common exercises do have an effect. (Obviously, customary exercise can likewise be incorporated, for example, running or high impact exercise.) Get free of vitality sparing gadgets and put resources into human vitality that will assist you with expanding your day by day exercises. • Use a hand-push yard trimmer instead of a power one. • Take the stairs instead of the lift.

MAKE EXERCISE FUN

For specific individuals, this implies practicing with a companion, relative, or coach. It may be the one time you can talk unreservedly with a companion. Or then again, maybe your days are so crazed with requests from other individuals that a little isolation would add to your activity delight. One positive approach to remove the enjoyment from practice is to get harmed. Do make sure to begin gradually in whatever movement you pick. Some further proposals:

Be sure to choose exercises that you appreciate. Consider playing a group activity, for example, volleyball, ball, or tennis.

To participate in an assortment of exercises—you need not devote your life to only one game. By broadening, you'll likewise diminish your opportunity of wounds and increase your satisfaction factor.

If you practice at home on stationary wellness hardware, include fun by getting a VCR and taping your preferred drama or TV film or perusing a decent book or magazine (instead of business-related papers).

Make your walk increasingly pleasant with a compact CD player. Tune in to books on tape or your preferred music.

MAKE EXERCISE A NON-NEGOTIABLE PRIORITY

Ask yourself, "When can I reliably create an opportunity to work out?" Make a meeting with yourself to work out and respect it as you would some other gathering or arrangement. If you travel a great deal:

Pack your strolling shoes. (It's a fascinating method to become more acquainted with another city.)

Pack a skipping rope. (It's a lightweight bit of hardware that conveys a cardio-workout in a short measure of time.) • Choose lodgings that have exercise offices. (They are expanding in number.)

Take a bit of leeway of air terminal delays and stroll around the air terminal. (It, for the most part, feels great after sitting.)

BE COMFORTABLE

Exercise clothing need not be an expensive fashion show material. Yet, it is essential to wear clothes that allow you to inhale and enable you the ease of flexibility with your movements. This likewise implies dressing for the climate. Overwhelming sweats can make you awkwardly hot when you wear them to mask your body. A larger than average lightweight T-shirt and stockings will, for the most part, be perfect for ladies. Or on the other hand, bicycle shorts with a larger than usual shirt functions admirably for many people. Remember about comfortable shoes too. Not only will they feel better, but they are also an investment in preventing injury.

IN CONCLUSION

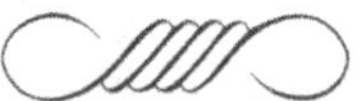

This might be the end of the book, but if you decide to turn into an Intuitive Eater, it turns into a fresh start for you. Take the voyage to turn into an Intuitive Eater, and you will experience a process that will undoubtedly challenge a portion of your most settled in contemplations and maybe work up some profoundly shrouded sentiments and fears. You realize that living in a universe of dieting tumult with its self-blame and disappointment doesn't work. It doesn't work metabolically or inwardly, and it doesn't work profoundly. Customers talk again and again about feeling pounded, crushed—as though their spirits are stinging. When they result in these present circumstances, many have surrendered any expectation of consistently being ordinary eaters.

However, turning into an Intuitive Eater requires an exceptionally conscious choice and responsibility. It implies relinquishing the old method for enduring and opening up to another technique for a renewed life. It may take some soul searching and contemplation work to choose whether counting calories has been keeping you from your most profound energy. Making this perspective change can be hard to achieve at first, yet it can, at last, become a method for living your best life.

To start this change in perspective, you'll have to think about the numerous tradeoffs in the eating scene. Having the "resolve" to remain on a diet can give you a fleeting feeling of intensity and control;

however, being an Intuitive Eater gives you a long-lasting feeling of self-strengthening. The demonstrations of slimming down and bounce back gorging can offer energy. So does eating the anti-diet foods. Be that as it may, when fervor never again originates from food or counting calories, different parts of life are liberated. When you are utilizing food or the fixation that dieting makes to numb yourself or to occupy yourself from your emotions most of the time, you may feel quieter and less pushed. However, your life can appear as though an obscured, out-of-focus home motion picture. You know you're alive and hustling through life; however, you experience its highs, lows, and subtleties of sensation. When you strip off the layers of counting calories and gorging deadness, you'll find extravagance in life that, for sure, has been covered for quite a long time.

When you become an Intuitive Eater, who reacts to those intrinsic organic and food inclination signals, you connect with your body, musings, and sentiments. Eventually, this affectability can change an amazing remainder. You additionally figure out how to work to straighten something up as opposed to judgment. When dieting, each straying from the food plan turns into a chance to condemn yourself.

Furthermore, analysis can be dangerous and irresistible. It's not irregular for this essential perspective to overflow into different practices or even to relatives and friends. As an Intuitive Eater, you see the food experience as a chance to get familiar with your considerations and sentiments. You may find that this interest triggers different investigations throughout your life. You may even choose to roll out genuine improvements in other parts of your life that have been making you angry or miserable. Either way, becoming an intuitive eater might be the best thing that has happened to you! The fact that you can monitor your body and weight while eating and exercising the right way is the best gift life has to offer. I hope to see you on the other side, living your best life!

INTRODUCTION

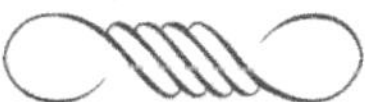

Deciding what to eat is not an easy task. It's so complicated that, in the United States, there are worries about diet and weight obsessions that have reached epidemic proportions, with serious health problems, emotional problems, and economic consequences for a large part of the population. We desperately need something new that could help us overcome these problems, and mindful eating could the answer.

Meaning Of Mindful Eating

Mindful eating means simply being fully aware of the food you eat and eating for the right reasons. Mindful eating can also mean sharing food on a plate, sitting down and enjoying every bite. Chew slowly, take time, pay attention to textures, these are good practices.

Mindful eating is derived from the word mindful and eat, which can be defined as:

Mindfulness means paying attention in a unique way on purpose, in the present moment, and nonjudgmentally.

Mindfulness means giving attention in a special way, intentionally, in the present moment and without trial.

The best way to think about mindfulness is to be more than just an activity. Almost any activity can be done with conscious awareness.

Initially associated with Buddhist psychology, the term "attention" comes from the sanskrit word smṛti, which literally translates as "what one remembers."

From there, we can understand reason by reminding ourselves that we must pay attention to our present moment experience

Mindfulness has three main characteristics:

- objective: mindfulness involves directing attention deliberately and intentionally, rather than letting it wander.

- presence: mindfulness means being fully involved and attentive in the moment. Thoughts about the past and future that arise are simply recognized as thoughts that occur in the present.

- acceptance: mindfulness means not judging everything that is happening at the moment. This means that thoughts and feelings are not considered good or bad, pleasant or unpleasant; they are simply recorded as "happening" and watched until they finally pass.

Research on mindfulness and its applications has grown exponentially in the last two decades. Although originally a Buddhist concept, mindfulness is now being considered to be an innate quality of consciousness that can be empirically measured. It is also understood that attention does not require religious, ethical, spiritual or ideological commitment

The scientific interest in mindfulness is largely attributed to the work of Dr. Jonah Kabat-Zinn, founder of the stress reduction clinic at the university of Massachusetts school of medicine. Kabat-Zinn, a molecular biologist trained at MIT, began his research on mind-body medicine in the mid-1970s, focusing on the clinical application of mindfulness meditation in people with chronic pain and illness. From this research, he developed mindfulness.

A History Of Mindfulness.

Mindfulness is a practice that is involved in various religious and secular traditions, from Hinduism and Buddhism to yoga and, more recently, to non-religious meditation. People have been in the practice of mindfulness for thousands of years, alone or as part of a broader tradition.

In general, religious and spiritual institutions have become popular in the east, while in the west, their popularity can be attributed to private individuals and secular institutions.

Even the secular tradition of mindfulness in the west owes its roots to eastern religions and traditions.

It is important to include some commentators who argue that the history of mindfulness should not be reduced to Buddhism and Hinduism, which also has its roots in Judaism, Christianity and Islam.

That being said, most modern western practitioners and mindfulness teachers have learned mindfulness in the Buddhist and Hindu traditions. This should not be interpreted as a denial of conscience rooted in other religions, and interested readers are encouraged to seek more information regarding these other religions. Leisa Aitken, a clinical psychologist and Christian practitioner, is a possible starting point, though this is just one of many options.

A brief history of Hinduism.

Hinduism is widely regarded as the oldest religion in the world, but its history is difficult to trace. This is due to the fact that it was originally a synthesis of many religious traditions throughout the historical region that now makes up India.

In other words, Hinduism has no founder or specific starting point.

In fact, its religious tradition was not even referred to as Hinduism, nor was it considered a single entity until the British writers began to call the Vedic traditions "Hinduism" in the 19th century.

The oldest traditions, which have since been integrated into Hinduism, were born more than 4,000 years ago in the Indus valley, now Pakistan. These religious traditions continued to develop in the vedic scriptures 2,500 to 3,500 years ago. These writings included the rites and worship of the gods common in modern Hinduism.

Idols in Hinduism.

About 1500-2,500 years ago, other texts were included that are included in current Hinduism, including texts that introduce the concepts of dharma and worship in the temple. Several hundred years ago, Hinduism in India experienced some competition with the rise of Islam, but nineteenth-century reformers revived Hinduism and helped it connect with identity from India

This proved successful, as middle-class Indians began to identify with Hinduism in the mid-19th century. This connection was strengthened a hundred years later by the Indian independence movement.

Mindfulness has been closely linked to Hinduism for thousands of years. From discussions of bhagavad gita yoga to vedic meditation, the history of Hinduism is partly read as a story of reflection. Of course, this is only a partial story: Buddhism is another key player in the history of mindfulness. It should be noted that even Buddhism owes much to Hinduism.

A little history of Buddhism.

Compared to Hinduism, the history of Buddhism is much more

accurate. Buddhism was founded around 400-500 BC C. Ad of Siddharth Gautam, who became buddha, is thought to have been given birth to and raised around modern India and Nepal. Depending on where and when Gautama was raised, it is believed that Hinduism informed him of his education.

Buddhism and Hinduism have many things in common: they are both born in the same region and are very interested in the term dharma. A difficult concept to define or translate, it involves a way of life in accordance with the natural order of the universe.

Despite the common presence of dharma in these two philosophies or religions, Buddhism is not a subsector of Hinduism, since Buddhism is not interested in the scriptures of the vedas.

Buddha as the spiritual center of Buddhism.

In general, Buddhism is a religion that aims to show its followers the path of enlightenment. Since its creation, Buddhism has been divided into several traditions, including teravada Buddhism and zen Buddhism.

Today, Buddhism is most commonly evoked by non-practitioners in terms of Tibetan Buddhism and the Dalai lama, one who is believed to be an enlightened teacher of Tibetan Buddhism.

Mindfulness is perhaps even more involved in Buddhism than in Hinduism, because mindfulness (sati) is considered the first step towards enlightenment. In fact, some sources even consider the word "mindfulness" to be a simple translation of the Buddhist concept of sati.

The fact that mindfulness is a key aspect of Buddhism, combined with the fact that many western influences on mindfulness have been studied by Buddhist teachers, shows that western attention is mainly due to Buddhism.

How much attention is paid to yoga

There is a lot of connection between mindfulness and yoga, both historically and today. Many yoga practices involve mindfulness, and some meditations, such as body scans, are very similar to yoga because they both involve body awareness.

Researchers found that people who did yoga regularly had higher levels of awareness than those who were not involved in yoga.

This indicates that yoga correlates positively with the level of consciousness and that some forms of yoga and some forms of consciousness are directed toward the same goals.

It is interesting to note that, although the origin of yoga coincides with Hinduism, the recent increase in the popularity of yoga in the west also coincides with attention. This emphasizes the intertwining nature of Buddhism, Hinduism, mindfulness and yoga.

How consciousness moved from east to west

Jon Kabat Zinn may have been the most important influence lately in raising awareness from east to west. Kabat-Zinn founded the prudence center at the University of Massachusetts school of medicine and the oasis institute for awareness-based education and training.

This is where Kabat Zinn developed its mind-based stress reduction program, an eight-week stress-reduction program.

Kabat-Zinn studied mindfulness with several Buddhist teachers, including Thich nhat hanh, an influential and popular figure of western attention. This gave him an oriental basis in the full awareness that he had integrated western science into the development of MBSR.

This integration with western science was a crucial element of awareness for gaining popularity in the west.

MBSR was the inspiration for the second program of mindfulness therapy, cognitive therapy based on cognition. This therapy aims to treat major depressive disorders.

This integration, like other science and mindfulness, has helped to popularize mindfulness in the west, especially for the public accustomed to western science and unknown eastern practices.

One of the reasons that prompted westerners to adapt and popularize the eastern tradition for the western public is the different worldview prevalent in each hemisphere.

In addition to academic science, Jack Kornfield, Sharon Salzburg, and Joseph Goldstein played a crucial role in raising awareness in the west with the creation of the Insight Meditation Society (IMS) in 1975.

IMS helped introduce mindfulness meditation in the west, and the combination of mindfulness meditation and MBSR helped popularize awareness in the west, both in the clinical and non-clinical populations. Of course, IMS is just one of many organizations that helped popularize mindfulness meditation in the west, especially in the United States.

The Benefits Of Mindfulness

Mindfulness is a practice of the body and mind that has been found to be beneficial for both mental and physical health. The major psychological change that occurs while practicing consciousness is a greater awareness of the thoughts and feelings of the present moment. Over time, mindfulness practice can help you become aware of the space between the realization of experiments and their reaction, allowing you to reduce speed and observe the processes of your mind.

The ultimate goal of mindfulness practice is to use this space to make more deliberate decisions: get out of your life by autopilot, based on unproductive mental habits.

It's easy to see how mindfulness can be helpful in dealing with stress or other difficult emotions. For example, we were all in a situation of anger or stress and said or did things we did not want to say. At that moment, we would feel that we had no control over our words or actions, as if we were responding to situations without thinking.

If such arises, attention can help in many ways. First, awareness can help you be more aware of your emotions before they transform and control you. Instead of recognizing your anger only after you attack someone, you can capture your anger when it is still soft and take steps to spread it. In addition, mindfulness can help you examine your thoughts and emotions with more objectivity. Instead of having small events cause negative thoughts, mindfulness allows you to move away and recognize that you are feeling stressed or anxious and that anxiety can affect your thoughts.

So how can mindfulness help you respond to your emotions?

Emotion regulation problems fall into two categories: depression and over reactivity. Instead of completely ignoring emotions or acting impulsively on every emotion, reasonableness offers a third option: "to be with" emotions. By keeping your emotions conscious, you can separate your raw emotions and feelings that accompany them from the thoughts you have about them. It would be the difference between thinking about all the reasons you are upset and just recognizing that you are upset. Being with your emotions this way allows you to observe your emotions up close as they flow naturally, and this allows you to make deliberate decisions about how to respond to information that provides your emotions.

According to the American psychological association, some

empirical benefits of mindfulness include the following:

Psychological benefits

- increased awareness of the mind.

- significant reduction in stress, anxiety and negative emotions.

- increased control of thinking (one of the main causes and symptoms of depression and anxiety).

- greater mental flexibility and concentration.

- more working memory.

- reduction of distractions.

- reduced emotional response.

- increased ability to act intentionally and receptively.

- greater empathy, compassion and awareness of the emotions of others

Physiological benefits

- improved functioning of the immune system.

- increased brain density and integration of neurons in some areas responsible for positive emotions, self-regulation and long-term planning

- reduced blood pressure.

- reduced blood cortisol levels (one of the main stress hormones).

- increased resistance to stress-related diseases such as the heart disease.

Spiritual benefits

- better self-perception and self-acceptance.

- greater acceptance of others.

- greater compassion and empathy.

- increased sense of morale, intuition and courage. Change

- increased control of automatic behavior.

How To Start Exercising Mindfulness

Mindfulness is a habit; it's something more that we do. It's more likely that we're in this mode with less and less effort.

It is a skill that must be learned, something we already have. Care is not difficult. The hard part is not forgetting to be warned.

With the practice of mindfulness, learning to be aware is just the tip of the iceberg. Most of this practice is to become familiar with the sense of awareness and to improve our brain for full awareness.

This means that almost all activities can become mindfulness practices if they involve these basic components:

1. Direct involvement of at least one of your five senses: focusing on one of your senses puts you in the present moment. It also gives you the opportunity to separate the sensory experience from the thoughts you have about it.

2. An anchor serves as an object of attention while practicing mindfulness. For example, if you are aware of your breathing, you should try to remain aware of the physical sensation of your breath entering and exiting your body. This can mean feeling the air in the nostrils and out of the nostrils or even the feeling the lungs expanding and contracting.

The exact feeling doesn't matter as long as you can stay focused on it. Other common examples of anchoring include a bell sound or the taste and texture of food. The range of possibilities is almost limitless. Feel free to experiment.

3. Back to anchor: this is where the strength of exercise comes from. You can most likely stay focused on your anchor for just a few moments before distracting yourself. When you realize you have lost focus, turn your attention back to the anchor. With time and practice, your mind will begin to calm down, and you will be able to concentrate longer. Initially, you will notice that you are moving away from your anchor long after you have started daydreaming, and over time, you will start to notice distractions (such as thoughts or feelings) as they arise. Instead of separating you from your anchor, it will be easier to simply notice and let them pass. A useful metaphor to keep in mind is that your abominations are like passing clouds.

Sky: watch them without judging them then let them leave no trace. Experiment by creating your own mindfulness practices throughout the day. Being fully aware of the feeling of your feet as you move around in the car or the taste and texture of your morning coffee can turn routine moments into deeply satisfying processes. However, ritualized and structured practice can be helpful. Below are guidelines for two common mindfulness practices.

Mindful Breathing

1. Holding: take a comfortable, straight but relaxed attitude. There is no need to sit on the floor, and sitting on a chair is completely acceptable. The key is to choose a good posture that will allow you to be comfortable and alert.

You may decide to keep your eyes open, but if you are a beginner, it may be easier to keep your eyes closed so as not to interfere. If you choose to let your eyes remain open, let the view rest a few feet away from you on the floor without focusing on any particular object.

2. Grounding - take a few minutes to notice that there is tension in your body.

Let your face and jaw relax. Let your shoulders get relaxed. Feel your body in resting position on the floor or chair.

3. Observe your breathing: once you begin to feel connected to your body, try to capture the sensation of your breathing. Some feelings you might focus on include air as it enters and exits the nose, the expansion and contraction of your lungs, or the sound of air in your throat. If you have difficulty breathing, it may be helpful to put your hand on your stomach, so you can feel it move up and down as you breathe.

4. Hold your breath: now that you've focused your attention on the breath, try to hold it as long as possible. Remember to stay relaxed with your posture and attention. If you feel stiff or fall asleep, do not hesitate to restart.

Hold on and release the tension you feel. If you notice that your attention is moving away from your breath, gently guide it to feel your breath in an instant. If you notice thoughts, try not to judge them! Just acknowledge their presence and let them go.

Mindful Walk

1. Holding - stand upright and cautious but not rigid. Spread the weight evenly between your legs. You can relax your hands or

hold them behind your back if they interfere with you. Please take a moment to feel your body rest on the earth. Soften and lower your eyes slightly if this helps you focus.

2. Choosing a path: if this is your first time trying to walk consciously, you can feel more comfortable choosing a short path (no more than 30 meters) and going from side to side from this path. When you feel comfortable in practice, do not hesitate to choose a more complicated trail or even try to walk consciously during the day.

3. Walking: when taking the first steps, focus your attention on the feeling that your weight is changing in the soles of your feet. If you are barefoot, try to record the textures of the soil. Keep a steady pace as you walk; it can also be helpful to walk a little slower than usual.

4. Follow the steps: as you progress through the rhythm, focus on the sensations that come from your feet. If you are fluttering, gently draw attention to your feet. Again, the important aspect of this practice is not the length of time you stay focused, but rather your mind wandering and re-focusing.

Common Problems And Tips For Staying Mindful

Finding the time it takes to maintain a "mindfulness practice" can be one of many difficulties in today's hectic world, but keep in mind that even ten minutes of exercise can help. Here are some other common problems and tips to help.

I keep thinking. The key to managing mindsets, while exercising mindfulness, paradoxically, is not to resist them. Instead, the idea is to record thoughts without identifying with them, as if you were observing your own thoughts from afar, resting in the quiet space of your mind.

I get too upset to be aware: it's normal to be upset when you try to stay calm, especially when you spend most of your time running in a very stimulating world! You can often feel the need to move and do things while trying to practice mindfulness. The best way to solve this problem is to continue practicing until your body and mind have time to slow down. When they slow down, anxiety naturally spreads.

I feel too tired to be awake. Slowing down and checking with yourself can make you realize how tired you really are. If you constantly feel tired while trying to exercise mindfulness, you may want to control your sleep patterns. However, if you think drowsiness comes from boredom, you can try more physically active care, such as conscious walking.

How to deal with unpleasant emotions that arise: often, emotions that are ignored throughout the day occur as attention moves inward. Sometimes, these emotions can be uncomfortable, and you may feel the need to resist them. Instead, if you allow these emotions to occur without judging them or following the stories your mind creates about these emotions, you will find that your emotions will naturally flow. To do this, you can observe the physical sensations that accompany your emotions, such as contractions in the chest that can cause anxiety. Of course, if these emotions are very strong or particularly disturbing, it might be helpful to seek the support of professionals.

MINDFUL EATING

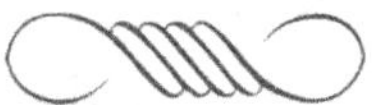

Meaning Of Mindful Eating

Mindful eating means simply means being fully aware of the food you eat and eating for the right reasons. Conscious eating means sharing food on a plate, sitting down, and enjoying every bite. Chew slowly, take time, pay attention to textures, these are good practices.

Eat with care. If you are busy and hurrying to eat to get back to work or some other activity, you can still eat "consciously". As long as you are sharing food, be aware of what you have eaten. You can count it as a conscious diet.

On the other hand, mindless eating is eating for other reasons than to feed one's body and satisfy one's hunger. We have endless opportunities to eat every day. Our pantries and cabinets in storage; grocery stores or cafeterias can offer samples; there may be leftovers from your child's dinner.

If you eat well enough, exercise, do not lose weight (or maybe even lose weight) and do not know why, mindless eating could be the cause. A little peanut butter when preparing a baby meal or a handful of chocolate chips may seem trivial, but it all adds up. Like most things worth doing, it takes work to eliminate the need for mindless eating.

Here are five steps to stop eating without meaning:

The Basics Of Good Eating

Nutrients found in our food

Food provides the body with the raw materials it needs to perform the metabolic processes of life. All foods contain at least one and often two or three macronutrients: carbohydrates, proteins and fats. These macronutrients give us energy to nourish our daily activities. They also fulfill unique roles throughout the body. Carbohydrates provide the fastest form of energy that any cell can utilize. Proteins provide the basic components of all our tissues and organs: skin and muscle, bone and blood, liver and heart. They also form a myriad of small cellular and messenger mechanisms, such as enzymes that digest our food and neurotransmitters that send signals to the whole body from the brain. Fats are woven into the membrane of each cell, isolating nerves and serving as precursors to life-sustaining hormones.

It also provides us with vitamins and minerals, called micronutrients, essential nutrients in small amounts that are used to make tissues and catalyze chemical reactions in the body.

Nutrition science in the early twentieth century sought to understand what macronutrients and micronutrients are needed to prevent deficiency diseases, such as kwashiorkor (protein deficiency) and rickets of vitamin d. Nutrition science has shifted its focus to complex chronic diseases, such as diabetes, heart disease diseases and cancer, diseases that develop over time, have no cure, and end life prematurely . With the level of advances in science, we now know a great deal about what to eat and drink and what not to eat to prevent chronic diseases. But you do not have to be a scientist to eat well.

After all, nutrients are in the food. And you just need to follow some basic dietary recommendations. And you just need to follow some basic nutritional recommendations to maintain your health and well-being.

Nutritional recommendations for adult

1 carbohydrates, proteins and fats

The Atkins Diet Zone books indicate that carbohydrates are the enemy. Other diet gurus offer low-fat and carbohydrate diets for weight loss and disease prevention or a high-protein diet as a way to maintain good health and healthy weight. However, the truth about macronutrients and health is that the type of carbohydrate, protein, and fat that one chooses is much more important than their relative abundance in our diet.

Carbohydrates can be found in many types of whole and processed foods, from apples to ziti, but not all carbs are the same. The healthiest carbohydrates come from whole grains, legumes, vegetables and whole fruits. Unhealthy carbohydrates come from white bread, white rice, pasta and other refined cereals, sugary foods and drinks and potatoes.

Whole grains, vegetables, whole fruits and legumes are good choices, like carbohydrates, and rich in vitamins, minerals and fiber. Whole foods, such as whole wheat bread, integral oats, brown rice, millet, barley, quinoa, etc. deserve special mention as more and more research shows that whole grains will become a daily habit. Research has shown that people consuming an average of two or three servings of whole foods per day have a 20 to 30 percent lower risk of heart disease and diabetes than people who rarely consume whole grains.

Consuming whole grains may also provide some protection against colon cancer, but further research is needed on this link between diet and disease.

Why whole grains so good for your health

The question of how whole grains protect against heart disease and diabetes remains an open-ended question. What most people do know is that whole grains contain fiber that slows down your digestion and increases blood sugar after a meal. The soluble fibers in whole grains, especially those found in oats, also help reduce the low-density lipoprotein (ldl), the "bad" cholesterol. Whole grain seeds provide folic acid and vitamin e. Whole grains are also a source of magnesium and selenium. Vitamins and minerals can help protect against diabetes, heart disease and some cancers. However, some studies have shown that the benefits of whole grains go beyond what is attributable to the particular nutrients they contain. It seems most likely that the health benefits of whole grains come from their particular combination of nutrients. The whole thing is really greater than the sum of its parts, the interdependent aspect of nature.

It is similar to protein. Foods of plant or animal origin can provide the body with the necessary protein. But when choosing protein-rich foods, you have to be careful about the other nutrients that come with protein. The healthiest source of vegetable protein (beans, nuts, seeds, whole grains, and foods derived from them) also contains fiber, vitamins, minerals, and healthy fats, as well as organic products. Some animal protein sources contain healthy fats or relatively little harmful fats (chicken, eggs). But red meat and high fat dairy products contain a lot of fats that are harmful for our heart.

Processed meat and dairy products can increase the risk of certain types of cancer. Red meat and dairy products are also harmful to the environment.

So, to choose the healthiest sources of protein, for both your well-being and the planet, choose vegetable proteins made from nuts, legumes, seeds and beans. If you have to eat animal food, choose fish or chicken. If you have to eat red meat, it is better to limit yourself to one or two times a week. Whole eggs can be a healthy source of protein but should be consumed in moderation, as eating one or more eggs a day can be harmful.

Drink moderately. Heavy consumptions can increase the risk of diabetes and the risk of heart disease in people who have diabetes. If you have heart disease or diabetes, you should eat less than this number per week.

Vegetarian and protein:

There is a difference between vegetable protein and animal protein, which is important for us, especially vegetarians. Our body absorbs proteins in food of plant and animal origin and breaks them down into smaller components, called amino acids, which it then uses to build and repair tissues and fulfill many functions. Some amino acids are referred to as "essential", which means the body cannot produce them and must obtain them from food. Others are not important, and the body can build them by rearranging essential amino acids. Proteins in food of animal origin are called complete proteins, meaning they contain all the essential amino acids. Proteins in plant foods are called incomplete proteins, which means they tend to have a little of one or more essential amino acids. However, plant protein can meet your daily protein requirements, provided you choose a variety of plant foods and eat enough calories throughout the day. As a result, vegetarians should ensure they consume a variety of high-protein vegetarian foods (beans (including tofu), nuts, seeds, and whole grains) on a daily basis to ensure they eat enough essential amino acids.

Fats and oils

Some fats are so useful that you can eat them every day, while others are so harmful that you should seriously limit them or avoid them altogether. There is an easy way to distinguish healthy fats from unhealthy fats. Most healthy fats, monounsaturated and polyunsaturated fats, originate from plants and are liquid at room temperature. Rich olive oil, oil that rises to the top of natural walnut butter and fatty oils are examples of good unsaturated fats. Unhealthy fats (saturated fats) and very unhealthy fats (trans fats) are usually solid in room temperature, such as the fat on a steak or that is contained in a stick of butter or margarine. Meat and integral dairy products are the main sources of saturated fat in the western diet; tropical palm and coconut oil are also rich in saturated fat. Trans fats in the western diet are derived mainly from partially hydrogenated vegetable oils, a chemical process that makes the oils stronger and more stable at room temperature and makes them extremely harmful to health.

What is the impact of these different types of fats on our health?

Many studies have shown that when people replace carbohydrates with monounsaturated and polyunsaturated fats, their offspring cholesterol in the blood improves the heart, reduces ldl cholesterol, and hdl cholesterol (hdl). Meanwhile, saturated fats increase hdl and ldl, so unsaturated fats are a better option for heart health. Trans fats are the worst and most dangerous types of fats, harmful even in small amounts. They reduce the protective hdl, increase the harmful ldl, and damage the lining cells of our arteries. Research also suggests that trans fats trigger inflammation, a red sign for our immune system that may underlie a number of life-threatening illnesses, such as heart disease, stroke, and possibly diabetes. A diet rich in trans-fatty acids can promote weight gain, though more research is needed on the relationship between trans-fatty acids and obesity. In addition, eating low in trans fats and healthy fats can reduce the risk of age-related macular degeneration.

Trans fats are all the more easily avoided. As rumors of its harmful effects circulate and manufacturers have to include them in their food labels in the united states, many food manufacturers and restaurants have begun to eliminate them. However, it is almost impossible to stay away from all saturated fats because even healthy sources of unsaturated fats, like peanuts and olive oil, contain a small amount of saturated fats. So, for good health, consume healthy fats, limit saturated fats, and avoid trans fats.

Weight control

Calories are important. If there is increasing evidence of the best options for carbohydrates, proteins and fats for health, then the best options for weight loss are discussed. Of course, to lose weight, dieters need to eat fewer calories than they burn. The big question is whether the relative amounts of carbohydrates, proteins and fats in the diet have a particular benefit for controlling calories and losing weight. Some scientists advocate a low-fat diet, while others follow a low-carb approach or a Mediterranean-style meal plan with moderate amounts of healthy fats and lots of fruits and vegetables.

You may be wondering how many calories you need to eat each day to maintain your weight and how much you need to reduce to lose weight. There is no answer to this question, as calorie requirements vary depending on age, gender, size, and level of physical activity. Some need only 2,000 to 2,500 calories to maintain weight, and some less to lose weight, while others are larger in size or very active.

Others who are taller or very active can eat more calories while losing weight. As people lose weight, their daily calorie requirements decrease. There are many websites that offer a calorie calculator based on your current goals and weight. It is also helpful to consult a healthcare professional, especially a dietitian, about their caloric needs. As a practical guide, an energy deficit of about 250 to 500 calories per day can result in the loss of two to four pounds per month. A surefire approach to creating this energy imbalance is to moderate your calorie intake and increase your activity, which means reducing your consumption of sugary sodas by about a can of beer a day and adding a brisk walk every day.

Coconut oil is less harmful than other types of saturated fat because it increases HDL ("good" cholesterol). Therefore, it is good to include a small amount of coconut oil in your diet.

Margarine can be a healthy option for fats as long as it contains no trans fats and is partially hydrogenated.

Check the trans-fat label for nutrition facts and look at the ingredient list to make sure the margarine does not contain partially hydrogenated oil.

Healthy fat - omega-3

When choosing healthy fats, make sure you include omega fats, polyunsaturated fats that are extremely beneficial for the heart. Omega fatty acids seem to protect against the wrong heart rhythms that can cause sudden death. They can also benefit people with inflammatory diseases, such as rheumatoid arthritis. Omega-3 fatty acids are essential fatty acids, which means our body cannot create them, and we need to get them from foods or supplements. It is therefore advisable to take at least one meal that is high in omega-3s every day.

Plant-based foods containing alpha-linoleic acid (ala) are an environmental source of omega-3s: mainly walnut oil, rapeseed and soybean oil, ax and ax oil, dark leafy vegetables and chia seeds. For those who consume fatty foods such as salmon, tuna and mackerel, they are rich in two types of omega-3 fatty acids, eicosatetraenoic acid (epa) and docosahexaenoic acid (dha), also known as omega 3 long chain fats.

Our body can convert the herbal form of omega-3 into a long chain, but it happens very slowly, and there has been a lot of scientific debate about whether these different forms of omega-3 fatty acids act as beneficial for the body in the same way. Still, vegetarians can be encouraged: the latest research shows that omega-3 vegetables can also play an important role in protecting the heart, especially in people who do not consume fish regularly.

Go with the plants

A conscious diet for weight loss should be a healthy diet for you and the planet. And the other basic principle of a healthy diet is to switch to a plant-based diet. Asians, especially vegetarians, have been practicing for thousands of years. The benefits of a plant-based diet are just as good for your health.

Decades of research have shown that a diet rich in vegetables, fruits, whole grains and healthy fats and a little unhealthy fat can reduce the risk of heart disease and diabetes.

Studies even suggest that people who eat little or no meat live longer than those who are richer in meat.

Vegetarians and vegans tend to be less overweight and have lower blood pressure, lower cholesterol, and therefore a lower risk of heart disease than people whose diets include some or all types of heart disease.

Some products may also have a lower risk of cancer, although studies are contradictory and more research is needed.

For optimum health, vegans should be careful to consume the right amount of vitamins, vitamin d, and other nutrients they may lack to avoid animal foods.

There is also strong evidence of health risks associated with the consumption of animal food. The center for science in the interest of the public estimates that saturated fat and cholesterol in red meat, poultry, dairy products, and eggs cause 63,000 deaths each year in the United States and 1,000 more deaths per year for food poisoning. People who consume meat and processed meat have a higher risk of diabetes than those who follow a vegetarian diet. High consumption of red and processed meat increases the risk of colon cancer. Consuming meat, especially meat cooked at high temperatures, can increase the risk of pancreatic cancer. Meanwhile, the nurses ii health study followed nearly 40,000 women over seven years to determine the association between consuming red meat and the risk of early breast cancer. They found that, for every 3.5 ounces of red meat consumed daily, a portion of medium-sized burger meat, the risk of breast cancer before menopause increased by 20%.

You do not need to become 100% vegetarian to enjoy the benefits of a plant-based diet for health. Several studies have shown that following a "cautious" diet rich in vegetables, fruits, whole grains and healthy fats, but including poultry instead of a high-meat diet can reduce the risk of different types of diets. A similar line of research has shown that following the Mediterranean diet, which is also herbal but includes dairy products, could reduce the risk of heart disease, stroke, Parkinson's disease and Alzheimer's disease, cancer as well as the risk of dying from heart disease, cancer or any other cause. Therefore, you can benefit from a part-time vegetarian diet.

Fill your plate with vegetables of different colors

In terms of fruits and vegetables, the basic message is two words: eat more. People who consume a diet rich in vegetables and whole fruits can reduce their blood pressure and risk of heart disease, stroke, diabetes and maybe certain cancers. A diet that is rich in vegetables and fruits can reduce the risk of cataracts and degeneration and help you protect your vision with age.

The benefits of eating whole fruits and vegetables probably stem from the nutrients they provide, as well as the lack of less healthy or more calorie foods that you can replace on your plate. Fruits and vegetables are full of vitamins, such as vitamin c, which boosts the immune system and acts as a powerful antioxidant in preventing free radical damage to cells. Vitamin k is for strong bones, and beta-carotene, Vitamin a is an antioxidant. They are rich in minerals, including potassium, which can help lower blood pressure, and magnesium, which can help control blood sugar levels. This are also a great source of healthy carbohydrates. Special phytopharmaceuticals, also known as phytochemicals, which give vegetables and fruits a bright color, can also play a useful role in protecting against disease. For example, lycopene, a pigment that helps tomatoes and watermelons turn bright red, helps in prostate cancer protection. Lutein and zeaxanthin, other members of the carotenoid family, can help prevent age-related macular degeneration.

To utilize all these protective nutrients, try picking vegetables and fruits in all colors every day. Include dark green varieties, such as broccoli, kale, brussels sprouts and kale; orange-yellow, such as sweet potatoes and apricots, carrots and melons; red such as tomatoes, watermelon, strawberries and red peppers; white, such as onions, garlic and cauliflower; and purple blue, such as red cabbage, beets, and blueberries. Make sure you take at least five servings of vegetables and fruits a day.

The more, the better. One serving is about half a cup of cooked vegetables or chopped fruit or cups of lettuce. For easier serving, devote half of your plate to vegetables or fruits at each meal.

Remember to taste all the fruit without drinking it like a big glass of juice. Fruit juices: as many as 100% fruit juices are rich in easily digestible sugars. A glass of orange juice contains as much sugar and calories as a glass of Coca-Cola. Fruit juice also lacks the benefits of whole fruit. In fact, a health study by nurses found that the risk of diabetes was 40-50% higher in women who drank one cup of fruit juice per day than those who drank less than one fruit juice daily. Once a month, however, whole fruit consumption was associated with a lower risk of diabetes.

To maximize the benefits of fruits and vegetables beyond your own health, buy fruits and vegetables at a local farmers market or buy a community-supported farm. It will support the local economy, consume fresh fruits and vegetables, and use less fossil fuel to make the transition from farm to plate.

Limit potatoes, refined cereals and sweets

You may notice vegetables that are missing from the rainbow vegetable list: potatoes. Although studies revealed the benefits of eating fruits and vegetables, potatoes do not seem to play a role in these protective effects. Indeed, potatoes, whether their skin is brown, red, yellow or purple, have more in common with white bread and white rice than with broccoli or peppers. Potatoes contain fast-digesting starch in large quantities.

Eating lots of this starchy food can send blood sugar to the rail. First, when your body quickly converts starch to glucose and absorbs glucose from the gut, your blood glucose levels increase; the pancreas pumps insulin to quickly remove glucose from the blood, but this can slightly outweigh the effects and cause a slight drop in blood glucose. This sequence of events can make you hungry again shortly after your meal is over. Over time, a starch-rich diet if digested quickly can increase your risk of heart disease and diabetes, and there is evidence that restricting this type of food from your diet can help you lose weight. Consume your potatoes sparingly, and if you think so, don't count them in more than five servings of vegetables a day.

Consuming large amounts of refined and sweet cereals, similar to many potatoes, can result in a rapid increase in blood sugar, an increase in insulin, and an equally rapid drop in blood glucose. In addition, refined cereals that fill the shelves of our supermarkets: white rice, white bread, and white pasta are nutritional substitutes for whole grain bankruptcy. The grain refining process eliminates bran and germs, eliminating almost all the benefits only starch medium or endosperm remains. The law requires food producers to add some nutrients lost to refined grains, but they do not replace everything that has been eliminated.

Vitamins and minerals

Take a multivitamin supplement daily to get a nutritional safety net

If you live in places with higher latitudes, spend a lot of time indoors. If your skin is dark, if you are overweight, you may suffer from vitamin d deficiency without you reporting it. Vegans and others who knowingly restrict the consumption of animal products may also lack certain nutrients, such as vitamin b group.

That's why nutritionist at the Harvard school of public health recommends that adults must take multivitamins daily as "nutritional insurance."

No need to buy a stylish accessory. Even the standard brand supplement contains enough vitamins and minerals you need. It is also not necessary to take a supplement that provides more than 100% of the daily value of vitamins or minerals, with the exception of vitamin D, nutrients essential for bone health, and scientists think they can also play a role in the prevention of chronic diseases, such as heart disease and some types of cancer, infectious diseases, and multiple sclerosis.

An estimated one billion people worldwide suffer from vitamin D deficiency, and scientists now believe that our daily vitamin d needs are much higher than expected. Only a few foods are naturally rich in vitamin d, and even foods fortified with vitamin d (like milk in the united states) do not provide much. In addition, during the winter months, people living at high latitudes cannot produce enough vitamin d by sun exposure. This is why many people can benefit from the daily consumption of 1,000 to 2,000 international units (iu) of supplemental vitamin d. Because a standard multivitamin usually only provides 400 iu, you can ask your doctor to evaluate whether you need vitamin d supplementation with your multivitamin.

Finally, be sure to look for multivitamins that get most of your vitamin a, if not all, beta-carotene instead of retinol. Consuming high levels of retinol can increase your risk of fracture; pregnant women should also avoid taking retinol in high levels, as this can cause birth defects.

Limit sodium intake

Sodium is a necessary nutrient, but most of us take it much more than we need every day. A high-sodium diet can exacerbate high blood pressure in some people. Reducing sodium can lower blood pressure and reduce the risk of heart attack and other heart problems in the long run. It is best to limit sodium content to less than 2,300 milligrams per day, an amount in about a teaspoon. People with high blood pressure or at high risk of high blood pressure (including people over the age of 40, African Americans or people with hypertensive hypertension) should reduce to 1,500 milligrams a day. In fact, the AHA now recommends that most adults reduce their sodium intake to 1,500 milligrams per day. A new study estimates that 70% of American adults are at that high risk, sensitive to salt group.

One way to reduce the intake of sodium in your diet is to reduce processed foods. Food manufacturers add a lot of sodium to frozen foods, soups, spices, cheese, breads and chips to satisfy our taste for salinity, but also to improve texture and extend shelf life. Fast food restaurants and seating also offer extremely salty foods.

Reducing your consumption of processed foods and eating at restaurants can also help you limit the amount of extra high-sodium food additive, msg that improves taste, and recent research suggests that consuming msg could be related. With weight, a small study in China found that people who consumed the most msg were almost three times more likely to bc overweight than people with the lowest intake of msg. The results are preliminary and researchers have not yet discovered how msg can be linked to weight. It may be that the improved taste of msg foods makes people eat more; it is also possible that msg has an effect on brain centers or hormones that control hunger.

Ingest enough calcium

Calcium is an essential mineral for strong bones and teeth, constant heartbeat and many other bodily functions, which has been the subject of much scientific debate. The US government recommends intake of 1,000 milligrams of calcium per day, while the UK recommends only 700 milligrams of calcium per day. Some critics have suggested that US recommendations are based more on lobbying the powerful dairy industry than on scientific evidence.

The best way to get calcium was also discussed. The US Department of Health and Human Services and the dietary guidelines of the Department of Agriculture recommend it to Americans.

Adults consume about three glasses of milk a day. However, milk and dairy products are rich in unhealthy saturated fats. Even skim milk contains about eighty calories per drink, and three glasses can raise the calorie budget of someone trying to lose weight.

This discussion of milk becomes even more complex when examining the relationship between dairy, calcium, and chronic diseases. Consuming dairy products can protect against colon cancer in moderation; however, it seems that high consumption of dairy products does not provide protection against breakage of premature duration. To avoid harm in consuming large amounts of dairy products and calcium would be a purely theoretical debate. But studies raise the worrying possibility that high milk or calcium intake is associated with an increased risk of prostate cancer in men, and that high lactose intake is associated with an increased risk of breast and ovarian cancer in women.

Milk production also has a significant environmental impact, as described in chapter 3. And consuming milk has an ethical impact, since the treatment of cows at dairy farms is often not very sympathetic, and if cows cannot produce milk, they are slaughtered. The dairy and meat industries are closely linked. Even if you don't eat cow meat and don't use leather made from it, someone else will.

So what is the best way you can get calcium? If you plan your diet carefully, you can get enough calcium from sources other than dairy products, including green leafy vegetables, tofu and tahini. However, some people following a vegan diet may consider taking calcium supplements or consuming soy drinks, calcium-enriched cereals or nuts, a small glass of juice fortified or fortified with calcium. If you want to consume dairy products, eat a modest amount of no more than one or two servings of cold cereals a day, and eat a healthy diet rich in vegetables and legumes. An added benefit of calcium supplements is that they are often enriched with vitamin d, which facilitates calcium absorption.

Choose healthy drinks

Water is the best drink option for health and weight loss. Sugar beverages are the worst solution because their excessive intake adds to the risk of obesity, diabetes, and possibly heart disease. However, sometimes it is not obvious that the drink contains a large amount of sugar and calories. If you read the nutrition label carefully, you will find that 100% natural fruit juice contains as many calories and as much sugar as soda. Grape cocktails and cranberry juice contain more sugar and calories than soda. If you like juice, keep a small glass a day, the size of an old "glass of juice" (4 to 6 ounces). Energy drinks and sports drinks also contain a lot of sugar, although beverage manufacturers try to cover up their drinks as "healthy" by releasing vitamins, electrolytes, antioxidants or herbs. Don't be fooled. Remember that many types of sugar are added to beverages: cane sugar, honey, high fructose corn syrup, fruit juice concentrates, but for the body, all sources of extra calories and sugars, diet drinks sweetened with artificial sweeteners may not be the best alternative because their long-term effects on weight and health are unclear.

Limit alcohol Consumption

From a health standpoint, alcohol should be restricted if consumed. Excessive consumption increases the risk of chronic diseases, such as hypertension, cirrhosis, esophageal, breast and colon cancers;

alcoholism also affects families, communities and nations. It is estimated that worldwide consumption of alcohol could cause one in twenty-five deaths, and the cost of alcohol for society is estimated at 1% of gross domestic product in high- and middle-income countries. Although moderate consumption can reduce the risk of heart disease and diabetes, it can also increase the risk of breast and colon cancer.

If you do not drink, there is no reason to start drinking, as there are many other ways to improve your heart health and reduce your risk of diabetes. (Reducing sugary drinks is one way; more exercise is another.) Scientifically, moderate drinking is determined not to exceed one drink a day for women and no more than two drinks a day for men, as the risks outweigh the benefits. However, even moderate drinking for some people can be the beginning of alcoholism. Although you can always be careful not to become addicted to alcohol and occasionally drink a glass of wine without making you happy, this may not be the case for your children, grandchildren, and other loved ones. Whenever you drink in front of them, you can increase your likelihood of drinking in the future. And they can grow up and become addicted to alcohol.

By completely abstaining from drinking alcohol, you become a role model to them and can protect them from using alcohol as a habit or in times of stress and difficulty. Alcohol is a substance. The first drink can lead to the second and third. As a society, when we consume alcohol, we run the great danger of avoiding drinking the first glass of wine as a manifestation of your enlightenment. You do it for all of us.

We need to look deeply to understand that, when we practice conscious consumption, we practice not only for ourselves but for others. The way you live your life is about your ancestors, future generations, and your entire society. Even if we completely refrain from drinking, a drunk driver can still kill us; helping someone to stop drinking makes the world safer for everyone. When we can get rid of the shell of our little self and see our interconnectedness with everything and everything, we realize that each of our actions is connected to all of humanity, the entire cosmos. Being healthy means being nice to your ancestors, parents, future generations, and your society.

In terms of care and compassion, we encourage you not to consume alcohol.

Dare to refrain from alcohol. As with meat consumption, reducing alcohol consumption can affect world hunger, because cereals and foods used in alcohol production can be used instead of direct human consumption. If you can't stop everything, reduce the amount you drink by one third, one half or two-thirds. None can practice perfectly, including the buddha. Even vegetarian dishes are not completely vegetarian. Cooking vegetables kills the bacteria that live there. Although we can't be perfect, because of the real danger that alcoholism poses to our society, destroying many families and causing much suffering, we must practice to reduce or completely stop drinking. We must live in such a way as to avoid the tragedy that alcohol abuse can create. Therefore, even if you can be healthy while enjoying a glass of wine every week, we recommend that you take a closer look at the harmful effects of alcohol on our society and do your best to reduce its consumption.

Now that we have come to the basics of healthy eating, let's focus on how to eat consciously to appreciate our food and eat with compassion and understanding. To eat mindfully simply means to eat or drink, noticing every morsel or sip. You can practice it at any meal, when you are alone in your kitchen or with others in a crowded restaurant. You can even consciously drink when you take a sip of water at your desk. Conscious eating allows us to appreciate the sensory pleasure of eating and become more aware of the amount and nature of everything we eat and drink. When we do maximum exercise, eating consciously transforms a simple meal into a spiritual experience, a deep appreciation for everything that has come during the meal, as well as a deep understanding of the relationship between the foods at our table, our own health and the health of our planet.

THE BENEFITS OF MINDFUL EATING

1. Mindful eating reduces stress

Much has been written on reduction of stress through time management and training the mind and body to relax. These are absolutely necessary tools for stress management. Did you know that another important player in your stress equation is what you eat and how?

Let us explore some simple yet powerful tips that can make your eating habits an ally for stress management.

Let's start by talking about your "stress equation". You feel stress when you feel that the requirements you are meeting exceed the skills and resources you have to meet these requirements. To better control your stress, you can increase your resources or reduce your workload. Nutrition may help you on both sides of this equation.

Let's start with how "what" you eat affects the stress you feel. Everything you eat can help boost energy and resources or increase toxicity and physiological stress. For example, fresh foods close to their natural state usually contain more vital energy and nutrients. These foods provide you with essential resources to help improve your health and energy and make you feel stronger. They give you what you need to make the demands of life.

Highly processed, genetically modified foods and those containing chemical additives can be depleted of vital energy and nutrients and include substances or structures that are toxic to your body. This second group of foods can put stress on your body while providing a little bit of what your body needs to be healthy, relaxed, robust and comfortable. In fact, these foods increase the load on your body, so you have less energy to use for whatever you need to do.

Therefore, it is a general good practice to choose fresh organic foods as natural as possible. Many people will have a variety of organic vegetables and non-fat protein as well as raw fruits, nuts and dairy products to provide the energy and essential nutrients you need to meet the demands of your life. For example, you are likely to get more energy, nutrients, and positive feelings from fresh fish salad than from an energy bar and protein shake. You are more likely to get more vital energy and useful nutrients from fresh broccoli, strawberries and blueberries than a packet of powdered vitamins. Fresh food contains not only more vital energy, but also a natural organic structure that is easily absorbed by the body.

Bearing in mind that each person's body chemistry is different, so it works well.

Maybe someone else can't serve you so well. A good way to measure the fuel your body prefers is to keep a "food and mood register" for three days. Write down everything you eat and drink, then write your energy and mood fifteen minutes, and then an hour later. Choose foods and quantities that give you a positive, energetic feeling, rather than being heavy and lethargic.

Another important way to absorb energy and nutrients from food is "how" you eat. If you eat slowly, chew every bite, and focus on the taste and texture of your food, it will better absorb what your food has to offer. Similarly, if you eat small, frequent meals, your body can more easily absorb what you eat. A good phrase to keep your energy in balance is, "never be hungry, never be complete." Eat every few hours to maintain your blood sugar level, but do not eat to the point that you feel full. When it is "full", your body will consume a lot of energy for digestion and will not be able to absorb the amount of nutrients at the same time.

Finally, take a seat, take a deep breath, and relax while you eat. A state of relaxation allows blood to flow through the stomach and intestines to facilitate digestion, absorption, and distribution of vital energy and nutrients in the body. If you are stressed or munching on the run, your body works according to rival plans, and digestion will suffer.

When you sit down to eat, remember that you will supply your body with essential resources that you can use to manage stress. Feeding your body well will reward you with positive energy and feelings that will help you meet the demands of life.

Improves digestion by healthy eating

Eating healthy does not mean good health. Real food comes when our bodies digest what we eat. Good digestion depends on the type of food we eat and on our body. Some people have fast digestion; others do not. What we eat is important, but the quality of our digestion is equally important.

Sometimes the body cannot break down the food we eat. That undigested food starts to rot. As a result, we produce gas that causes bloating. Now, small episodes of farting are normal because sometimes we have pockets of trapped air. But if the bloating is exaggerated and comes with an unpleasant odor, something is wrong.

For good physical fitness, we should not only eat healthy foods, but also improve the way we eat. We need to chew the food properly. When we chew, our mouths are full of saliva. This speeds up the digestion process. If we eat all our meals, the digestion process takes longer. Remaining undigested food presents problems.

Instead of three large meals, we should eat small meals at regular intervals. Small meals can be digested faster. In addition, with the right meals, try taking vitamin supplements as vitamins are important for our body. We usually suffer from a form of vitamin deficiency, given our lifestyle and dietary choices.

Water is important too. Drink at least 6 to 8 glasses of water daily. Water removes toxins from our body. Less water consumption leads to constipation, which is very painful.

Many nutrients are lost during cooking. Having cooked food is a good option. Steamed foods retain natural elements and are more beneficial. You can also add digestive enzymes to your dishes. Add a lot of fiber and go for high fiber integral bread, dried fruits, green leafy vegetables, fruits, etc. The fiber content of the food absorbs the fat that adheres to the intestinal walls and then removes it, which greatly detoxifies our body.

The digestion process takes time. Ideally, there should be an interval of 4 to 5 hours between meals. Do not lie down immediately after eating. Some things, like meat and poultry, are harder to digest, so keep that in mind before making a diet plan. A vegetarian diet is much easier to digest, but some items, such as sugar and pepper, make it difficult to digest. Peppers are especially irritating, as well as too much tea and coffee. These stimulants contain toxins that interfere with the digestive process.

Healthy eating should exclude canned and processed foods because it contains preservatives, artificial colors, and artificial flavors that are harmful to our bodies. Processed foods contain a lot of fat. When we eat such foods, the fat content usually sticks to our intestines and causes constipation. Try adding food from live culture to your diet. Probiotic yogurt is a very good option. Good bacteria greatly help the body digest food. Once you make these healthy decisions, you can feel the difference.

Mindful eating and yoga lower blood glucose in gestational diabetes.

When diabetes develops during pregnancy, the medical goal is to keep blood glucose within normal limits. Thai nurses have noted the practice of conscious diet and yoga in pregnant women with gestational diabetes to determine whether overeating and control of blood sugar can be improved.

A study published in February 2014 in the Journal of Applied Nursing Research, randomly divided women with gestational diabetes into groups. One group received usual care while the other received instructions on conscious eating and yoga. The second group had significantly lower blood glucose and hba1c levels than the control group.

From these findings, it was concluded that conscious diet and yoga can help control blood sugar in gestational diabetes.

Conscious eating is a way to eliminate overeating. It is based on the Buddhist idea of becoming aware of everything that surrounds you at a given moment.

It fights stress, high blood pressure and indigestion.

It has for a long time been known that people who eat slowly have less problems with being overweight or obesity than those who eat faster. It will take about 20 minutes from the time you eat until your brain receives the signal you ate. If you eat too fast, you will tend to continue eating after eating enough because your brain has no time to tell you that your stomach is full.

While studying a conscious diet, students can take 20 minutes to eat tangerines or 3 raisins, thinking about food and how they feel all the time.

Try to prepare a small meal and sit down to eat without a computer, television, or phone. Decide to spend 20 minutes or more at the table without distraction. Think of every morsel of food and try to imagine your journey from the sun's rays by warming the seeds, soil and water, during the growing, harvesting, market, returning home with you, washing, preparing and placing on the market.. Take time to enjoy the color, aroma, texture, and taste of each bite. Eating with a stick or knife and fork can slow it down if they are not your usual accessory. Eating with your less dominant hand instead of your favorite hand can also make you less skilled and need more time to eat.

Eating is believed to cause digestive problems when the body is preparing to fight or run. This could explain the desire caused by poor absorption of the required nutrients. Try to clear your mind from stressful thoughts while at the table. When you want a bite, know why you want it. Are you hungry, bored, or angry?

Mediation and mindfulness can stop a binge eating disorder.

Food anger is called "disorder" for a reason. All too often, the outside world is in a hurry to make judgments and comes to the uneducated conclusion that people who suffer from this type of disorder are "lazy" or "may choose to eat less if they want." It could not be further from the truth.

Bulimia binge eating disorder (bed) is a diagnosed disorder characterized by the inability to control certain impulses coming from the brain. It is not the individual's fault; previously it was caused by faulty wiring at the bottom of the brain. People who suffer from overeating have difficulty controlling their impulses. Once the impulse strikes, they are often helpless. It is part of the spectrum of obsessive-compulsive disorder (ocd) in which, once you have a particular thought in your head, you cannot avoid performing a specific action that you find that will make you "feel better". Only when that action is taken (in this case physical act of overeating), the person finally feels calm.

Unfortunately, this sense of calm usually does not last long, and the cycle continues. Once the person has eaten and the initial calmness is established, which allows him to feel fulfilled and full, the feeling is quickly replaced by shame, guilt, and the question: "How could I lose control that way?" Eating too much is only a very short-term solution; anxiety is then quickly extinguished, the person feels a deep sense of anxiety and shame, and in return, the coping mechanism is adjusted, which adjusts to get rid of these unpleasant feelings (overeating), thus the vicious cycle continues.

It is possible to interrupt this cycle. Meditation and mindfulness can calm down the quick triggering signals in your brain that make you eat too much. Your brain tells you that this is the only way to achieve a sense of inner peace. But with a calmer mind, you can begin to see aspects of your life in a calmer, clearer way, and you can "train" your brain to act as you wish.

You can achieve true inner peace, a peace that is not dictated by the power that food has on your life. It takes a lot of hard work and dedication, but you can do it. No one can promise that it will be easy, but the end results (better physical and emotional health, happiness and tranquility) will be precious. In the long run, the benefits of this hard work far outweigh the efforts.

Meditation and mindfulness are simply ways to calm the mind and become aware of our inner being. The most important thing to remember is to be "aware" of focusing on the present. It is crucial to leave the past behind in these times of reflection and ignore your fears about the future. These things no longer matter here and now. The most important thing is to calm your mind and listen to your inner self in real-time but without prejudice. Do not be ashamed of past events and do not worry about things that might or might not happen in the future. They don't matter right now.

Interestingly, with practice, you can completely change the dynamics of your brain. Signs of fast messages in your brain that cause stress (and therefore lead to overeating) will diminish over time and reinvent the trapped person, the one who is overcome.

The real measure of "success" through mindfulness and meditation is to let out the wonderful person in you as one portrayed from the outside. Awareness of your thoughts and feelings and how they manifest in harmful behavior can be the first step in changing your life and unleashing the true potential of the amazing person you know.

Mindful eating motivations

Emotional eaters will find a list of emotional dishes full of simple, yet effective, tips to help you practice mindfulness while eating. A separate list of conscious dietary commitments will motivate you when you need additional support. Finally, tips for applying the four basic principles of mindfulness are divided into practical and concise segments

Ways To Exercise Mindful Eating

Participating in a conscious diet, even if it only takes a few minutes, can help you understand how mindfulness practices cover all spheres and activities, including ordinary tasks. Drink a glass of water. If we are fully aware that we drink water and think of nothing else, we drink it with our whole body and mind. As we eat, we can also be aware of how we feel and what we eat, whether we are really hungry and making the best decisions for our health and the health of the planet.

Eat with care every day

We may not all be able to have lunch with Chef Sati, but we should try to follow his precious example as much as possible. Book an hour for dinner at home. Turn off the television. Put away newspapers, magazines, mail, and homework when you eat.

Work with others to prepare dinner. Each of you can help wash the vegetables, cook, or set the table. When all the food is served, sit down a few times and practice mindful breathing to reach your body and mind and recover from a busy day. Be fully present to one another and to the food in front of you.

After a few conscious breaths, look at yourself with a friendly smile and recognize each other's presence. If you eat alone, remember to smile. Breathing and smiling are easy to do, but their effects are powerful in helping you and others feel comfortable. When we look at food in a moment of peace, food becomes real and reveals our connection to it and everything else. How much we see our interaction with food depends on the depth of our consciousness. We may not always have the chance to see and enjoy the whole universe every time we eat, but we can do our best to eat as consciously as possible.

When looking at our food on the table, it is useful to name each dish: "pea soup", "salad", etc. To call something by name helps us to touch it deeply and see its true nature. And mindfulness reveals the presence or absence of toxins in every meal, so that we stop eating something that is not good for us. Kids love to name and identify foods when we show them how. Being with our family and friends enjoying the food is wonderful. Many are hungry and have no family. When we eat with all our attention, we create pity in our hearts. With compassion and good understanding, we can strengthen our resolve to help feed the hungry and lonely people around us. Conscious eating is a good education. If you exercise this for a while, you will find that you will eat more carefully and that your conscious consumption practice will be an example to others. It is the art of eating so that we draw our full attention to our lives.

Six ways to exercise mindful eating

One way to incorporate mindfulness into your feeding is to use your breath. Before eating, rest. Inhale and exhale several times to become one with the food you will eat. Conscious eating requires dedicated practice. You can develop seven practices to help you eat consciously for good health.

Complete all six sessions.

When serving and eating, observe the sounds, colors, smells, and textures, as well as the reaction of your mind to them, not just the taste. When you put the first bite into your mouth, pause briefly before chewing and observe its taste as if you had tasted it for the first time. With more practice of engaging all your senses, you will notice your tastes change, increasing your enjoyment of what you once experienced as "boring" healthy foods.

Serve in modest portions. Moderation is an essential component of conscious eating. A conscious effort to choose smaller portions not only helps you avoid overeating and gain weight; it is also less wasteful of your household's food budget and our planet's resources.

Using a small plate no larger than nine inches and filling it only once can help you eat more moderately.

Consciously picking smaller snacks and chewing them well can help delay your meal and allow you to feel the taste of your food. It can also help improve your digestion as the process of breaking down our food starts with enzymes in the mouth. Chew every morsel until the food enters your mouth; it can be twenty to forty times, depending on what you eat. Chewing well allows the tongue and palate to taste better. After you swallow this morsel, you can still feel the wonderful taste that your food offers.

Eat slowly

Eating slowly can help you notice when you feel comfortable, so you can stop before eating too much. There is a difference between feeling that you have eaten enough and feeling that you have eaten everything you can eat. Conscious eaters first exercise to avoid overloading their bodies or overloading the planet's resources by eating more food than they require. In Chinese medicine, it is a recommendation to eat only until you are 80 percent full and never "cover your stomach" because it weakens the digestive power of your stomach and intestines, which puts pressure on them in the long run. Scientific research is ongoing on the effects of calorie restriction on longevity, although the results are far from conclusive in humans. Of course, avoiding overeating is half the secret to weight control.

One way to reduce speed is to think about your body as you eat. When we eat carefully, we are relaxed and calm. There is no rush to solve other tasks, no hurry. There is only the present moment. To help you practice, be sure to take plenty of time to enjoy your food. If your lunch time is short, for example, during your lunch break at work, plan a smaller meal instead of quickly preparing a large meal.

Do not skip meals

Skipping meals can make it difficult to make conscious decisions.

When hunger swallows us, the strong forces of habit can lead us to take any food at our fingertips, whether at a vending machine or fast food restaurant, and these foods may not promote our goals of eating healthy or losing weight. So-called grazing that moves from one food item to another, some snacks, without even sitting down for a regular meal, may be at odds with your healthy weight goals, as you can consume more food than you think without ever feeling satisfied. Then you have the opportunity to make conscious decisions throughout the day; plan regular meals and healthy snacks between the two as needed. It is also good to eat at the same time each day to help your body adjust to a steady pace. And take the time to enjoy the food and all the sensory pleasures your meals offer.

Eat a healthy and planned meal. When conscious eaters peek deep into the food they are about to eat, they see it very well across the edge of the plate. They see that the dangerous costs of consuming certain types of animal foods can affect their bodies, for example, an increased risk of colon cancer caused by red meat and processed meat or an increased risk of heart disease caused by saturated fat. It is found in meat and dairy products. And consider prices as dangerous and destructive as meat production and milk production in our environment. University of Chicago researchers believe that, when it all comes together, the average American could do more to reduce global warming by becoming vegetarian than from switching from a Camry to a Prius. Simply switching from red meat and dairy products to poultry or eggs one day a week could have a measurable impact on global warming and a greater environmental impact than choosing locally sourced foods.

Watch out for the blind traps

We talked about what to eat and how to eat. We would all like to eat healthy, but we also have our inner knots, the usual powerful energies that keep us from being careful. People are more likely to eat healthy if they think they can; if they believe it will have beneficial health effects, if they have the support of family and friends, and if healthy eating is the norm for most family members or colleagues. People are also very likely to eat well if their community or workplace makes it easy for them, for example, if they live near supermarkets or if their cafes and vending machines provide healthy food.

Similarly, there may be obstacles to a healthy diet in the person or environment in which they are immersed. You don't want to discard your favorite foods, you don't like the taste of healthy foods, you don't rely on the seemingly changing diet tips, of all this can hinder our efforts to stay healthy. People living in "desert restaurants" without easy access to the supermarket may have difficulty eating fresh fruits and vegetables, and it may be less easy for people living in fast food restaurants to choose fewer calories, less nutritious foods. Food prices can also be a barrier: lower calorie and more nutritious foods, such as fruits and vegetables and fish, are more expensive than more caloric and less nutritious foods, such as cereals and vegetables. Agricultural policies, food advertising and labelling can affect the food we can buy in supermarkets or restaurants if we are aware of their nutritional benefits (or disadvantages) and if we choose to consume them.

Habits That Can Interfere With A Healthy Diet

Once you have identified these personal barriers to healthy eating, you can begin to overcome them and make every meal healthier.

Do you skip breakfast or other meals?

In the United States, fewer and more people start their day with breakfast, and our growing inability to take breakfast can contribute to obesity. Research suggests that people who skip breakfast have a tendency to weigh far more heavily and gain weight over time compared to people who have breakfast. The national weight control registry collected data on breakfast habits of nearly 3,000 people who lost and maintained significant weight and found that nearly 80% of them reported having breakfast. Every day, 4 percent say they skip breakfast. Scientists are still discovering the nature of the connection between breakfast and weight. Breakfast can help control starvation later in the day and, as a result, the amount of calories we eat, especially if breakfast includes protein or fiber, such as whole grains and fruits.

Diet books give you all kinds of tips for eating: eat six small meals a day, eat three meals a day and avoid snacks, do not eat after 8pm, etc.

The truth is, there is no "perfect" type of food that suits everyone's lifestyle or provides weight loss. However, it is a good approach to allocate meals throughout the day. This can mean three meals, including breakfast and a snack or two or four.

If skipping breakfast or other meals is a habit, consider these suggestions for changing your habit:

If you find yourself skipping breakfast or lunch because you do not have enough time in the morning to prepare, plan the breakfasts and lunches you can prepare before going to bed. For lunch, keep the leftovers in a bowl, add a roll of whole wheat and a piece of fruit or baby carrots and place them in a bag in the fridge, so you can get them in your bag.

Some skip breakfast simply because they do not appreciate traditional American dishes, like cold cereals and milk or eggs and toast. There is no reason to have such a limited palate. Try whole hot cereals, which combine whole grains and seeds like sesame seeds, whole oats, whole rye, whole barley, millet, quinoa, and whole buckwheat. For convenience, you can cook the batch for some days. Or even try an

Asian breakfast, with tofu or fish, vegetables and brown rice. Prepare a burrito with beans, salsa and corn tortillas ground with stones. Even last night's leftovers can make for a nutritious and satisfying breakfast.

Do you eat fast?

It has become common to advise dietitians: "Eat slowly and chew your food," and that certainly has an intuitive meaning. The theory, popularized nearly forty years ago, is it takes our brain twenty minutes to realize that our stomach is full, and that when we eat too fast, it speeds up the physical and hormonal process

Eating slower can also give us more enjoyment with food as we take the time to feel every bite. Many researchers have tried to prove this notion, sometimes with conflicting results, but recent support for the theory comes from a small body of research at the University of Rhode Island. Researchers asked about 30 women who eat fast and, a few days later, eat slowly (or vice versa), and measured the amount of food they ate and their satisfaction at the end of each meal. When women ate slowly, they consumed fewer calories and drank more water than when they ate fast. After a slow meal, they reported more satiety than after fast food. Although they ate less than the fastest food, they felt more satisfied. It is interesting to note that Japanese studies of food speed control and weight control have shown that people who say they eat fast tend to be heavier and more likely to be obese than those who say they eat slowly.

Do you eat too much?

Often, people eat too much without realizing they are eating too much. They eat too much because they eat a big bag of potatoes, serve them a plate of food, watch tv while eating, or because of external signals that have nothing to do with hunger. Dr. Cornell University's Brian Wansink calls this type of food an "insignificant diet." He and other researchers have shown numerous ways in which our environment can lead us to overeating. Certainly, there are many options for overeating: portions have grown enormously in restaurants, supermarkets and homes over the last few decades, even in the classic American cookbook Joy of Cooking. These large portions lead us to unconsciously redefine what a "normal" portion quantity is and make it difficult to estimate how much we eat. Having food temptations in sight, jamming the magazine and offering a variety of foods can lead to overeating without thinking. If you are used to eating with your eyes instead of your belly, follow these tips to help you carefully monitor the size of your portions.

Use small plates and service devices. Reducing the size of your plates, bowls and serving spoons can help reduce your portions.

Avoid being distracted by anyone.

Watching tv during a meal can lead to less attention to what you eat and to satiety and, therefore, lead you to overeat without thinking. Other distractions, such as film, socializing, workplace demands, could have a similar effect. Separate your food from watching tv or other activities. When engaging in a fun activity that revolves around food, like dinner, you realize that you should pay more attention to what you put in your plate and in your mouth. Breathe in regularly and carefully during your meal to remember to get back in your body and control your stomach. Relaxing your whole body with conscious breathing while eating is a good way to keep you in tune with your food and avoid overeating.

Can't stop eating after dinner

People who strive to eat healthy often complain, "I make good decisions all day, but after dinner, I can't stop eating snacks." For some people, eating at night means chewing without thinking about a bag of chips while watching tv or serving an ice cream bowl as a reward for a stressful day. For others, eating at night is a more serious disorder of their circadian rhythms, in which they consume at least 25% of their daily calories after dinner, or wake up at midnight to eat, leaving little or no appetite for breakfast. Night-syndrome is not technically classified as an eating disorder, but it is estimated that between 6 and 16% of those involved in weight loss programs suffer from it and may interfere with weight loss attempts. You may not have complete nighttime syndrome (if you think so, consult a professional), but if you feel that night has become synonymous with unhealthy snacks, consider these tips:

Find anything to work with your hands. Knit, make an album, read a book aloud to your kids, play chess. Do something to keep your hands occupied and your mind occupied, so it doesn't tempt you to turn to food.

Stop television. As we will see, people tend to eat without thinking while watching television and tend to eat what they see in commercials, mostly unhealthy snacks. Turning off your television and finding another night's activity can help break your eating and watching habit.

Know where you work. Checking your email at the kitchen table after dinner may mean you are too close to the temptation of snacks. Move to another room. If you have to work in the kitchen, keep the most enticing foods out of sight.

Reduce stress. There is evidence that stress can trigger night food syndrome and that stress reduction can help stop it.

Muscle relaxation bandages before going to bed indicated less hunger and nocturnal foods and less stress compared to no-stress nocturnal eats. It's a good time to try meditation or other relaxing activities, such as listening to light music, reading a book, or taking a bath.

If you choose to carefully respond to your body's invitation to eat something nightly, do so with vegetables or fresh fruit. They come full of fiber, fill you up quickly, and most don't have that many calories.

Do you enjoy fast food or in a restaurant?

Americans spend more than 40% of their budget on out-of-home meals, and research has shown that meals prepared outside the home are usually less healthy than those prepared in our own kitchens. The best way to lose weight is to cut the fast food completely. Even "healthy" options are generally not as healthy. Consider these tips for making the healthiest decisions when visiting fast food or regular restaurants:

Make your research before time. Many restaurants now offer nutritional information online, which may surprise you. In some fast food restaurants, for example, a small sandwich may contain fewer calories than a large salad soaked in cheese and toppings.

Ask for smaller parts. When we eat in a restaurant, once the food is on our plate, it is very likely that we eat it, and the larger the portions, the more we eat. Therefore, order a small snack instead of the main course, share the main course with your catering partner, or ask the waiter to bring you a "take away" container for your meal, so you can put half the meal in the bowl before eating. And avoid extra bread and butter, sugary drinks at will, to save the appetite and calories needed for more nutritious and satisfying foods.

Do not buy fast food. Going to the fast food menu might be a little more expensive, even buying less food, but does one really need to try fifteen hundred calories of total foods with big fries, big burgers, and thirty ounces of soda? You will be surprised how filling a sandwich and smaller fries can be, especially if you eat slowly and taste them.

Ask for coffee or tea after food in the place of dessert. Wansink emphasizes that the relaxing atmosphere of a candlelight restaurant can make a meal more enjoyable, but it can also cause people to spend more time at the table and eat more. Suggestion: get a cup of coffee instead of a high-calorie dessert.

Don't have time to prepare healthy meals?

The pressures of work and family time can make us feel limited, and the lack of time to prepare a meal is considered a barrier to healthy eating. But with careful planning, a healthy diet can be achieved.

Division of the dinner function. Involve family members or roommates in food preparation; even young kids can help. If you live alone, consider creating a healthy diet with four friends or colleagues at work. Ask everyone to create a healthy five-day weekend getaway and split the lots into portable containers. Bring them in and exchange them on Mondays, and everyone will have enough lunch or dinner for the week.

Be very careful with practical food. Prepared meals can be used while preparing meals, but they may have their drawbacks. Some processed foods are either filled with salt or added sugar or contain high unhealthy fat. Look for frozen foods containing less than 300 milligrams of sodium, less than two grams of saturated fat, and zero grams of trans fat and at least a few grams of fiber per meal. To add a meal, add fresh fruit or salad. Or prepare your own "healthy" food. Cook large quantities of whole grains, dried beans, or grilled vegetables on Sundays and use them in meals throughout the week or freeze them in small portions to get one for a light lunch or dinner.

Do you eat more on weekends?

Weekends are a time of relaxation, socialization and, for many of us, overeating, and these small indulgences can lead to weight gain or weight loss. The national weight control registry has determined that the following people follow the same eating habits on weekends, holidays or public holidays.

Employers on weekends, holidays or vacations, such as working on weekdays, are usually more successful in maintaining their weight loss.

If you stray with your intention of eating healthy on the weekends, consider these suggestions:

Keep a food journal. Research suggests that people who consume what they eat are better at losing weight and avoiding weight gain, because self-control is a key element of weight control. Write down everything you eat and what you eat and drink on your calendar, on your smartphone, or on one of the many websites that offer free online registrations. You can even try to take a digital picture of what you eat; a picture is worth a thousand words, and there is evidence that photographing what you eat can make you more aware of your food choices. Don't worry about the details of the food diary. Maintaining tickets can be just as effective for losing weight.

Place when you change if you go shopping all day, put healthy snacks in the fridge, and use the time for a thoughtful lunch break. If you are having lunch at a restaurant, visit the restaurant's website before departure. Most have nutritional information available to help you choose the healthiest options.

Make your social time an active time. Instead of getting a glass of coffee soaked in sugar, meet for a short walk. Or go dance on a Saturday night instead of going out for dinner.

Do you eat when you are angry, bored, sad, or stressed?

The connection between food and emotion is complicated. At a particular end of the spectrum, there is someone who has a stressful day at work and finds solace in a chocolate bar on the way home. On the other hand, some people struggle with anorexia, bulimia, eating drinks or any other messy diet. Stress, as well as various emotions, including anger, anxiety, boredom, loneliness and sadness, can cause a person to turn to food to feel comfortable. There are various techniques for changing your behavior or your thought process to cope with emotional eating. If you think eating emotionally can interfere with your attempt to eat healthy, consider the following tips to avoid using food to control your emotions:

Understand the difference between physical and emotional hunger.

Before going to the fridge or supermarket, stop, take a deep, slowly breathe and ask yourself the following question: am I really hungry or do I want comfort foods to alleviate stress or to alleviate other emotions? If you keep a food diary, recording your mood and hunger while eating can help you determine if your emotions have led to overeating and when.

Find out other ways to respond to stress and emotions. Walking, practicing yoga, mindfulness meditation, singing with an mp3 player, gardening, bathing, an herbal bath, talking on the phone with a friend are just some of the many activities that you can choose to make it easy.

If you are under pressure at work, replace the candy jar on your desk with a pressure ball or a Zen office fountain.

If you cannot reduce your emotional eating habits on your own, you can seek out a psychiatrist or therapist who specializes in eating problems. Your doctor or worker assistance program can provide you with a reference.

Knowledge translation at work: we've come up with a menu of options for healthy changes to your daily diet. We looked at the best nutritional options for health, common barriers to healthy eating, so you can really taste your food, the connection between mindfulness and food. Now is the time to put everything into place and come up with a practical strategy that allows you to be careful with every meal and achieve your goal of achieving a healthy weight. We call it your nutritional strategy, where it means being in the present moment. With your dietary strategy, you can set healthy and conscious eating goals and avoid overeating, discover ways to avoid obstacles that can prevent you from achieving your goals, and establish steps to reach your goals.

Why do you want to eat healthier and more conscious? Think about why you want to choose healthier foods and choose smaller portions. And think about all the reasons you pay attention to your meals. They can go through all parts of your life. It would be helpful to write these reasons in a newspaper so you can think about it later.

However, for something so rich in positive aspects, this is not the easiest step. We all live in a society that spends so much time and money promoting unhealthy foods and insignificant foods and restricting access to healthy foods. Focusing and selecting food requires a special and conscientious effort. The steps in this chapter give you the tools to listen to your body, relive the moment, and become truly conscious and healthy dining.

1. Keep a food journal. Make a note of absolutely everything that goes into your mouth. Even if only two smarties were able to reach your lips (these crafty smarties!), write it down. No matter how insignificant, its monitoring creates an awareness of the food you eat.

2. Plan each meal in advance. Don't leave anything to chance. Plan for absolutely every meal and snack throughout the day. If you go out in the afternoon, plan where to go for lunch and what to order.

3. Ensure that anything and everything you eat comes from your

plate or bowl. It's an easy way to eliminate "eating options": eat only because the food is in front of you. It also means you will say goodbye to taking a few handfuls of French fries in the bowl off your coffee table or eating snacks directly in the drawer. Instead, you are obliged to divide the portion on the plate to know how much you are eating.

4. Eat according to hour and hunger. Waiting too long to eat makes it difficult to plan your meal. Eat before you become sharp, dizzy, or unable to concentrate on eating. At the same time, if you are used to spending the whole day without eating and are not hungry, eat by the hour. Your body will soon get used to eating frequently and will begin to show signs of hunger.

5. Build a support network. Having support can be the most important step in combating unnecessary food consumption. Regularly check with your coach or accountability partner to keep in the right direction.

Mindful Eating Exercises

Informal, thoughtful practices for those of us who do not have five minutes to think about grapes.

Eating consciously, as during withdrawal or awareness, is not realistic for many of us, especially with the families, jobs, and the myriad of distractions that surround us. Not to mention that our loved ones, family, and even colleagues may not have the patience to eat with us, as we take each bite for five minutes. So take pity on yourself and think about formal conscious eating during withdrawal and special occasions, as well as informal conscious eating in your daily life.

Especially in times of madness, stress and extra food for the holidays, which go from Halloween to new year's, where they eat more often without thinking. Here are six simple steps to keep in mind to detect meaningless eating and (more) conscious eating and to unite our body and mind.

1. Start with a shopping list. Consider the integrity value of each item you add to your list and keep it to avoid impulses when shopping. Fill most of your cart in the produce section and avoid the center aisles, which are packed with processed foods, fries and sweets at the counter.

2. Come to the table with a great appetite but not when you're hungry. If you skip meals, you may be so eager to put something in your stomach that your first priority is to fill the void instead of enjoying your meal.

3. Start with a small section. You may find it helpful to limit the size of the plate to nine inches or less.

4. Appreciate your food. Stop for a minute or two before you start eating to consider everything and for anyone who needed to bring food to the table. In silence, express gratitude for the opportunity to enjoy the delicious meal and the entourage you enjoy.

5. Bring all your senses into the food. When cooking, serving and eating, be aware of the color, texture, aroma and even sounds of the various foods being prepared. While chewing on food, try to identify all the ingredients, especially the spices.

6. Keep small snacks. It is easier to taste the food when the mouth is not full. Leave accessories between snacks.

7. Chew well until you feel the essence of the food. (you may need to chew each bite 20 to 40 times, depending on the food). You may be surprised at all the flavors posted.

8. Eat slowly. If you follow the tips outlined above, you will not lose food. Spend at least five minutes consciously eating before speaking with colleagues.

9. Let your body reach your brain.

Eat faster and ignore your body's signals, rather than slowing down, eating and stopping when your body tells you it's filled.

Slowing down is one of the ways for our body and mind to communicate what we really need to feed ourselves. The body actually sends its satiety signal about 20 minutes after the brain, so we often unknowingly eat. But if we slow down, it can give your body a chance to reach your brain and listen to signals to eat the right amount. Here are some easy ways to bring down your speed: sit

down to eat, chewing every snack 25 times (or more), placing a fork between two bites, and all those old habits that aren't possible.

10. Know the personal hunger signals of your body.

We often hear our minds first, but like many notification procedures, we can also discover more wisdom by giving ourselves first to our bodies. Instead of eating only when we receive emotional signals, which can be different for each of us, whether it be stress, sadness, frustration, loneliness or even boredom, we can listen to our body. Too often, we eat when our mind signals us to do it, instead of our body. True, conscious eating hears the signals of our body's hunger. Ask yourself: what are your body's hunger signs, and what are your triggers for emotional hunger?

3) Develop a healthy diet in the environment.

Another way to eat without thinking is to walk in the cabinets, eat at random times and places, and not think proactively about our meals and snacks. This slows us down for a reason but prevents us from developing healthy environmental signals about what to eat and in what amount and connects our brain to new signs of eating that are not always ideal.

Of course, we all take snacks occasionally, but it can also improve the health of your mind and body, not to mention that it's great. It helps your mood and your sleep schedule to eat in constant hours and places. Yes, that means sitting (at the table!), putting food on a plate or bowl, not eating it from a bowl and using accessories other than our hands. It is also helpful to eat with other people, not only for sharing and a healthy relationship, but also for slowing down and enjoying more food and conversation, and for dinner, we take our partner's signals, with no excess or less emotions.

When we store food in cabinets and in the fridge, we are more likely to eat healthy amounts of healthy foods as well. Think about what is around you, where it is located, and if it is in sight. If we limit our food to the kitchen and dining area, we are less likely to eat without thinking or eat as we perform more tasks. When there is food, we eat it. And food, not always the healthiest, is usually present at parties.

There are many reasons the grapes we consume are such a powerful exercise, but one of them is that when we slow down and eat healthy foods like raisins, we often appreciate them more than the story we tell ourselves.

You don't have to plan your meal for every snack, and it's important to be flexible, especially on special occasions, but keep in mind that you may be able to change your eating habits at different times. And when you plan ahead, you are more likely to eat the amount your body needs than not to eat later and indulge or overeat and regret later.

Exercise of raisins by Jon Kabat Zinn

Perhaps the most popular mindfulness exercise is Jon Kabat Zinn, a prudence specialist. Raisin meditation can be found to be on the Greater Good Science Center website, but we will also describe it here.

Here is how it works:

Hold: take the grapes first and hold them in the palm of your hand or between your finger and thumb.

Look: take the time to focus on it; watch the grapes carefully. Imagine you have just arrived from Mars and have never seen such an object in your life. Have your eyes explore each part of it, exploring reflections where light shines, gaps, creases and darker edges, as well as any asymmetry or unique features.

Touch: cover the grape between your fingers to explore its texture. You can do this even with your eyes closed if it enhances your sense of touch.

Odor: keep the currant under your nose. Take with each inhalation any odors that may result. In doing so, observe anything that may interest you in the mouth or stomach.

Put in your place: now slowly bring the grape to your lips, noting that your hand knows exactly how and where to place it. Gently place the grapes in your mouth; without chewing, notice how this enters the mouth first. Take a moment to focus on the sensation of having it in your mouth and explore it with your tongue.

Tasting: when ready, prepare to chew the grape, noting how and where to chew it. Then, very consciously, bite off one or two snacks and watch what happens afterwards, feel every wave of taste that comes from it as you continue to chew. Without swallowing, observe the naked sensations of taste and texture in your mouth and how they may change over time, moment by moment. Also note any changes to the object itself.

Swallowing: when you feel ready to swallow, see if you can first discover the intent of swallowing, so consciously experience this before swallowing the grape.

Then: last, see if you can feel what is left of the grape that lands on your belly and feel how your whole body feels after you are done with this exercise.

Strategies For Creating Conscious Eating Habits

If the challenge seems too intense at this point, you could benefit from implementing simple and proven strategies to build a more conscious diet.

- Make catering an exclusive event instead of multiple tasks.

- Check your stress levels before eating, as you might turn to food even if you really aren't hungry.

- Recognize the gift of food and effort devoted to its cultivation and preparation and enjoy your food.

- Eat slowly, place a fork between bites, chew food, and allow each meal to last at least 20 minutes.

- Observe the taste, texture, shape and smell of your food. Enjoy it.

- Think of the parts to make sure you value quality, not quantity.

- Remember how hungry you are to make sure you only eat when you are hungry.

- Eat before you get hungry or you can make impulsive decisions.

- Take into account your protein and make sure you choose vegetable proteins (such as beans and legumes) often.

- Test your calorie budget to make sure you are eating the right amount to maintain a healthy weight.

- Determine if your food is worth the calories and eat only a few snacks, if any.

- Eat special foods or desserts, so you don't feel like you're missing out, but don't feel guilty about eating too much.

Useful tips can also help you develop a more conscious eating habit

- Think about how you feel before eating.

- Sit instead of eating on a trip.

- Turn off your tv, phone, tablet, computer, etc. (all with a screen).

- Serve a reasonable portion instead of eating out of a bag or box.

- Select a smaller plate to facilitate portion control.

- Take a moment to take a break and cultivate gratitude for your food before you eat it.

- Chew several times: the default value is 30, although some foods require chewing more or less.

- Leave a fork or spoon between each bite and do not lift them until you have swallowed the last bite.

- Give up the "clean eating club"; remember, you don't need to eat everything!

- Try to eat in silence. Recognize when your mind wanders, but bring it back to eating every time you notice it.

7 simple conscious feeding exercises every day

Like meditation, conscious eating is a skill that must be developed over time.

Here are some simple diet-conscious exercises you can do at your next meal.

Remember, it will take time to get used to these exercises. That's why doing everything one hundred percent from the beginning is not the goal. Over time, you start to build your "conscious diet muscle".

1. Reduce speed

Do you remember your grandmother telling you to chew each bite fifteen times before swallowing? The moment has come to obey her. Although you don't want to count every bite, take the time to chew slowly and deliberately, rather than swallowing almost all of the food.

If you usually eat in 10 minutes, prepare a 15-minute timer and reduce the speed enough to eat for another five minutes. Easy? Try for 20, 25 or 30 minutes!

You may not have enough time to chew your sandwich for thirty minutes. It's good. You can take the first five bites slowly and eat the rest as usual. Or finish slowly in the last three snacks. Whatever works for you.

2. Enjoy the silence

Meals are a good time to communicate with friends, family and colleagues. But having a good conversation will distract you from your food. If you want to develop the habit of eating more consciously, eating quietly regularly can help.

Do you feel uncomfortable being the only one at the table not talking? You can train silence instead of calling or texting the next time you eat alone. This way, you will be able to adjust and focus on your food.

This exercise can be fun for families as well. If you want to exercise in silence but do not miss the opportunity to hear about your children's school day, become a game where you have to be quiet for five minutes at the beginning of a meal. Who can do it wins. The speaker comes to do the dishes.

3. Share your experience of mindfulness

If you do not like to eat in silence, you can talk about what you eat. Pay special attention to what you like, whether it's texture, taste or temperature, and share it with people around the table.

Listening to what others notice about your food will often make you revisit your plate, and you may find something you have not noticed before.

It's also a great activity with kids. This will help them understand what they like and why. It is also an opportunity to practice new food-related words with them, so they can better express their experiences.

4. Ditch technology

As for distractions, you probably waited for this one. Yes, please leave your phone, tv, and other electronic devices you normally use at lunch.

As we spend more time on screens, meals are a great opportunity to escape. Take time to eat and take a break from the stress of your job.

Think honestly: if you don't get back to email right away, will you get fired? Will you have other opportunities to hunt for friends on Facebook and Instagram after you're done eating? Do you see what I mean?

5. Stop and listen

As you eat, stop and rest periodically to see how your body is feeling. Are you complete? Are you tired? Want more? By subscribing to yourself, you avoid overeating and will learn to understand how food affects you.

You may find out what foods will make you bloated, drowsy, or energized. You may notice that chocolate does not make you as happy as you thought. Or you could even see your taste buds changing and now you prefer healthier options than unhealthy foods.

6. Accept your choice

The guilt and negative feelings about food stem from the fact that we do not have our own food choices. We say to ourselves that we no longer have the right to eat treats or French fries and when we have them, we feel bad.

MINDLESS EATING

Types Of Mindless Eaters

The following broad categories describe five types of mindless eaters:

1. The occasional mindless eater

2. The chronic mindless dieter

3. The mindless undereater

4. The mindless overeater

5. The mindless chaotic eater

This book covers the whole range of meaningless meals. The breadth of this approach is one of many that is so exciting and unique in the conscious consumer. Anyone can benefit, from the person who eats without thinking, sometimes in a restaurant where something like this exists

She longs for the person who has been fighting it for twenty-five years to eat and feel trapped. If the characteristics described in the following sections seem familiar to you, you probably have some form of pointless eating. However, it must be emphasized that we are all unique. People may show similarities in their eating habits, but the specific characteristics and expressions of meaningless eating determine life, culture, and family experiences. Therefore, you do not have to log in with all of the features listed. It most likely identifies with certain aspects of each type of absurd diet. Again, keep in mind that the categories below are not a diagnosis but a way of grouping certain types of eating habits.

The occasional mindless eater,

Characteristic

Mostly aware of how much he eats, but he slips from time to time.

From time to time in a diet like trance, often in the case of stress or fatigue. Serving size awareness becomes a challenge for your favorite foods. Dinner with friends who eat without thinking.

You usually stay at a fairly constant weight; if weight is increased, it is very slow or abrupt. You may notice changes in your body during the holidays or holidays.

The tendency to feel excessively satiated in a restaurant. He is vulnerable to eating new things or eating comfort foods from childhood. He is usually hungry, but can sometimes lose his head when busy.

Think about what to eat, but you can fall into your usual or usual eating habits when you are overwhelmed.

You may have thoughts of guilt after eating too much. He can criticize himself when he eats too much.

He usually uses healthy activities to make him feel better, but sometimes he eats to relieve stress.

You can eat too much when you feel extremely anxious or nervous.

You get frustrated when you eat too much, because that's usually not a problem.

You can use food to celebrate or socialize.

The chronic mindless dieter

Characteristics

Beware of food, review food labels.

Classify food as "good" or "bad".

Choose foods based on expected weight loss, not health.

Eat well before starting a diet and believe the diet will last for a short time.

Participate in a yoyo diet, which results in constant weight gain and decline, which is very unhealthy in the long run.

Follow the eternal diet and try all the new tips for losing weight.

Fast and reduce food consumption to unhealthy levels.

He does not listen to the desires of his body.

Knows lots of information about calories, food portions. and diet tips.

Neglects nutrient requirements.

He thinks he has the "ideal" weight to reach.

Talk and think about food often.

Think more about the caloric value of the food than the experience or joy of eating it.

He feels fat; disapproves and / or is threatened by his own body.

Experiences mood swings based on diet.

You feel guilty about "breaking the regime".

Examines the bodies of others; check mirrors frequently.

You feel overwhelmed when you eat something that is not part of your diet.

He has trouble accepting the shape of his own body and wants the wishes of another person.

The mindless undereater

Characteristics of the undervalued without meaning.

Limit your food intake or eliminate whole food groups, like all red meat,

Cheese or wheat products.

Participates in food rituals or have strict and repetitive eating habits.

For example, eat only frozen meals or eat at the same time every day.

He has a strong desire for perfection.

Experiences significant weight loss.

You have a slow metabolism (your body burns food very slowly).

Experience various physical consequences, such as a decrease in heart rate.

Body frequency and temperature and loss of menstrual cycle.

It gives up most of the time, has problems with concentration, has little energy.

Worried about the look.

Feeling fat or having a negative body image.

He has an unrealistic perception of his own body.

Determine self-esteem by weight.

He is involved in inflexible and extreme thinking, whether black or white.

He constantly makes critical judgments about weight and self.

You feel fat; does not approve and / or is disgusted with your body.

Experiences intense mood swings based on diet.

Feels guilty when breaking a diet.

Examines the bodies of others, checking mirrors frequently.

You want to "cheat" yourself when you eat something that is not part of your diet.

You have trouble accepting your body shape and want to look like another person.

The mindless overeater

Characteristics

He knows his diet is uncontrollable. He thinks he can't stop eating.

Lives an intense craving.

Eats more than what is considered "average" in a given period.

Eats, chews and swallows very quickly.

Earns or changes weight often.

You have high blood pressure, fatigue, shortness of breath, high cholesterol, etc.

He is aware of the fullness, but still continues to eat.

Avoid scales or discussions about weight loss or weight loss.

Believe that weight is associated with success and failure.

Participate in supercritical thinking about yourself and your weight.

Feel anxiety about your excessive drinking behavior.

You feel shame that causes you to eat small amounts of food when you enter

public but in large quantities.

Social exclusion seems to be overweight.

The mindless chaotic eater

Characteristics

Buy large quantities of the food you eat secretly.

Overeating and then elimination (vomiting, over-exercise, laxatives and / or diuretics).

Experience extreme weight fluctuations.

Bleeding foods: make long visits to the bathroom after eating excessive amounts of food.

Exercise

Buy large quantities of food, diuretics, and / or diet pills.

You have an unusual swelling around your jaw.

You have negative physical reactions, such as gastrointestinal problems,

Swelling, gas, headache and / or sore throat.

Think of yourself very critically and negatively.

Experiencing self-esteem determined by its severity.

Participate in rigid thought.

Experience intense mood swings.

Afraid to be or to grow.

Does not cope well with stress and anxiety.

Feels temporary relief after purification.

Now that you've identified what nonsense food can be relevant to you, let's get started. It's time to learn how to eat consciously.

Practical Solutions For Everyday Mindless Eating Scenarios

What specifically can I do when I'm really struggling? The following scenarios guide you through some useful steps.

1: Eating excessively makes no sense.

Sit at your desk for several hours working on a project. You start thinking about the chocolate reserve hidden at the bottom of your desk drawer. You immediately forget what you are working on and can't think of anything but chocolate. In the past, opening a desk drawer led to eating without control and without meaning.

Practical solutions

Pause, stop everything you are doing (leave your pen, unplug your phone), and pay full attention to this problem.

Breathe in slowly and do a quick breathing exercise. Focus and become aware of your body and environment. Ask yourself what breathing tells you how you feel. Focus on breathing to concentrate and increase your awareness.

Ask for hunger. Ask yourself, "Am I very hungry?" Examine the physical cues and facts that will help you decide whether or not you have them. When was the last time you ate? What does your body tell you?

Find another fuel. If the answer is "No, I'm not hungry", examine your feelings. Are you feeling bored at work or worried about the project you're working on? What's happening? What else can you do to manage what you feel? Imagine what could complement you other than food. Will it help you to get up from your desk and take a walk? Has your body been still that long? Need to reach out? Would it be helpful to call a friend or talk to a colleague for a few minutes?

Examine your wishes. If yes, think about your options. Identify what you really want to eat and how much you need to satisfy your hunger.

Use your senses; give all your senses as you eat. Stay in touch with your diet and your body's reactions to food. Make conscious bites.

Using pictures you know that the onset of chocolate consumption has led to a slippery slope of overeating in the past. So imagine the big yellow and black danger sign that locks the drawer handle on your desk. Meditate on this image.

2: Without thinking

You tried to lose weight and skipped breakfast this morning. Your stomach rings and your head kicks. Although you want to eat something, there are many thoughts in your head like, "You are too fat to eat." You have trouble listening to your stomach and having a critical voice in your head.

Practical solutions

Don't expect too much between meals. If your stomach is

thundering, consider it a big huge flashing red neon sign: "I need food." When your stomach makes noise, it means you've waited too long. That is why you run the risk of pointless eating. Stop what you are doing and focus fully on the physical signals your body sends you. Be careful and watch. Record the feelings you feel next time. They will tell you that you are very hungry.

Plan carefully as you think about what might be good for your body and what you need now. Spend time being inside your body and figuring out what it needs. Observe your thoughts

Meditation: study the signals of your body with care.

Stop critical thoughts. Listen to the comments that come to mind. Observe your thoughts and feelings as you understand them. When they appear, call them what they are, like "just thoughts" or "just feelings." if you are being attacked personally, pause and think about the physical and emotional consequences of your actions. Turn your critical language into calm and relaxing words. Talk.

Be compassionate to yourself. Think about what you would say to someone else. If you have trouble empathizing with yourself, call someone who will. Avoiding criticism will help you explore the situation with an open and thoughtful attitude.

Ask what else is going on. Examine the broader context of what is happening now. Obviously, you're hungry, but what's going on internally? Think about what happened during the events that surrounded this moment. First, think about the present moment, then think deeply about your feelings from the previous moments. What caused this fight?

Accept yourself. Eating can lead to many negative feelings about you and your body. At this point, recognize that, at some level, you simply have to accept your body as it is. You have control over making that decision. It is not necessary to love every aspect of your body to respect and treat it properly. Imagine how food will improve your body's work. Your headache will stop.

3: Chaotic food makes no sense

A group of friends gathers for a night at home to watch a movie and eat pizza. They are looking for their favorite pizza ingredients. Everyone eats a few slices, which makes you eat two more pieces than you would normally eat. After they leave, you eat another slice without being hungry. You begin to feel the need to get rid of heavy pizzas and feel full.

Practical solutions

Sorry and accept. When you are still eating without thinking, it may seem that you are embarking on the journey again or, worse, that you are completely out of the way. This is not true that after you have learned the attention, you will not forget it. It is about reapplying principles. In this period, you have to forgive yourself. Most people advocate "forgive and forget." Carefulness does not do this. Instead, "forgive and accept." Do not try to withdraw your feelings. Accept whatever you feel.

Explore. Feeling full is a common reason people feel the need to eliminate food. A much healthier way of dealing with unpleasant feelings is to deepen them. Stop and meditate on the emotional components of your physical emotions. Making contact with your feelings will be helpful to avoid overeating next time.

Discover compulsive triggers. The need to refine food is a quick way to manage the anxiety that comes from consuming unnecessary calories. It is important to be careful and meditate all night. What feelings made you eat without thinking, especially after your friend's departure? What tendencies can food cause when you are not even hungry? Is that a motive?

Understand the physical consequences. Cleaning is caused by the negative emotions that come when you realize that you have eaten without thinking. Cleaning is dangerous. When people first cleanse themselves, they are more aware of their negative feelings and physical reactions. Over time, the individual is disconnected at any time from the inconvenience of cleansing and plans to feel better, calmer, or relieved to lose extra calories. Recognize the effects of purification on your body without prejudice.

Redirect activity. The need to feel better faster with food purification is tempting and sometimes difficult to control. Therefore, it is important to direct your mind to other things. Get out of the house. Take a walk, listen to music, or visit someone. Find a relaxing activity to participate in that will reduce your anxiety during the experience.

4: Return in the midst of temptation

You are in your kitchen and having trouble trying to get a bag of cookies. You think, "I just want the taste," but you're afraid you'll be able to eat the whole bag.

Practical solutions

The return: imagine actively withdrawing from a situation. Why is it important to give up? When people are stressed or overwhelmed, people tend to return to autopilot. This means eating or behaving in the usual way. Basically, you respond automatically instead of exploring all relevant and critical information. Taking a step back helps you to be thoughtful and aware of all the information you need to identify different solutions. To distract means to react cautiously by thinking, not to reacting in a robotic way. Determine your normal reaction.

Say it. Draw what is happening to you inside and out. Use details, descriptions, and many adjectives. Trust your senses: sight, smell, sound, taste and touch. Use striking details as if you were describing a scene to someone with their eyes closed. For example, say, "I really want a cookie. I'm in the kitchen in front of the closet. I'm afraid to eat too much and finish all the cookies in the box. I feel nervous, and my hands are shaking. I'm sweating and walking around because I don't know what to do. "

Turn on your sixth sense. The sixth and most important sensory organ is your mind. Describe how you feel and think. Think about the situation objectively without inserting a critical statement. Do not distort the description by saying that what is happening is "bad" or "wrong". Be sympathetic to yourself. For example, say, "I'm very hungry and frustrated. It's a really difficult situation for me. In the past, I know this situation has hurt me a lot. It's good to feel that way."

Specify what you want. Verbalization is obviously like translating a foreign text into your own language. Read the situation, rest and describe it in your own words. For example, say, "I want to eat a cookie, but I don't want to overeat. How do I feel?"

Think about the future. Describe your options. Think about each scenario. You could say, "I could get drunk or I could leave the room, eat something else, bring a cookie and stop, call someone, watch tv, or go for a walk."

Describe your choice. Make a decision. Visualize this decision. Imagine making your decision. Then say it out loud, "I'm only eating one cookie and I'm going to leave the kitchen so I don't eat." Close your eyes and imagine leaving the room.

Let it go. Please tell us what you need to release. One might say, "I may not be completely satisfied at this point, but I feel better about myself after the swing."

Effects Of Mindless Eating And Compulsive Over-Consumption

High cholesterol

High levels of cholesterol can lead to dangerous accumulation of cholesterol and other deposits in the walls of the arteries (atherosclerosis). These plaques can reduce blood flow to the arteries, which can lead to complications such as:

Chest pain: if the arteries that supply your heart with blood (coronary arteries) are affected, you may experience chest pain (angina) and other symptoms of coronary artery disease.

Heart attack: if the plaques break or rupture, a blood clot can form at the site of the plaque rupture, blocking blood flow or releasing and obstructing the downstream artery. If blood stops circulating in a part of your heart, you will have a heart attack.

Stroke: similar to a heart attack, a stroke occurs when a blood clot blocks blood flow to a part of your brain.

Diabetes

Diabetes mellitus, commonly known as diabetes, is a metabolic disease that causes high blood sugar. The hormone insulin moves the blood sugar for storage or use as energy. In addition to diabetes, your body does not produce enough insulin or cannot effectively use the insulin it produces.

High blood sugar not treated with diabetes can damage your nerves, eyes, kidneys and other organs.

Heart disease

Although cardiovascular disease can indicate various problems with the heart or blood vessels, this term is often used to refer to lesions of the heart or blood vessels due to atherosclerosis (ath-ur-o-scle Roe-sis), accumulation of fatty plaques in your arteries, and hardening of the arteries, which can prevent blood flow through the arteries to the organs and tissues.

Atherosclerosis is the main common cause of cardiovascular disease. This can be due to correctable problems, such as poor diet, lack of exercise, being overweight and smoking.

Kidney disease

The kidneys are two bean-shaped organs. Each kidney is the size of a fist. The kidneys filter water and waste from the blood and create urine. Kidney disease means your kidneys are damaged and unable to filter blood as they should.

If you have diabetes or high blood pressure, your risk of kidney disease is increased. If you have kidney failure, treatment includes kidney transplantation or dialysis. Other kidney problems include acute kidney damage, kidney cysts, kidney stones and kidney infections.

Arthritis

The most common type of arthritis, osteoarthritis, involves lesions due to wear of the cartilage of the joint, a hard and slippery wall at the ends of the bones where they form the joint. The cartilage cushions the ends of the bone and allows the joints to move almost without friction, but enough damage can cause the bone to implant directly into the bone, causing pain and limited movement. This wear can occur for many years or can be accelerated by injury or infection of the joints.

Osteoarthritis also affects the entire joint. This causes changes in the bones and deterioration of the connective tissue that binds the muscles to the bones and maintains the joint. It also causes inflammation of the joint mucosa.

Practical Ways To Overcome Emotional Eating

Chewing gum. If you have trouble eating emotionally or are hungry all the time, even after eating, try chewing gum. According to a study published in Appetite, chewing gum for at least 45 minutes can reduce your appetite, make you feel less hungry for snacks, and increase satiety. This will not help you limit your diet. Instead, chewing gum gives you activity that you adapt to your body and observe how you feel and think.

Prevent roaming. Roaming is another sign that you are close to an insignificant diet. You may notice that you walk in the kitchen, open the closet, look at it without really looking at it, then close and repeat the steps with the refrigerator. If so, sit down. Imagine being hooked to your seat. Take the time to think clearly about what you are looking for.

Decipher your physical hunger. A gradual increase in the desire to eat in relation to an impulse that suddenly appears, a void in the stomach (grunting, sounds, etc.), a moment (the last meal or snack you ate there for three hours). Ask yourself if it's time to get some food.

Feed a good thing. Put feelings and hunger in separate corners. If emotions make you want to eat, be very specific about your feelings. Assign emotion very clearly. This will help you find the right solution. For example, eating a sandwich or reading a book is not likely to alleviate anger. But inviting a friend to let the money go will be enough.

Reverse hindsight for foresight. Ask someone after the fact why he ate too much, and he can often explain it quite clearly. "I ate cookies because I'm bored." Therefore, the idea exists in you. However, understanding is often sought only after the fact, when it is already too late. Throw in some attention and ask yourself, "Why am I going to eat this cake?" It doesn't matter if it's "right" or "wrong." Just inject reason. If you hear yourself saying, "I just want it," try to think more deeply. This type of answer avoids the question.

Turn a meaningless choice into a conscious choice. It's easy to pick up without thinking about a bowl of French fries or another serving of baked beans. You can even feel your hand have its spirit. Fingers are extended without real thoughts. To change this, focus on the position of your arms and body. Pay attention to the position of your body and observe it carefully. If you find that you are naturally at the table or in the snack storage area, imagine wearing a lead vest (the kind you would use for an x-ray) or walking underwater. Notice how these feelings slow down your automatic and sometimes unconscious movements. If your hand likes to touch the food, imagine wearing a heavy bracelet or watch. Or use one to remind you to take your movements into account.

Energize consciously. Some emotional meals are the result of excessive fatigue. Determine if you eat when you wake up or receive an increased amount of energy. The most obvious intervention is to sleep more. If that doesn't work or you can't tighten it, try vigorous exercise. Running or walking fast can raise your blood pressure. Black tea with caffeine instead of coffee or soda can be beneficial; it helps to reduce cortisol, a stress hormone that often causes you to eat with stress, and it works soothing. However, in the long run, it is worth noting that, if you use food to deal with fatigue, then you will find ways to rest more.

Relax consciously. After work, one of the most common times of the day is when people struggle to overeat with no emotional meaning as soon as you walk in the door, go straight to the kitchen. Sometimes you are hungry. But in reality, it's often just a way to relax and unwind. This is a good case for finding a healthy way to get rid of business. It can be something like taking five minutes to close your eyes to the table before running. You can also take extra time to listen to a relaxing song before going home. You can also try changing clothes as soon as you enter the door to make it easier to leave work mode and feel comfortable. If you are really hungry, grab a snack before leaving the office. This gives your body twenty minutes for your brain to record eating and reduce the intensity of hunger as it enters the door.

Use a napkin. Moving from the fast-paced rhythm of everyday life to the careful state of mind on the table may seem like a real penny. Put a towel in your lap. It is slowly expanding. Pay attention to the color of the towel and its weight on the knees. Imagine putting all the problems in your head under this towel. Begin eating only when you are physically and mentally present and careful at the table. Use a towel ritually to change your mental state.

Listen to critics about internal food. We all have a food critic living in our head. Your internal food critic makes decisions about what to eat and what not to eat. In order not to get caught up in your demands, learn to listen without paying attention to all your wishes. Just because you think about it that doesn't mean you must to do it. So, if your mind tells you to eat, recognize this message and know that you do not have to obey all the orders of the food critic.

Cook enough. After dinner, there is a significant amount of pointless food. Because? This is part of the cleansing ritual. You say to yourself, "If I take another bite of garlic bread, I don't have to put it in a bowl or toss it." Reducing the size of your cooking is an easier way to solve problems than trying to avoid cutting leftovers. Try for one night. If four people eat, cook only four meals, not enough for extra meals. This is not to take away your food, but to break the cycle of overeating without meaning. If you want more later, you can still make extra portions. Or pack the leftovers right away. Keep your mind focused on eating less tomorrow if you consume it now.

Resistance to magnetic force. Many of my clients describe the appeal of eating as a magnetic force. For example, suppose there is a bag of French fries in the cupboard. Take your fist out and then leave. Then you chew the fries, and when you finish in the same place, you take a handful and move away again. This cycle can be repeated several times. It is a sign of emotional eating. Exit the kitchen.

Take a mental break. Eating senselessly sometimes plays the role of delaying. Do you use foods that you think are useful for avoiding or delaying an unwanted task, such as eating or doing homework? Instead of eating, give yourself permission to take a five-minute mental break. At the end of the five minutes, re-evaluate whether you are ready to complete the task or need to take five more. In the long run, it is more beneficial to give yourself permission to relax than overeat.

Watch out for the slippery slope. Think about activities that will inevitably lead you directly into eating without making any sense. Does a Mexican restaurant inevitably lead to over-fried tortillas? Nine times out of ten, maybe you buy a box of donuts instead of picking one. Avoid the inner battle with cakes by not reducing the slippery slope in the first place. In other words, stay away from a bakery or restaurant until you feel more secure. Make a list of events that seem to be related to getting a slippery slope.

Be careful when eating socially. Most people tend to reflect the way their friends, family and loved ones eat. If you do, don't be too hard on yourself. This often happens unknowingly. Be careful. Make sure you agree with your food partner's bite. If so, try to spread your bites. Watch your pace and try to chew a little slower.

Eat before a meal. Too much hunger can cause you to eat too much. Before reaching an extreme level of hunger (shivering, headache, lack of energy, etc.), choose a healthy snack. Deliberately choosing to eat consciously can help you eat too much later. Choosing a healthy snack is like an over-the-counter insurance policy at your next meal.

Review the portions. It is good to eat snacks. You may just need to find ways to control portion size. Get a six-hole muffin pan (or just use muffin pans). When you want a snack, fill one, two or three of these holes according to the degree of hunger. This can help you visually see the size of your portions. The muffin pan is also a great tray.

Snack all the time. Immerse yourself in your snack routine by designating a particular bowl as a "snack bowl." Make it small and put what you want to eat. This will help you eat the same amount all the time.

Train to measure hunger and satiety. Knowing signs of hunger and satiety is a key task in conscious eating. Try exercising to know how full your stomach feels when you are in a good mood. Don't try it when you're fighting. Estimate your hunger level from 1 to 10, 1 extremely hungry and 10 extremely full. Then drink a glass of still or sparkling water and re-evaluate your hunger and satiety. Keep drinking the fluid. Observe different levels of fullness. You may want to repeat this exercise at different times of day and when your mood will be different. Does your mood prevent you from knowing how full you are?

Sleep deprivation, unhealthy substances, and stress are a recipe for emotional overeating. Feeling tired, too much stress and drinking or using drugs can make your body function at a lower level. During stress days, consider SOS: a safe place (choose the safest possible environment to reduce the risk of pointless eating), observe (watch how these conditions affect your mood and your conscious diet), calm your senses (focus on calming senses while you sleep, applying a warm handkerchief to your face, reading a fun book, meditating, etc.).

Plan carefully. We often unknowingly differentiate ourselves from our desires as if the child being played follows the leader. To stop this autopilot behavior, plan your meals for the rest of the day before leaving home. It gives you the opportunity to throw a snack in your bag or gather the resources you need, so you don't eat later without thinking. It is always useful to have a contribution at your fingertips. We tend to eat whatever comes close to us when we feel hopeless. This is when vending machines and fast food take over. It is best to have a bite you choose in advance rather than an impulsive option.

Find snacks. When people try to quit, they often confine themselves to a specific area, such as outside their home, in a spot outside their workplace, or in their car. This allows for behavior, but locates it to reduce other variables. It also reduces the ease and comfort of behavior. Try the same with snacks. Allow yourself a snack, but in a place that is outside the kitchen and a little uncomfortable. This way, you won't eat without thinking, and you may need to think twice if you really want to eat something.

Take small steps. Dieting is like trying to empty a large pool in minutes. To eat consciously means to empty the pool one bin at a time. What is a good little step? Try to leave only one or two snacks on the plate. Small conscious steps are important.

Prepare. If your mind keeps telling you, "I want to eat healthy, but I can't right now," that's fine. Respect this feeling. Ask yourself, "What can I do to prepare myself when I'm ready? ... Cutting vegetables for later? Take off my sportswear? Pack a bag of snacks?"

Play the detective. If you are not sure that you are hungry, examine the body for signs. Start with your fingers and end at the top of your head. When you focus on each part of your body, recognize how you feel at that moment. Then ask yourself if it is hunger. For example, "Is hunger on your feet?" You can answer, "Partially, yes, I realize I'm looking for something to eat." This exercise has two purposes. First, it helps you become more familiar with your body and better read the signs when you are really hungry. Second, it is a distraction.

Adjust your blood sugar. One of the best ways to prevent emotional eating is to eat certain foods that will maintain stable blood glucose levels. Whole grains, vegetables, and some fruits prevent blood sugar peaks (caused by sweets and chocolate, for example) and accidents that cause bad mood. These foods keep blood sugar levels more stable, which helps to avoid the emotional feeding cycle. Notice how your mood changes after consuming certain foods. Take care fifteen minutes after eating. Come back an hour later. What did you notice?

Review meals. Do you eat every day at the same time, hungry or not? You can eat during your favorite tv show every night. In a week, see if you set your meal schedule by time. Mixing common routines can help break this cycle. For example, walk the dog before breakfast instead of after. Record your favorite show and watch it earlier in the day when you are normally not eating. The goal is to eat more according to hunger than what is called "dinner time."

Have healthy food. Think for a moment about where you store healthy foods. It's easy to forget them when you can't see them. So keep healthy snacks in your visual journey: at your desk, in the bowl at the counter, in the basket by the door to grab it as you go. Refurbish your refrigerator. Put healthy foods in them, without hiding them in a vegetable tray where you will never see them.

Eat like an athlete. Athletes view food from a completely different angle than most people. When they pick up a piece of food, they perceive it as energy. Before eating, ask yourself if the food is worthy of a marathon (it will keep you fed), best for running (it will feed you until your next meal), or whether it is ideal for sprinting (yes, you will be breathing energy very quickly). Think about how long this meal will keep you active and full of energy.

Love it or leave it. Stop chewing without thinking of mediocre foods by focusing only on the treats you love so much. Consume only desserts and treats that represent 9 or 10 on your list of delights. Some guests agree that they only eat really unique or homemade treats. Maybe for you, it's the release of any non-cheesecake gift.

Think of comfort, not pleasure. Is your first reaction to insisting on the desire for sensory pleasure in the language to improve things? When you notice the need to eat with stress, think about comfort, not pleasure. What kind of things bring comfort? Sleeping, scented candle, sports pants, relaxing cup of tea, warm bath? For more ideas, see my book: 50 Ways to Calm Down Without Eating.

Create breakpoints. Packaged foods often have a natural breaking point built in. These are the places you pauses to ask, "Do I want more?" For example, the tipping point of a sandwich cookie container is usually at the end of the queue. For a bag of chips, this could be the bottom of the bag. However, these built-in stopping points often come too late. You may need to create your own to avoid overeating. You can do this by placing food in smaller bags. The bottom of the bag creates a new breaking point. When you are done with your bag, strain your belly. Ask yourself, "Do I want or want more or am I happy?

Eat something new. Are you afraid to order a new meal or eat unfamiliar healthy foods? Don't say to yourself, "Just for that meal, I'll investigate what happens if I don't eat onion rings," or "I'll order something different this time for dinner."

This does not commit you to a long-term commitment. Use this test to see how new feelings emerge.

Recalibrate the palate. Do you want extremely sweet food? Don't like healthy meals? This may be because many processed foods are hundreds of times sweeter than natural foods. Then our taste buds are distorted by exaggerated aromas that do not occur naturally. Eating whole foods can help your tongue be satisfied with healthier and more natural foods. As sugar and salt consumption decrease, the palate changes and sensitivity to these elements increases. Try eating locally grown foods that are fresh, so they are not full of artificial flavors, preservatives, added sugar, extra salt, and so on.

Consider your carbon footprint. What you eat has an impact not only on you, but also on the environment and the world. This is not to produce guilt but to help you get out of your plate. What you eat also affects your environment, from your spouse to someone on the other side of the world. If you can't motivate yourself, take a moment to pause before eating. Look carefully at what's on your plate. Consider the origin of all objects. Local farming? Another state? Another country? Before you eat a banana, check the label to see where it comes from.

Scroll consciously. If the word "exercise" is a fever, stop using this trigger word. Instead, focus on movement. Sign up for a kilometer local walk or run a 5k (or more if you already have experience) for charity: breast cancer, autism, diabetes, etc. If not, check the national eating disorders website (see resources) for national markets. Participating in an organized event has many benefits. It takes you into training mode, gives you a measurable and defined goal, and sets a permanent end date.

Calm the body. A stress-induced diet is partially fueled by the physiological response you have when disturbed. Your body changes in response to a fight or theft. If you feel the urge to eat with stress, try different ways to calm your body: take a deep breath, stretch, relax, practice self-massage, reduce further stimulation (such as lowering music or light). Soothe all your senses. Then examine if you want to eat.

Dinner instead of eating. Think for a moment how you eat, especially things like fast food. Do you eat them in a paper bag? Standing over the sink? Don't have boxes? To switch to power conscious mode, use a placemat or a good plate. This can help you remember that eating is important, special and deserves your full attention.

Can vs can't. Your mind keeps saying, "I can't eat that!" If this is the case, you may cause more meaningless meals than prevention. By constantly moving your finger towards yourself, you run the risk of compromising your food or feeling deprived. Instead, direct your mind to look at foods with the "I can eat" attitude. Remember it is a choice. "I choose to eat it or I choose not to eat it." Remember that it is better to make a conscious decision to eat without thinking than to make an unconscious decision.

Practice gratitude. Before you bite, take a moment to enjoy the food in front of you. Think about where it came from and how long it took to get on your plate. Say a short sentence or just say "thank you". Gratitude can change your mind in a grateful and caring way.

Create a selectmyplate.org tablecloth. Don't know how your plate should be? In 2011, the government rejected the food pyramid and created a tool that can help you become a more considerate consumer. Instead of specific quantities, the icon indicates the proportions of usable portions. Print a photo and turn it into a single tablecloth.

Believe in change. Many want to change, but they do not secretly believe for a moment that something could be different. Imagine eating consciously, eating when you are hungry and quitting when you are full. You see yourself doing something you don't feel like, like eating a cookie or cooking a healthy meal. If you see yourself doing it, you can!

Pay attention to the internal signals.

If you use internal or external signals. Outside signals are things like a waitress taking a plate (implying it's over), the bag is over, it's time to get back to work. By internal signals, you are satisfied with the food or you realize that your thoughts are saying stop or "I'm done." See if you rely on external or internal signals to know when to stop and start eating. Focus your attention on internal signals. They are much more accurate to help you know when to leave the fork.

Turn it around. Many of my clients have trouble opening their food containers. This can be a bag of chips or a plastic container with debris. Once the lid is closed, it is often difficult to stop eating until nothing is left. You may notice that your hand still enters the open bag. If that sounds like you, do an experiment. Open the container and pour all the contents into a paper towel. Notice how different the food looks. This impedes the spending process. If you look at the whole quantity at once and not in a shot, it can help you eat better. Now try taking a few bags and splitting the food into portions that will leave you satisfied.

Change your goal. Try to eliminate hunger instead of feeling satisfied or full. They probably made you think that "full feeling" ends the meal. If you wait for this signal, you may not eat anything. Learn to feel good instead of getting tired.

Consider dessert first. Have lunch and then ask, "Do I have room for dessert?" You usually have to be full enough to turn down dessert, right? Sometimes it is useful to put the car in front of the horse. First think about dessert, then adjust your diet accordingly. Don't find a place for dessert; make room.

Avoid thinking in black and white. Nothing leads you to overeating like extreme thought. Whenever you hear it, it says, "I took full advantage of it!" or in other phrases that start with "I should" or "I always" or "I can never do this", follow your thoughts. Notice how many times you decide on food, whether it's all or nothing.

List more neutral ways to talk about your diet. Staying away from the absolute is a useful practice for life in general.

Be realistic. Emotional sails are often unknowingly preparing for guilt and disappointment. They set their expectations too high and make great promises, such as: "I will never eat junk food again." If you constantly feel disappointed, make your expectations more realistic. Think about what you really do now and challenge yourself. If you usually eat three cookies, targeting two may be more realistic than one or none.

Leave food to whom. Eating emotionally often removes all feelings. You may be slapped as if you were touched by anesthesia, a diversion of thoughts, feelings and sensations that would otherwise force you to solve the problem. When you get into a food coma, you feel nothing. But you don't even hear your thoughts about stopping or feeling full in your stomach. If you notice that you feel nothing, give yourself a gentle pinch to help you stay awake and present. Pay attention to the sensation. It's probably a little awkward. Notice how this changes your consciousness. Eat conscious again.

Drop the piece. Can't decide to eat something or not? If so, remove the food fight by tossing a coin (face to face or cross), tossing only one of the dice (1 to 3 means to eat, 4 to 6 means no) or stealing the ticket (black card means eat, red means no). Watch your reaction when making your decision. How do you feel? Relief? Anger? Disappointment? Rebellion? This feeling is important because it gives you a lot of information about your difficulties. Explore that.

Remove distractions. In a recent study, respondents who were distracted while playing alone at lunchtime were less full after eating than those who did not play while eating. They also ate much more than participants who were not distracted. So, take care to avoid overeating.

Ask yourself ... Complete this statement: if I eat, then I will feel ... This technique can help you understand the emotion you are trying to calm with food.

Minimize eating comfort. If you continue to move towards a comfortable diet, reduce its negative impact. For example, eat a healthy snack, like carrots. Choose the healthiest and most affordable option; if chocolate candy is your weakness, drink chocolate milk.

Keep small snacks. Eat what you want in slow, conscious snacks. Eating at a slow pace can significantly reduce the amount of food you eat, especially for larger meals. To reduce speed between bites, consult a skill builder slowly but surely, slow down your diet, one moment for a moment.

Eating delay. Promise yourself that you will eat the food you want after doing something else in five minutes. You may find that your desire decreases slightly or disappears during this period. It is a sign of emotional rather than physical urge.

Cherish your senses. Choose a meal that changes your senses radically: try something hot, fresh, spicy, crunchy, etc. Notice how all parts of your body respond to sensations, from what you feel in your tongue to what you hear and feel. Repeat this with new, different foods next week.

Use your slow cooker. You eat a lot without thinking about the end of a long day when you are tired. Cooking a healthy meal and being prepared for dinner will help you avoid unhealthy snacks or fast food. Turn on the slow cooker after breakfast and dinner for a few hours.

Who can help with mindful eating?

Mastering a mindful diet is not an easy task. The earlier you change your eating habits and mentality, the more likely you are to get professional help. Although friends and family can be very helpful, sometimes it can be difficult to talk to them about weight problems. When they talk about their own problems and fears, it is often difficult for friends or family to be sufficiently detached from their fears and anxieties to really listen to what you say.

If you are unable to change your eating habits on your own, or if meditating on the underlying issues of your eating problem triggers overwhelming emotional reactions, it is important to call an expert. A professional can evaluate what other factors to consider. Professional help can be obtained from psychologists, psychiatrists, doctors, nurses and nutritionists. A team of professionals is highly recommended. Each specialist provides specialized training in one aspect of the mind, body, thought, or feeling, which together creates a holistic treatment. A healthcare provider is especially helpful because some people need antidepressants or other medications. There are many options, including hospital treatment, for those who need to devote their full attention to this time.

Fluctuating calorie intake is heavy on your body and your mind. This can seriously affect your concentration. A professional can tell you how to regain concentration. It is crucial to seek additional help if you have mood, alcohol or drug problems. It also matters if you feel suicidal, if you have lost a lot of weight, if you have physical symptoms, or if you act impulsively. These symptoms can seriously inhibit conscious eating due to competing emotional demands.

Counseling is basically a way to break down your "standing" thinking patterns. It helps you express your feelings about food, identify patterns, and connect the dots between important events in your life. As a counselor, I have led many people to overcome a wide variety of eating problems. I feel honored for their confidence, and they have allowed me to help them solve their difficult problems.

How to eat mindfully at work

At work, eat consciously.

So you made it. You graduated! Fortunately, you have a degree

With security in hand. A small piece of paper indicates that you have endured years of hard work and mental sweat. Better yet, you have

a square business. Thank God!

In preparing for your new life, you probably have thought about all the little things in university life that you would miss.

It's a safe bet that cafeteria food is not part of it. In fact, you are most likely breathing a sigh of relief. More crazy people in the cafeteria line, mass produced by food, taco bell runs at 3:00, or eating while studying late into the night. Finally you are safe.

Don't get too excited. The road ahead will actually bring a thoroughfare,

a new series of conscious food challenges. Foods make no sense.

They are likely to accompany you directly from the room and directly at headquarters, internship or graduate school. It doesn't matter where you go or what kind of work you do, there are pitfalls to eating that make no sense everywhere. Get a solid education on healthy and conscious eating; enjoy everything you do in college.

1. Nine to five challenges: when you start this business from nine to five,

most of the working hours will be in the office. So at work, you will eat one or two meals a day. If you travel in the morning or work late, it can mean breakfast, lunch and dinner in the office.

Your options are to go back to brown paper or eat out. The key is to plan ahead. Make sure you have enough food with you so you are not very hungry, which is great

but you will be encouraged to eat mindlessly. Pack an extra snack in case you have to stay up late. It is up to you to eat a healthy and balanced diet.

Feed yourself on weekdays. It's pretty hard to work with and focus on an empty stomach.

2. Job interviews: as part of the interview, many employers include a lunch interview. It's partial to see how you react in a social setting. However, nothing is more difficult.

Eat carefully during a high stress interview. When you're nervous, it's hard to be present with your body. You can eat not to talk or check in with your

body. It is good to eat a light snack before leaving. Don't leave for a lunch meeting or meeting too hungry.

3. Business account: do I want dessert? Of course, why not! When someone else is paying for dinner, free speech can interfere.

Eat with care. It is tempting to order this expensive and gigantic product, steak especially, when someone else pays the bill. To avoid mindless eating, remember to eat exactly what you can pay for.

4. Eating opportunity: for one of my clients, every Wednesday morning was office day in the office. She was looking forward to it and eat two or three donuts. Normally, she wouldn't eat more than one bagel. But there was a perception that it was free.

This motivated her to make the most of it. Plus, it seemed to make up for some things she didn't like about work.

If the food is free, we tend to eat it, hungry or not.

Never underestimate the power of a free bagel to incite some meaning.

Eat to stay fit

6. Office dining: you mean you don't have time for lunch?

This is unfortunate. Because of this, you can take multiple tasks at the same time.

You eat maybe cookies, you write a note,

and talk on your cell phone at the same time. When you're at work, your body does not treat anything at all.

You eat. Often, your brain does not completely capture food as well.

You could still be hungry.

7. Stress: you can have that awful colleague who loves them.

You walk down the hall, you hear the music of Darth Vader as it begins.

People hide and start to bend under the tables.

Stress is reflected throughout the office. Eating stress is a common reason people eat too much at work. They don't know how to deal with stress at work. Let's consider alternative ways to handle stress at work. Send a quick email, walk around.

MINDFUL EATING APP

Using external influences, like your phone, can help us refine some of the central components of conscious eating. We know that eating slowly, focusing on food and the experience of eating, and adjusting to the signals of hunger and satiety can be extremely helpful in creating healthier relationships with food.

What makes a good diet app?

The best apps are focused on raising awareness of the eating experience by observing the speed at which we eat and our emotions or making food decisions.

Two questions to ask before downloading a mindful eating app:

1. Is weight loss reported in the application information? - If so, the application is not exactly based on care. Mindfulness and careful eating are focused on approaching the present, not the future. Because weight loss goals are part of the future (and not useful to many at all), they don't really fit the notion of mindfulness. The same goes for counting calories.

2. Is there developer information and additional "support / assistance" information? Accessing more credible help for your personal situation is very important (and helpful), so check it out.

Ten mindful eating apps

I'm hungry? ®: this application is based on the conscious dietary cycle of Dr. Michelle May. Am I hungry ®. Whenever you want to eat, the app guides you through a series of conscious decisions.

Mindful bite: mindful bite is focused on the time we eat. It blinks every 30 or 60 seconds and then you bite. It also gives you periodic instructions to think about your hunger and satiety.

Before I eat (a moment in the zone): this app is useful for people who have had bulimia attacks or cravings that do not feel useful. It focuses on identifying what you feel before eating (e.g., hunger, anxiety, sadness, boredom, etc.) and guides you through strategies for each sensation. It also includes some components of health training and goal setting.

In the moment: much like before I eat, this app guides you through strategies for managing your senses, not using food to control your emotions.

Mindful eating tracker: based on mindfulness, this app allows you to bring in an idea or thought of food (and decide what to do with thought), evaluate and track levels of gratitude, hunger, thirst, and pleasure and enjoyment of food.

Eat drink and be mindful: this app allows you to record your hunger level and type of hunger. It also shows how you respond to food (mind, body, thoughts and feelings) and includes reminders to eat consciously.

Rise up and recover: although it is specifically designed for people with eating disorders (and, in addition, there are great eating disorder apps, such as a recovery record), this app still contains really useful tools for everyone. Meals can be recorded, followed by emotions and behavior, which includes a large portion of resources and additional support.

Mindful meal timer: currently available only on google play, this handy app guides you to eat slowly and has a time span for eating and major snacks (with a halfway alert).

Mindful eating: encourages you to photograph the foods you eat with hunger, sensory perception, satisfaction level, etc.

Eat, chew and rest: according to the concept of slowing down, applications guide you into 3 feeding phases according to each color that may occur in the next food step: 1) put food in your mouth (green), 2) chew (yellow), and 3) leave accessories for cooking, reflecting and expressing gratitude (red).

CONCLUSION

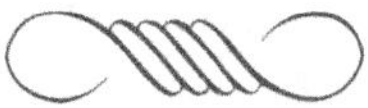

Mindfulness involves special care, intentionally, in the present moment and without prejudice. It also means paying special attention, intentionally, to the present moment and without judgment.

The best way to think about mindfulness is to be more than activity. Almost every activity can be done consciously. Originally associated with Buddhist psychology, the term "attention" comes from the sanskrit word smṛti, which literally means "what one remembers."

Mindfulness involves directing attention intentionally, rather than letting it wander. This means being fully involved and careful at the moment. Past and future thoughts are simply recognized as thoughts that occur in the present.

This means that feelings and thoughts are not considered good or bad, pleasant or unpleasant; they simply register as an "event" and are watched until they finally pass.

The benefits of mindfulness

Mindfulness is a practice of the body and mind that has been found to be beneficial for both mental and physical health. The major psychological change that occurs while practicing consciousness is a greater awareness of the thoughts and feelings of the present moment. Over time, mindfulness practice can help you become aware of the space between the realization of experiments and their reaction, allowing you to reduce speed and observe the processes of your mind.

The ultimate goal of mindfulness practice is to use this space to make more deliberate decisions: get out of your life by autopilot, based on unproductive mental habits.

How to get started with mindfulness

Mindfulness is a habit; it's something we do. We are more likely to be in this mode with less and less effort. With the practice of mindfulness, learning to be aware is just the tip of the iceberg. Most of this practice is about becoming aware of the meaning of consciousness and improving our brains for mindfulness. This means that almost all activities can become conscious if they include these basic components.

Mindful eating means simply being fully aware of the food you eat and eating for the right reasons. Mindful eating can also mean sharing food on a plate, sitting down and tasting every bite. Chew slowly, take time, pay attention to textures, these are good practices. While on the other hand, mindless eating means eating for other reasons than

feeding one's body and satisfying one's hunger. We have countless options to eat every day. If you eat well enough, exercise, lose weight, and do not know why, an mindless diet could be the cause.

Poor eating habits include overeating, or eating too little healthy food that we need every day, or eating too much fiber and low fat, salt and sugar. These unhealthy eating habits can affect our food intake, including energy (or kilojoules) of proteins, carbohydrates, essential fatty acids, vitamins and minerals, as well as fiber and fluids.

Mindless eating means eating for other reasons than feeding

one's body and satisfying one's hunger. We have countless opportunities to eat every day. Our pantries and storage cabinets, supermarkets or cafes can offer several food items.

The following broad categories describe five types of mindless eaters, which includes the occasional mindless eater, the chronic mindless dieter, the mindless undereater, the mindless overeater, and the mindless chaotic eater.

Healthy eating includes eating lots of fruits and vegetables. This is one of the most important food items; vegetables and fruits are full of nutrients such as antioxidants, vitamins, minerals and fiber, which help in the maintenance of a healthy weight by holding you for a long time. Fill half a plate of vegetables and fruits with every meal and snack.

Choose whole foods, Whole foods include whole wheat bread, crackers, brown or wild rice, quinoa, oatmeal, and barley-free barley. They are prepared using whole grain. Whole foods contain fiber, protein and b-type vitamins to help you stay healthy and satiated for longer. Choose whole grain options instead of processed or refined cereals, such as white bread and pasta.

Eat protein foods, Protein foods include legumes, nuts, seeds, tofu, enriched soy drinks, fish, seafood, eggs, poultry, lean red meat, including game, skim milk, lighted yoghurts and lighted kefir and cheeses with low fat and sodium. Proteins contribute greatly to the formation and maintenance of bones, muscles and skin. Dairy products are a great source of protein. Choose low-fat, flavorless options.

Restriction yourself from highly processed and ultra-processed foods.

Highly processed foods, often referred to as ultra-processed foods, is food that has changed its sources and contains many additional ingredients. During treatment, important nutrients such as vitamins, minerals and fiber are often removed when salt and sugar are added. Examples of processed foods are fast food, hot dogs, French fries, cookies, frozen pizzas, sausages, white rice and white bread. Learn more about ultra-processed foods here. Some poorly processed food is fine. They are slightly modified foods, but they contain little additives in industrial production. Minimally processed foods retain almost all their essential nutrients.

Here are some examples, a bag of salads, frozen vegetables and fruits, eggs, milk, cheese, flour, brown rice, oil and dried herbs. We do not refer to these minimally processed foods when advised not to eat them.

Make water your favorite drink. Water promotes health and promotes hydration without adding calories to the diet. Sugar drinks, including energy drinks, fruit drinks, 100% fruit juices, soft drinks and coffee with flavors, have a lot of sugar and little or no nutritional value. It's easy to drink empty calories without realizing it, which results in weight gain. Avoid fruit juice, even if it is labeled 100% fruit juice. Although fruit juice has some of the benefits of fruits (vitamins, minerals), it contains more sugar than fruits and less fiber. Fruit juices should not be eaten as an alternative to fruit. When there is no drinking water, quench your thirst with coffee, tea, low fat milk and boiled water.

Mindful eating exercises, prepare a meal plan every week, this is the key to easy and quick meal preparation. Choose recipes with lots of fruits and vegetables. Your goal is to fill half a plate of vegetables and fruits with each meal. Choose bright fruits and vegetables every day, especially dark orange and green vegetables (click here for more information). Frozen or canned fruits and vegetables without sugar are the perfect alternative to fresh produce.

Avoid sugary drinks and drink water instead. Low fat and sugar free milk is also a good way to stay hydrated. Keep a reusable water bottle in your bag or car so you can refill it wherever you go.

Eat smaller meals more often. Eat at least twice a day with intermediate meals. When you wait too long to eat, you are more likely to choose unhealthy foods. Keep snacks easy to eat (like this one) in your bag or emergency bag.

How poor nutrition affects us, Poor nutrition can affect our health and wellbeing on a daily basis and impair our ability to live an active and enjoyable life. Poor feeding can contribute to stress, fatigue and our ability to work. Over time, it can also contribute to the risk of developing certain diseases and other health problems, such as being overweight or obese, tooth decay, hypertension, high cholesterol, heart disease and stroke, type 2 diabetes, certain types of cancer, depression, eating disorders.

Effects of pointless eating and compulsive over-consumption, High cholesterol, this can lead to dangerous accumulation of cholesterol and other deposits in the walls of the arteries (atherosclerosis). These plaques can reduce blood flow to the arteries, which can lead to complications such as: chest pain, Heart disease, although cardiovascular disease may indicate several cardiac or circulatory problems. This term is often used to damage the heart or blood vessels caused by atherosclerosis.

Kidney disease, the kidneys are two organs shaped like beans. Each kidney is the size of a fist. The kidneys filter water and waste products from the blood and create urine. Kidney disease means your kidneys are damaged and unable to filter blood as they should.

Arthritis, the most common type of arthritis, osteoarthritis, involves injuries caused by wear of the cartilage in the joint: a hard, slippery wall at the ends of the bones that make up the joint. The cartilage blocks the ends of the bone and allows the joints to move almost frictionless, but enough damage can allow the bone to implant directly into the bone, causing limited pain and movement. This wear and tear can occur for many years or can be accelerated by injury or infection of the joints.

The benefits of mindful eating include, Conscious eating reduces stress, Improves digestion by healthy eating. Mindful eating and yoga can lower blood glucose in gestational diabetes. It fights stress, high blood pressure and indigestion while meditation and mindfulness can stop eating disorders.

A healthy and balanced diet is one of the most important things you can do to protect your health. In fact, you can prevent up to 80% of premature heart disease and stroke through choices and habits of your life, such as eating well and being physically active. A healthy diet reduces the chance of having a heart attack and stroke, improves cholesterol level, lowers your blood pressure, helps you control weight, controls your blood sugar.

The significance of mindful eating cannot be over emphasized. The practice of mindful eating comes with its attendant health benefits, which is very important for physiological and physical wellbeing.

EMOTIONAL EATING

How To Develop Healthy And Guilt-Free Eating Habits

INTRODUCTION

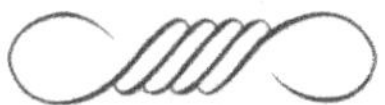

A good number of us have a general, rationale feeling of what to eat and when—there is no lack of ideas regarding this matter. However, there is regularly a distinction between what we know and what we do. We may have the facts; however, making choices must involve our emotions. Numerous individuals who battle with emotional struggles likewise struggles with an eating disorder. Emotional eating is a well-known term used to describe eating that is affected by emotions, both positive and negative. Emotions may influence different parts of your diet, including your inspiration to eat, your food choices, where and with whom you eat, and the speed at which you eat. Emotions incite most overeating as opposed to physical hunger. People who battle with obesity will generally eat in light of how they feel.

Be that as it may, individuals who eat for emotional reasons are not frequently overweight. Individuals of any size may attempt to get away from an emotional encounter by engrossing themselves with eating or by fixating on their shape and weight. Here are a few instances of what emotional eating may present as:

- Snacking when you don't feel physically hungry or when you are full

- Feeling an exceptional longing for a specific type of food

- Not feeling satisfied in the wake of eating satisfactory measures of healthy meals

- Restlessly picking more foods/snacks while your mouth is full

- Feeling emotionally calmed while eating

- Eating during or following a distressing encounter

- Numbing your feelings with specific foods

- Eating alone to maintain a strategic distance from others seeing you.

People who eat for emotional reasons frequently eat trying to self-alleviate or to find short-term relief from emotional trauma. A few people eat certain kinds of foods as a psychological approach to adapt to pressure. Emotional eating is identified with emotions of deficiency or inadequacy. Feelings may appear to be serious to the point that we believe we have to cope with them by getting away with choice meals, or we may feel we need other means to cope with emotional stress.

Consider your experience over the years. Do you experience valid or long-lasting relief while eating? Or on the other hand, is the relief temporary or halfway at the best-case scenario? Similarly, when we impulsively sit in front of the TV, drink liquor, or shop, we may wish to escape through eating. In later sections of this book, I will discuss some tried and tested methods to adapt to stress. In this book, you will figure out how to understand and deal with your emotions with the aim of feeling less averse to or overwhelmed by your feelings. These important tips will guide you into having perfect control over your eating habits as well as your emotions. However, you must take time to understand the problems before understanding how to pick the best solution that will work for you. Allow me the privilege to walk you down the path of guilt-free, emotion-free healthy eating habits!

CHAPTER ONE
UNDERSTANDING EATING DISORDERS

Emotional eating isn't a particular eating disorder worth losing your peace of mind over; however, emotional eating happens in eating disorders. Emotional eating is related to obesity, binge eating, and bulimia. You might or might not have an eating disorder, yet every now and then, I will refer to eating disorders to delineate the manners in which emotions influence eating disorder conditions.

To begin, I'll quickly explain how the Diagnostic and Statistical Manual of Mental Disorders—Fourth Edition (DSM-IV-TR) explains eating disorders. Anorexia includes over-evaluation of shape and weight. Individuals who battle with anorexia characterize their self-esteem to a great extent based on their weight. In this disorder, people keep an unusually low body weight (under 85 percent of average weight). To meet the criteria for anorexia, a lady must lose her menstrual period because of her dietary limitations.

Bulimia correspondingly involves an over-evaluation of one's shape and weight and inflexible struggles to control one's body size. Individuals who battle with bulimia intermittently "binge eat" or eat an enormous amount of food and experience loss of control at the same time. Notwithstanding binge-eating, individuals with bulimia participate in certain compensatory practices, or endeavors to "make up" for unnecessary caloric intake, by limiting their food consumption, intentionally inducing nausea, over-exercising, or abusing laxatives. Eating disorder not generally indicated (NOS) is the most widely recognized eating disorder. This classification depicts an eating issue of clinical seriousness that doesn't meet the criteria for anorexia or bulimia. For instance, a lady who is a heavy, however, ends up unreasonably engrossed with worries about her shape may meet the criteria for eating issue NOS. A man who is engrossed with his shape and restricts his food intake, but doesn't weigh under 85 percent of the normal human weight, would correspondingly get the eating disorder NOS diagnosis.

One type of eating disorder NOS is binge-eating disorder. Binge-eating disorder portrays intermittent binge-eating without extreme intentional efforts to control weight, and this issue regularly corresponds with obesity—however, it can likewise happen in individuals who are of average weight.

In contrast to anorexia or bulimia, which overwhelmingly influences women and young ladies, around 33% of individuals who binge-eat are males. We should pause for a minute to separate objective binges from subjective binges. An objective binge portrays devouring a considerable amount of food, joined by a sense of loss of control. An individual may consume a large number of calories in a sitting in an objective binge. An emotional binge includes feeling or thinking you ate excessively.

If you indulge yourself on Thanksgiving, this would be an emotional binge; if you ate what is normal on such a unique occasion, however, despite everything, you would have an inclination that you indulged yourself. Recognizing objective binges from subjective ones can assist us with starting to move away from seeing our practices in supreme terms or participating in pondering those practices. Feeling or thinking you ate an excess contrasts from losing control and quickly devouring unreasonable calories. Most eating disorders share specific center highlights, and numerous individuals who meet the criteria for one eating disorder wind up meeting the criteria for another eating disorder sooner or later. For instance, somebody who battles with anorexia may, in the long run, get a diagnosis of bulimia. For the most part, individuals who struggle with eating disorders over-evaluate their shape and weight and are strongly engrossed in fruitless attempts to manage their size. Binge eating likewise is prevalent among various diagnoses of eating disorders. Thoughtfully, this makes a lot of sense. If you characterize yourself by your weight, you may decide to restrict your meals, and limiting regular food intake brings about overeating, as your body's cells begin to feel denied of the required nutrients and energy to function. After a diet routine, individuals tend to indulge in foods and snacks they craved during the diet period. Individuals regularly likewise binge in light of negative states of mind or after having a stressful day.

EATING AND EMOTIONS

Individuals may either increase or decrease their eating rates because of stress. For instance, a few people experience an increase in craving when they feel discouraged while others experience a reduction. Restricting foods might be an approach to oversee feelings, as may binging. You may wind up reveling when you feel stressed out to calm yourself, and afterward placing yourself on harsh eating regimens trying to control your weight and your emotions. Psychologists conjecture that trouble in managing your emotions is the major issue behind both binge eating and bulimia. Binge-eating and different types of an unhealthy diet are regularly observed as social endeavors to impact, change, or control excruciating emotional states. Individuals who don't have an idea of how to manage feelings, either positive or negative, may depend on binge-eating, as well as cleansing, as an approach to oversee feelings. Anorexia is correspondingly determined by efforts to maintain a strategic distance from feeling any form of emotion. In particular, decreased awareness of emotions can happen in individuals with bulimia, and emotional shirking is normal for individuals who battle with anorexia. Emotions may influence eating in increasingly unobtrusive manners that don't enroll clinically. For instance, how many of us have plunged into a plate of cupcakes after a breakup or lost business deal? There is nothing amiss with appreciating good food during an unpleasant time; however, consistently relying upon food to deal with our emotions sends us the negative message "You can't adapt." Plus, what does a cupcake do to respect your emotions or to explain what matters to you? Research has shown that trouble recognizing and getting feelings, just as issues in controlling them, impacts gorging more than sexual orientation, food limitation, or exaggerating shape and weight do. At the point when individuals experience intense emotions or experience difficulty recognizing what their feelings are, they may feel they can't adapt to their emotions and may then attempt to keep away from the uneasiness by diverting themselves with food. You may see that you bounce from feeling any extreme emotions to eating, accordingly losing touch with your feelings. This may feel like a relief from the outset, yet it brings about your passing up on the chance to encounter the inclination for what it is (this is something you can work on doing effectively, as we will see in subsequent chapters). It is a must that we will encounter awkward emotions and reliably keep away from them, restraining our capacity to live with both wisdom and freedom. Specific individuals are all the more emotionally helpless, encountering feelings more strongly and feeling feelings for a more extended time than others.

If you are emotionally helpless and were brought up in a situation where you were not instructed how to adapt to emotions—or more awful, were rebuffed for showing your feelings—you may have figured out how to control emotions with food. When you experience a feeling and eat accordingly, you may encounter a normal feeling, just as different feelings that emerge because of emotional eating. Eating to numb your emotions doesn't completely assuage your emotions; instead, it only includes increasing mental (and caloric) weight to the experience. Likewise, if you eat because of your emotions, you may frequently neglect to value the message the emotions will teach you. Prominently, outrage and sadness are particularly identified with eating disorders; numerous individuals likewise see they will, in general, eat when upbeat, desolate, or restless.

Eating fried chicken may at first appear to be calming, yet overindulging in comfort foods when your emotions are unbalanced can give you significant emotional information, which will inevitably lead to disgrace and confusion. Food may likewise be utilized to increase the force of emotion. We may, for instance, use food to add to the standard experience of satisfaction, endeavoring to take our happiness up a notch.

Shirley, one of my clients, battled with an extraordinary bout of emotional trauma for a year. After a blend of intellectual, psychological treatment, and prescription meds, her state of mind improved, and she started to savor food. She depicted eating as relearning joy. At first, Shirley cherished exploring new wines and cheeses. In the long run, she chugged wines and ate cheeses, looking for an interminable divine understanding of what she tasted. Shirley had gone excessively far. A hyper insatiability exchanged for the straightforward delight of eating. The momentary advantages of turning into a cheese expert and an informal sommelier were presently being refuted by uneasiness and low self-esteem around her increasing weight.

CHAPTER TWO
ACCEPTING THE IDEA OF ACCEPTANCE

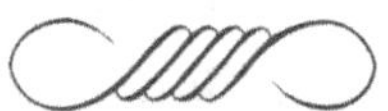

What is genuinely behind emotional eating? It is our reluctance to accept, or sit with, our feelings. However, when we eat for emotional reasons, we never really rid ourselves of our feelings. Or maybe, going into and tolerating our feelings is the entryway to opportunity and happiness, just as help from the cycle of emotional eating. However, this can be difficult to hear. Indeed, even my most charitable clients shiver when I state "accept" with regards to emotions and eating. Who wants to acknowledge difficult emotions or pain or acknowledge a burden that feels inadmissible? It can feel like I'm encouraging you to throw in the towel.

I submissively propose this procedure; a deep new worldview is a way into a new perspective and kinder association with food. Diets, food plans, blending and coordinating, enhancing, and denying may briefly help. Tolerating, minute to minute, is a long-term solution. A long way from being agonizing, acceptance is a type of graciousness: you recognize your facts and where you are at this time of your life. Will your weight go down as your psyche extends? Perhaps. Will your suffering decrease and become bearable? Truly. As you read further in this book, acceptance won't block change; rather, acceptance goes with change. Battling your body brings stagnation. Acknowledgment brings the flow into the best things life has to offer.

WHY DO WE HAVE EMOTIONS?

How about we step back for a minute and think about the various emotions we experience. Feelings give us a list of valuable information about our lives. The base of "feeling" is "motere," from the Latin for "to move." Emotions rapidly create changes in our mind and spinal cord to start an action—our conduct is frequently firmly attached to the feeling. An emotion is a precise signal that promotes survival instinct. Emotions spur our behavior, furnish us with significant information, and enable us to communicate with others in ways they will understand. How about we deliberate on two regular emotions and their functions. For example, say your partner becomes friends with an astoundingly alluring associate at your office, and you experience envy. Why? This emotion (envy) flags a risk, motivating us to plan ahead because our relationship may be in danger. At the point when we feel jealous, we are given information that our relationship is valuable and might be at risk. Our jealous disposition conveys our uneasiness to our partner; along these lines, envy guides us toward securing the relationship. If we eat to smother this feeling or to divert ourselves from it, we can't realize what the feeling is letting us know, and we can't respond in a fitting way, for example, communicating our emotions to our partner. Also, what is the incentive to feel cheerful? Bliss propels us to keep seeking after an action or esteemed bearing. The inclination gives data on what makes a difference to us. Satisfaction likewise conveys data to people around us, solidifying fundamental social securities. Would a friend be as excited to welcome you to a birthday dinner if you looked hopeless on the last occasion she hosted?

UNDERSTANDING ACCEPTANCE

Have you, at any point, eaten to cope with feeling fat? Time after time, individuals need to shed pounds and get baffled and somewhat frustrated when their weight reduction goals appear to go slower than expected. The process of weight reduction has become more like an ailment treatment than an experience to seek after. One may contend that obesity is a genuine medical condition, or eating for emotional reasons as opposed to hunger prompts, which may be hazardous. At the same time, would we energize an individual with disappointment to accomplish better psychological wellness by harping on how low his temperament is?

Or would we urge him to acknowledge his disposition—not in the soul of giving up on consistently improving, yet imaginatively and eagerly looking for unique arrangements? The idea of this continuous voyage requires continually coming back to an acceptance of self and mishaps and new challenges. The beginning of "acceptance" is the Latin for "to take." This is fitting because the best way to lessen the suffering is by taking the pain till you devise a means to living above the pain.

The fundamental equations are:

Pain = Pain

Pain + Non-acceptance = Suffering

Acceptance isn't abdication. It doesn't incorporate enjoying or approving the pain process. Yet, if "acceptance" is making you tingle, you may supplant it with a term like "extensiveness." Acceptance is deliberately receiving an open, nonjudgmental, responsive position, in any event, when faced with a challenge. This incorporates tolerating our feelings, contemplations, sensations, body shape, and reality, all in all, similarly for what it's worth at this time.

Non-acceptance—battling reality or our feelings—constrains our mindfulness and expands our struggles. Envision clutching one part of a scarf as I clutch the opposite end. If the scarf symbolizes your weight, what is your relationship with it? It is safe to say that we are loose as we hold the scarf together, or is there strain—would we say we are pulling in inverse ways? For a minute, consider the physical and emotional experience associated with a tug-of-war. It hoards our attention and vitality. Is it justified, despite all the trouble?

What is the other option? We could relinquish the fight, dropping the pull and opening our hands to receiving more energy. If we are eager to take an interest just in circumstances that give us great vibes, what will our life about? When we are reluctant to acknowledge our existence, we radically reduce our available options. That being stated, we can decide how to meet and acknowledge circumstances.

Acceptance, in a sense, is about empathy and dignity, not masochism. It is mind-boggling and dynamic—a continuous arrangement of decisions that relate our musings and activities to our profound qualities. Qualities depict what profoundly matters to you or what you need your life to represent. You may decide to acknowledge participating in a difficult relationship with a friend or family member if doing so identifies with your estimation of supporting your friends and family ("I will visit Mom at Christmas and assist her with getting out the loft"), while additionally doing what you have to do to in the administration of your benefit of securing and thinking about yourself ("I'll remain at a lodging, so I have my own place to go to if things start getting harsh").

If you can acknowledge the reality of a circumstance, instead of trusting or fantasizing things will, by one way or another, be different this time, you can take actions that respect the two sets of qualities. Correspondingly, you may acknowledge both your present shape and the emotional and social responsibilities required to transform it. You may acknowledge your emotions and, at the same time, change how you react to them. You don't need to acknowledge steady yearning and self-inflicted pains. Frequently, when we experience pain, we tend to get furious with others, accusing ourselves or responding indiscreetly. When our feelings trap us, it very well may be a test to back off and see whether our emotions are situated truly and whether our actions are serving our well-being and our qualities. Acceptance involves perceiving reality for what it's worth, non-judgmentally understanding the reasons for this reality, and drawing in with it instead of battling against it. Acceptance implies powerful seeking practices instead of stalling out in decisions with respect to what is "correct" or "wrong," "reasonable," or "out of line."

RADICAL ACCEPTANCE

Radical Acceptance is a functioning procedure involving being available to the experience of what is at every minute. "Acceptance without duty is a shallow triumph, and responsibility isn't practical without acceptance." Acceptance is mental and social, including tolerating with both our brain and our activities; tolerating our world altogether—the main extremely viable type of acceptance is called radical acceptance. It is hard to acknowledge what is at the time altogether; be that as it may, just incompletely tolerating our world won't support our torment. Envision that you "acknowledge" your relative. However, when you see her, you unremittingly consider how terrible she is as an individual. What does this kind of acceptance achieve? You may mentally acknowledge her; however, despite everything, you feel tense and pushed when she's near, and you can scarcely remain to address her. If you unapologetically accept your present weight or shape, you are neither scowling when you look in the mirror nor surrendering to failing to address it. Acceptance implies seeing without judgment. This doesn't mean you are not permitted to have an idea like "I can't stand how I look"— it just means you can see it when you have it ("that is an idea"). This naming can enable you to have and see the idea without joining misery or disgrace to it. You don't stifle the idea, and you don't harp on it—you watch it come, and you watch it go. For this situation, you've made a conclusion, yet you didn't pass judgment—you simply saw it—and this dulls its sting and may likewise enable you to take a look at the substance of the making a decision about the idea. As you may envision, this is a training that nobody ever gets flawlessly—we are human—however, once you start doing it, it's consistently there and accessible for you to use as you are capable. Imagine yourself, once more, before the mirror. Acceptance additionally includes moving toward the circumstance with both an exacting and a non-literal stance of ability—maybe truly loosening up your neck and shoulders, smoothing your brow, and unfurling your arms as you look in the mirror. This can assist you with seeing the idea, "I can't stand how I look" without becoming tied up with it. There is an input circle between our physical stance and our cerebrum; once more, so as to push toward acceptance, it is essential to do as such with both personality and body. If your brain accepts something while your body tenses, flagging dismissal, would you say you are drastically tolerating your existence? The accompanying action will give you practice in seeing the connection between your body and your mind with regards to acceptance.

CHAPTER THREE
EXERCISE PROGRAMS AND DIETS WORKING TOGETHER

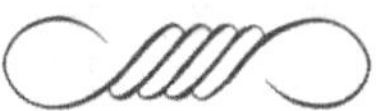

Throughout the years, I have remained friends with a considerable lot of my clients. It would astound you how, every now and again, they slip into the discussion some remark about being fat or humiliated or overweight. I recall one customer who had not physically met with me since she had recovered the weight she'd lost; she would just interface via telephone or by email. Goodness, we both felt like disappointments for various reasons. She felt she'd neglected to keep up her weight reduction, and I felt that I hadn't adequately met her mentoring needs. It was agonizing for the two of us.

This is the reason I composed this book: to decrease the pain in our relationship with food. Much of the time, the main question individuals ask me is, "Which program or diet functions admirably with results showing within a few weeks?" The appropriate response is straightforward. Journaling your experience is something that you can use related to any food or exercise program, and it will improve your goals. Regardless of what program you are following, since it is sound, it will work; please go for it and break the bad habits. Today, there is a variety of phenomenal programs and diets accessible to suit the necessities and desires for nearly everybody. They change contingent upon the individual and the particular needs of the person. Before beginning any food or exercise program, it is basic that you check with your doctor or your local wellbeing authority. If you have any wellbeing concerns, you should counsel with your primary care physician to guarantee which sustenance or exercise program is for you. You can likewise counsel your locale wellbeing authority; inquire as to whether they offer any programs in food direction or advising. A few programs do all the arranging and thinking and cooking for you. That sort of controlled diet is the thing that a few people need. In these programs, feast arranging and sustenance preparing come later in the program as the customers quit utilizing the readied menu and prepare dinners for themselves.

Different programs require a more elevated level of customer inclusion from the earliest starting point, figuring out how to design and prepare suppers. Still, other diet programs use a blend of thoughts and methods with fluctuating degrees of dinner arranging and food preparing. As far as I can tell, regardless of what a program offers, there is only enough accentuation on the upkeep part of the program. While customers accomplish transient satisfaction through weight reduction or legitimate conditioning for their body, an excessive number of individuals think they have every one of the appropriate responses and leave the program with practically zero help. The outcome: their weight immediately rebounds. I know; I have seen it too often. There is an inquisitive incongruity here. Indeed, they do have every one of the appropriate responses. However, memory can be short, and old propensities can crawl back. Procedures and systems for program support can gradually start to bomb as memory blurs. Is it safe to say that we are impeccable? No. Would we be able to get ourselves before things go sideways with our weight? Totally! Breathing devices, as a self-disclosure instrument, encourages us to remember the strategies we have learned and to incorporate them to the point where they supplant old habits.

OBJECTIVE SETTING: WHAT'S IN IT FOR YOU?

All through my counseling profession, when I have moved toward the subject of objectives and defining objectives, customers have over and over made statements like, "I can't envision what arriving at an objective will resemble. I can't see past my stomach, don't worry about it the promising finish to the present course of action." Some objectives are only too far away for individuals to envision. Since you are getting into the swing of things, how about we get into the point. It is fantastic to have objectives—a guide of what we need to accomplish.

Here are a couple of tips for fruitful objective defining:

Make the objectives achievable. Maybe characterize transient objectives for the present—until you can see that famous promising finish to the present course of action. Why? I have seen many customers define an enormous objective for themselves, such as being a sure weight for their wedding.

What's more, when the wedding has gone back and forth, so wants to keep endeavoring to keep up that weight. To maintain a strategic distance from untimely deserting of an objective, ensure that, when you are drawing near to achieving one objective, you set another one for the prompt future. While you're grinding away, set an objective for the removed future also. Record your goals. Update your diary as you arrive at an objective or need to change your objective.

- Goals don't need to be about a specific number or accomplishing a particular weight. They can be close to home objectives.

- Reduce your waistline with the goal that you can tie your shoes on the top to bowing from your midsection as opposed to holding your leg to the side!

- Be comfortable in your present belt and not have it hit your sides.

- Have the jeans that are too short, really get some length to them—bafflingly! (As individuals lose or put on weight, the trouscr legs don't abbreviate or extend. Individuals simply round them out increasingly, taking up more texture, so apparently, the jeans are shorter. When you get in shape, the texture isn't taken up to such an extent, and evidently, the jeans get longer.)

- Adjust your belt one step littler.

- Snore less.

- Get into the next smaller dress size.

CHAPTER FOUR
WHAT'S FOOD DOING FOR YOU?

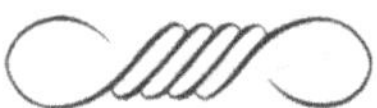

WHY WE EAT

The reasons we ought to eat are for sustenance and for fuel; in any case, we eat for numerous different reasons. We eat as a result of what our way of life lets us know is correct and appropriate behavior, and on account of exercises and thought patterns we learned in youth. We eat to fulfill social desires, without really thinking, because of feelings, for comfort, and to fulfill longings. We eat because we are enticed by the smell, taste, surface, look, and inviting nature of the served food. We eat to satisfy our creative mind, for self-satisfaction or discipline, and from impulse. Our essential purpose behind eating ought to be that we are hungry, having arranged our fuel admission to help with the exercises for the afternoon. This is rarely the situation.

In the last decades, our general public has changed significantly concerning action. Regardless of whether it is physical or mental movement, life in our bustling society here and there implies appropriate sustenance is impossible. We are attempting to pack such a great amount into our days that physical exercise goes as a second thought. The outcome? If our admission of food is more noteworthy and higher in calories and fat substance than would generally be appropriate, and our physical movement is lower or even non-existent, the main path for our waistline to go is out! The changing occasions influence all ages. In numerous parts of the nation, our kids have physical training as a choice in their schools as opposed to a compulsory course. Cooperation in sports appears to drop off in adulthood with the essential game movement a ride in a golf truck or sitting in the stands.

Since we have such a quick-paced way of life today, innovators are attempting to make everything simpler to achieve, so we are even less physical in what we do. At work, leaving our work area becomes restrictive with our connections to PCs; the time of the remote-controlled everything keeps us on the lounge chair for everything from tuning hardware to diminishing the lights to opening the window ornaments. However, for every one of the machines of comfort, we're accomplishing more while we take care of solid life-decisions less. These bustling components change the purpose behind "why you eat" and the decisions you make.

If you proceed on this hamster wheel, you will wear out. So take a DEEP breath and set aside some effort for you! Arranging your day around your exercises, your food prerequisites, and offsetting those components with time to rest is basic. Equalization! This is significant for your association with others also. You have to inhale effectively!

What's more, that takes us back to the genuine explanation of "why we eat"— it is for food, fuel, and rest—all to advance the parity of our real needs with the goal that we can live healthily. When your body appreciates balance, you appreciate life—and the others in your life. This is putting on your own breathing apparatus first! We should investigate a portion of the thoughts you have about offsetting your existence with your food, your eating, your exercises, and your rest times. Generally, when we have balance in our lives, we discover time to accomplish different things that we like doing.

SOCIAL DESIRES—HOW WE EAT

The various lessons from our social roots regularly form our relationship with food. Previously, the desires encompassing food utilization were more characterized than they are today. Individuals from various societies have different standards concerning food utilization. Where you are brought up on the planet, what religion you practice, can affect social thoughts, for example, the right blends of specific foods, the animals and plants that might be utilized for food, the significance of the individuals you share your table with, feasting with suitable refreshments, social graces, who eats first, sharing food, which foods might be eaten with the hands and when utensils are fitting. Social standards and desires assume a tremendous job by the way you characterize your relationship with food.

Numerous concepts and sayings began years ago, at various times and in various circumstances. When we hear these thoughts, we have to ask where they originated from and what was happening at the time. Was there a war? Was there a lack of any food? Did individuals need to shroud food to endure? Were there eight kids, and the best way to get a significant piece was to stack up your plate or you didn't get any food whatsoever? As children, we heard:

- Clean your plate.

- Don't squander food.

- Bread and spread with each meal.

- Pasta and potatoes with each meal.

- There are starving youngsters on the planet, so you need to eat the entirety of your food.

- Always finish with a sweet treat.

- You won't leave the table until you have completed your supper.

How about we address the value that you wind up paying for overeating?

Clearly, your wellbeing is endangered! What does it take to change this conduct? Abruptly, you may end up in a wellbeing emergency that will push you from 'I need to change how I eat' to 'I need to change how I eat!' Imagine a scenario where you were in the emergency clinic and not ready to deal with yourself or your children or your family or your pets. Or then again surprisingly more dreadful, if a wellbeing emergency would end your life? What cost would you say you will pay? You choose. Again, it's about what you realized in adolescence and have brought into adulthood as self-talk. What are you educating yourself regarding food that you learned as a kid, and how might you modify those thoughts?

COMFORT FOOD

Do you recollect what pacified you as a kid around food and eating? I remember how I would sneak treats off of grandmother's table when she was beating the batter before cutting the treats. I can nearly smell the bowl of chicken noodle soup that my mother or grandmother offered me to help with a cold or an irritated stomach. There were times when my father took me for a dessert to keep me at ease while thinking about a soccer match that my group lost. Did you sneak turkey cuttings off the platter at the special seasons as I did when my grandpa was cutting the feathered creature? I remember how I would sneak some pie crust off mother's counter when she wasn't looking as she prepared the mixture to make a pie. The smell of turkey and stuffing makes me remember my home. The smell of crusty fruit-filled treat makes me feel all warm inside, similar to a kid at grandma's—sheltered and warm.

Do you have fond memories that associate food with comfort? These are normal emotions. Food gives us joy and satisfies our hunger. It is essential to understand what your result is concerning food. Maybe you never thought of it that way. Once more, dive profoundly into your self-talk related to your relationship with food. When we speak about comfort food, what we truly mean is the food we eat to make us feel better when we feel pitiful or something has turned out badly in the day. It is food that will comfort us.

That is what our folks, grandparents, and grown-ups in our general public frequently thought when we were troubled: "How can I make you feel good? What about ice cream or chicken noodle soup...or hot cocoa?" Their consideration regarding us frequently came as food. Temporary comfort may originate from eating choice food; however, when we eat comfort foods in excess amounts or more every now and again, then our sound association with food decays and the blame and the negative cycle resumes. Mindful of the undesirable food decisions you've made and the sum you ate can prompt negative self-talk. You become disappointed over your inability to be fruitful with food. That is the point at which you start to deal with yourself, making statements like: "I'll simply begin once again on Monday...or next week...or one month from now." Eating solace food typically just sets aside a short effort to gain power. What amount of harm would you be able to do at this time?

GET-TOGETHERS

In the present fast-paced society, the expression "work hard, play harder" is by all accounts the standard. It is difficult to imagine a get-together without food and refreshments. The food business, from supermarkets to cafés, is intended to advertise food sources for each get-together from religious events to retirement parties, from Superbowls to chapel picnics, from private evening gatherings to Charity banquets. A major social event without food? Unimaginable, you would say, it isn't? Food and eating are customs fitted to get-togethers in our lives.

We hope to be properly fed when we play hard. In numerous societies, enormous and little get-togethers are not only defined by eating but by an excess availability of various food choices. Get-togethers are an opportunity to consider the types of food we are eating. It's an opportunity to consider our limits and our breathing space around the food that accompanies the occasion. It's an opportunity to set ourselves up to be aware of what decisions we can and should make about food.

Get-togethers are a major test for me! I frequently contemplate internally: "Free food...yummy. New plans and top choices I don't ordinarily have! Treats!" I get all energized—for a couple of seconds— then I return to strategies and boundaries that I have built for myself. I'll have just a sample of only one top pick, request the formula, and keep the social parts of the occasion as my core interest. I keep my hands full so that I won't be enticed to snack at the food.

Now and again, I have a mint before I stroll in the entryway, which will demoralize me from examining different foods. Or on the other hand, I eat before I go for any gathering, brush and floss my teeth, so I don't feel like I have to eat. I remind myself that the food does not deserve the struggle and pain to get the weight off or to feel wild. I remind myself how it feels to be in outfits that are my ideal size. I recollect the minute I put them on, and I feel like a million!

Almost immediately, distressing happens directly before the get-together that could factor into your choices. This is the point at which you will require your journal to help you to remember the motivations to remain on track and not let a person or thing influence your weight and your choices.

FOOD HABITS

A dietary pattern is something that we have become acquainted with doing, potentially out of routine or maybe even unwittingly. We routinely eat a few foods without a great deal of thought since it is simply programmed conduct. What is a food habit? It might be continually having potatoes with steak.

Or on the other hand, routinely eating bacon with your eggs or frozen yogurt with your cake. Without really thinking, you may consequently be adding salt to every one of your foods. These habits must be broken in a systemic way, not by forcing it or starving yourself. As they say, easy always does it!

FOOD REWARDS

Once I was in a dress store. I caught two individuals saying to one another that they merited a treat. Then they kept examining the sugary frozen yogurt and baked good treat that they got ready for themselves, portraying the foreseen food in such detail and with such eagerness that I hoped to check whether they were drooling. I was nearly drooling myself simply tuning in to them. Rewards don't need to be a sugary treat; it could be going out for supper and requesting what you wouldn't ordinarily request and afterward overindulging in that food too. We can treat ourselves every so often, however making food a reward is certifiably not a healthy habit. We have to concoct new thoughts regarding prizes and treats for ourselves. One of the genuine outcomes of utilizing food as a reward is that we can pass along with this negative behavior pattern to our youngsters.

SHOULDN'T SOMETHING BE SAID ABOUT YOUR METABOLISM?

In every one of the years that I trained individuals, I have always stumbled into many who didn't eat throughout the day—some of the time, holding up until 8 PM to have their first meal of the day. When individuals hold up until night to eat, they are upsetting their metabolism. They are either not eating enough regularly, or they may be compensating for it in a couple of days at the end of the week, or they are indulging each night because, before dinnertime, they are starving! Think about what befalls good judgment of your actions that occur when you are extremely hungry? It departs for good. You eat a great deal at the same time—and you feel qualified to eat anything you desire!

In this state, you are probably not going to settle on solid decisions. This is the most accurate explanation of why diet programs reliably caution individuals not to go shopping for food when they are hungry. The propensity is to purchase out the store and fill your truck with a ton of junk food and poor decisions since all food looks great! Would you be able to relate to that? So what job does your digestion play in why you eat? Think about your digestion as a fire in your body. If you put some fuel and paper on the ashes, a fire will start. If you continue including fuel and some littler logs, you will keep your fire consuming all through the entire day. During the night, or at whatever point you quit eating for a more extended timeframe, your body goes into a smaller than expected quick, and your digestion and processing will back off until you eat again in the first part of the day. That is the point at which you "break the fast" from the evening of not eating, hence what we call "breakfast."

So the sooner you eat at the beginning of the day, the more extended your digestion will work. The quicker your digestion begins toward the beginning of the day, the more productively you will utilize the food you have eaten to fuel your body. Your morning feast starts your digestion. In any case, it is essential to eat things that won't slow your digestion. A major heavy breakfast may not be shrewd. Rather, consider breakfast foods that you discover simple to process. All things considered, our assimilation needs to restart for the afternoon, so settle on decisions, for example, juice, yogurt, natural product, toast, and bubbled egg—foods that are gentler on the stomach.

If you don't eat your first supper until some other time in the day, that is the point at which your digestion will begin once more. Returning to my fire relationship, if you put on a major gigantic log—a major feast once per day by day's end—it will seethe and simply stay there. When leaving your food utilization until the day's end, two things can occur: you can be hungry to such an extent that you indulge, or you are enticed to devour all your everyday calories at one sitting. If you don't utilize that food vitality immediately, it gets put away as fat. Also, your digestion isn't working at its ideal. If you just eat once per day, your body will go into "fasting" mode, closing down for the evening and the daytime. Food is fuel for your body. You need great fuel, conveyed consistently, for your cerebrum to work appropriately. If you just eat once per day, either your body trusts you are fasting or shuts down, or your body trusts it is in starvation mode, and all food gets put away as fat. Tinkering with standard eating times undermines the manner in which the body should work. Eating 5–6 snacks or small meals a few times each day props up your metabolism.

If you are not acclimated with eating this regularly during the day, go gradually as you change your feast propensities. Ease into eating meals a few times during the day with the goal that you don't feel like you have tried too hard when you do eat. Cut back on your segments; space your dinners and snacks close to 3 hours apart. Much the same as those little bits of wood on the fire, littler measures of food eaten 2–3 hours apart keep your digestion working perfectly—and it starts toward the start of your day with that very significant dinner we call breakfast.

Don't overdo it; even a bit of dry toast in the first part of the day is superior to nothing. Later toward the beginning of the day, when you are more in a hurry, some wheat wafers with nutty spread would be a smart thought.

Here's an example day of what eating 5–6 little dinners and bites may resemble: Breakfast Whole wheat toast with jam.

- Snack: Whole-wheat wafers with some nutty spread.

- Lunch: Grilled chicken in a small plate of mixed greens with a balsamic vinegar dressing and a side of new natural product cuts.

- Snack: Yogurt with cut almonds and raisins.

- Dinner: Roast hamburger with pasta presented with a steamed veggie and an organic product cup.

- Snack: Celery sticks with light cheddar and an apple. (Note that I haven't put sums adjacent to the food things in this model.

Individuals will have distinctive vitality needs relying upon their movement, age, body type, sex, digestion, and wellbeing concerns). Notice I have put a protein—in this model, nutty spread, chicken, yogurt, nuts, hamburger, and cheddar—with pretty much every dinner. The explanation is because we digest sugars—organic products, vegetables, slices of bread, wafers, raisins, pasta, and so on first; then, we digest protein. We digest fats last; in this model, fats are a portion of the nutty spread, a plate of mixed greens dressing, a few sauces, margarine, meat fat, cheddar, and yogurt. By having a sugar with a protein, you get a transient vitality stretch and afterward have enough protein to last a couple of hours until the following dinner or bite. Plan out a day like what I have done above and report it in your journal.

Here's a recommendation: Set up a layout for your day like the one I have given you above and afterward swap out the foods every day. For instance, where I composed Lunch – Grilled chicken on a nursery plate of mixed greens with a balsamic vinegar dressing and a side of new organic product cuts, you can supplant the barbecued chicken with cuts of turkey or ground prepared hamburger for a taco serving of mixed greens or the meat with cheddar. You may supplant a nursery serving of mixed greens with cucumbers and tomatoes. You could substitute a light Italian dressing or a light cream for the balsamic vinegar. You get the image! You have the format for what you are eating; simply change the foods. This is only a proposal of how to begin; sooner or later, you will think of some more plans to have a fair day. (Bits will rely upon you as an individual and will consider the stage you are at in your weight program or wellbeing concerns. You can check with your food control, your eating regimen program, your exercise center, your locale wellbeing authority, your physician, or a neighborhood nutritionist for a progressively point by point rule.)

It is a great idea to have some gentle appetite signs just before you are expected to eat; this discloses to you that your digestion is working. Everybody is unique, yet some regular appetite signs are:

- Stomach protesting

- Cold nose, hands, and feet

- Slight crabbiness

- Slower response to things

- Decreased capacity to focus

- Drink water in the middle of dinners and bites - Water tops you off, yet water is significant for all parts of your body.

Water, water, water!

Much the same as the oxygen (O2) in your body, water (H2O) is fundamental for your organs, blood, skin, electrolytes, balance, and a large portion of all for consuming fat! Inhale, exhale, and relax! Slow down when you eat. It takes about 20 minutes for your stomach to tell your mind that you are full. What amount would you be able to eat in 20 minutes- in 5 minutes? The appropriate response is a ton! How to back off? Put your fork or spoon down when you are chewing. In the wake of gulping, get your utensils again and continue eating. Drink water between significant meal times. Take as much time as necessary chewing, savoring the taste your food, enjoy the different flavors and textures, and appreciate what you are eating—one piece after another.

CHAPTER FIVE
WHAT'S EATING YOU?

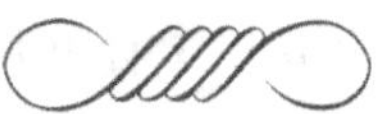

Knowing the various purposes for what you eat and what food is accomplishing for you was the subject of the last chapter. In this chapter, I will explore a portion of the reasons you eat. Recognize that what you eat might be pushed outside your ability to control by an assortment of variables. Beyond giving nutrition and fuel to your body, food is additionally associated with cultural, social, and social thoughts. Your food habits might be not quite the same as what your body and digestion require for ideal wellbeing.

Individuals are dependent upon passionate changes, testing circumstances, individuals, and conditions that make them go to food. For an assortment of reasons, yearnings and habitual practices may lose our control around eating. These elements—uniquely or in a blend—are genuine difficulties that can add to wild eating, which has nothing to do with fulfilling hunger or giving sustenance and vitality to our bodies. This piece of your self-revelation adventure might be especially uncovering, which is the reason I request that you give specific consideration to journaling your bits of knowledge and afterward moving your positive systems and ways to write a journal. Deep emotions encompass a significant number of our states of mind: stress, outrage, weakness, hunger, fatigue, pity, uneasiness, expectation, fervor, sadness, and delight. We, as a whole, encounter incredible emotions that can trigger passionate eating. What I mean by emotional eating is described by an out-of-control eating occasion that is utilized to battle, solace, or veil feelings that challenge our feeling of prosperity.

Put simply, emotional eating is bolstering your emotions, not your stomach. When you eat to fulfill something more than hunger, you are occupied with numbing pain or stress. A part of these behaviors can get neurotic—delivering such dietary issues as anorexia and bulimia—however, that isn't my core interest. Or maybe, how about we investigate a portion of the regular causes that a great many people involved in emotional eating. Feelings produce various responses in individuals; however, stress is, by all accounts, the most well-known factor in a poor diet. Stress can be communicated in an assortment of feelings and result in many harmful practices around food. Emotional eating can turn into your greatest test and even damage your weight reduction endeavors, so you must become mindful of what you are eating, yet additionally, why you are eating.

When you can perceive what is going on with your feelings and relate that to your conduct, you can modify what you are doing and defeat eating to fulfill awkward emotions. We all resort to eating for emotional reasons, yet when this turns into a primary focal point of our lives, which is the point at which the issue starts—we experience torment, battles, disappointment, and at last, weight gain. I had personal difficulties with enthusiastic eating: not minding what I ate when I got furious, irate, or tragic, eating out of weariness or dawdling. I ate when I was focused. Mindfulness and making an arrangement helped me escape the enthusiastic eating trench. I accept these two systems can help you as well, so relax! How about we take a shot at an arrangement!

When I have feelings that could lead me to eat wildly, I actualize the accompanying:

- Plan ahead for shopping for sound dinners.

- Plan to make additional foods early that can be solidified.

- Plan bites that have some assortment.

- Check my self-talk and alter it to be certain.

- Use my interruption systems to keep occupied.

- Eat little suppers and nibble 5–6 times each day.

- Slow down as I eat.

- Drink heaps of water, water, water!

Give myself the permission to have a few treats in minimal amounts and afterward change my day by day food admission: practice control as opposed to end.

EMOTIONAL DISTRACTION TECHNIQUE

Feelings can be strong to such an extent that we truly couldn't care less about our sound objectives any longer. It is essential to have an arrangement set up for when this occurs, so have your journal on you consistently. We don't create these feelings; they simply happen at the most awkward occasions. Any occasion can be ruined with a feeling that pushes you over the edge; outrageous feelings can drive you to settle on undesirable food decisions. What you need is something to remove your psyche from the feelings or worry until you can quiet down and settle on great food choices. Figuring out how to control your responses to profoundly charged emotions—regardless of whether it's satisfaction, pity, or weariness—and joining that control with a balance in your eating motivations will assist you with staying away from enthusiastic eating. During times when feelings brief you to eat or even gorge, ask yourself, "What is my motivation for needing to eat healthily?" This will help keep you spurred. Various programs offer an assortment of methodologies for turning away passionate eating. The system that has been effective for my customers has been an interruption strategy. The emotional distraction method starts with mindfulness. In the first place, list the classes of distractions that could keep you from emotional eating. Also, record exercises that relate to the classification that you think would help with diverting you from indulging as a reaction to enthusiastic pressure. Attempt to think of 4 to 5 great exercises for every classification that you would really take part in. Remember that, if the movement isn't appealing to you, what is the probability that you will expand your passionate eating? Keep it genuine for you!

Examples of classes of distractions:

1. Things that should be rapidly done at any time or place.

2. Your emergency distraction (which thoroughly removes your brain from food).

3. Things I can do while dressed up.

4. Things that are calming and relaxing.

5. Things I can do with others or with others present. A few instances of something that should be possible rapidly any place are:

- • Get the vehicle washed

- • Call a companion

- • Organize your day-clock or equalization the checkbook

- • Make game plans for a forthcoming occasion

- • Book a hair arrangement

- • Document your self-talk in your Journal

- A few instances of an emergency movement done any place would be:

- • Begin an art venture

- • Call your help person(s)

- • Organize a family carport deal

- • Repot your houseplants

- • Plan your youngster's birthday party

- • Go to the rec center

- • Get a nail treatment

- • Attend a game

This distraction process works a good number of times. When you have emotional difficulty, you choose which classification you need right then and there. Select one of the exercises in the classification that fits the condition and do that action. If you need more interruption, then select another action from that class. (Simply figure the amount you will achieve in your life when you are not doing enthusiastic eating!) Distraction methods remove your brain from food and grant you to jump on to greater and better things.

This urges you to settle on better choices and to like having that power. It additionally works you to inhale effectively in your relationship with food since you deliberately consider the circumstance. Knowing about your self-talk concerning your feelings can help you adjust self-talk if it is negative and settle on a savvy decision by maintaining a strategic distance from food or giving yourself authorization for control. You finish with power over your food admission and with an arrangement for the afternoon.

The following stage is to move your interruption classes into your Journal. Leave space to record new interruptions as thoughts arise for you. Take your Journal with you consistently, because we don't design these triggers, and the interruption arrangements you need will be readily available. That way, you remain on track, paying little mind to the time or spot. If you are finding that passionate eating is a major test right now, here is a progressively serious strategy for expanding your mindfulness and utilizing interruption methods. I consider it the envelope strategy and have thought that it was extremely successful.

Allude to the classifications you have distinguished and list everyone on the face of an envelope. Take bits of paper that will fit into the envelopes and record one interruption movement for each bit of paper. Spot that interruption action in the class envelope that compares with the movement. Convey these envelopes with you to assist you with traversing enthusiastic eating occasions; this is likely the most significant time that these interruptions work for you. I have utilized this envelope strategy with an assortment of individual difficulties. It works!

In the long run, you will move from the envelopes to your Journal. What's more, inevitably, you will do a diverting action; consequently, when an enthusiastic eating occasion comes around. You realize that you have the envelopes or your Journal to direct you—composed by you for you—helping you breathe easier about your association with food! Even better, place an additional duplicate in the ice chest or pantries to help keep you on track!

Home alone—that is presumably where we do the most harm to our eating plans and ourselves. When we are without anyone else's input, and in our very own homes, we give ourselves the authorization to eat any way. I know this as a matter of fact; when I have occupied with gorging, it has been in my home away from other observers. I felt truly senseless because I was acting like a child, avoiding everybody. It is miserable when individuals feel constrained to consume food hungrily. However, it occurs and is so harming to our self-esteem and to our prosperity.

What's more, a while later? The blame, shame, misery, and self-avocation that shows up in our self-talk isn't exceptionally beautiful, is it? Maybe, with our quick paced ways of life, we gorge significantly more in the protection of our own vehicles. Inexpensive food adds to the issue, yet it's not exclusively the fault for undermining our best eating goals. For instance, after grabbing some staple goods, we're frequently alone, and in the security of our vehicles, we enjoy eating anything we desire.

BINGE EATING IS THE ISSUE.

Binge-eating can prompt bulimia nervosa, a dietary problem for which there is no single recognizable reason. Gloom, eating less junk food, poor adapting aptitudes, and even hereditary qualities might be involved in gorging. Described by mystery and quick eating to the point of being awkwardly full, gorge eaters eat alone and regularly when they aren't ravenous. Regret and shame make bulimics cleanse their assortments of undesirable food by spewing or by utilizing intestinal medicines. If you are a gorge eater, what are you letting yourself know? "It doesn't make a difference any longer—I am a disappointment when it comes to food." If you state this, then it will work out.

If binging gets ceaseless in your life and you presume or have been informed that you have this dietary issue, you should look for help from a social insurance supplier: a specialist, analyst, or a doctor. There are numerous medications for bulimia nervosa. I encourage you to discover them. If you do have a passionate eating scene—since it will occur as it happens to us all—you can deal with it emotionally if you take some time, analyze the circumstance, and excuse yourself for settling on a poor food decision. It is essential to the point that when you understand that you committed a genuine error, or even basically decided to eat food to assist you with getting over awful or serious emotions, you should be sensible and take a look at your self-talk related with that occasion.

Hear what you are saying to yourself and change your affirmation if it is negative. Recognize to yourself that you settled on the choice to have that food and that you will alter your day by day food admission to be on track with your vitality needs. Say to yourself, "This isn't actually how I had arranged my day, yet I will change things for whenever and gain from this experience." Every opportunity that a test comes up, record it in your diary. Also, proceed onward. One scene is no major ordeal; it's a hindrance, much the same as we experience all through life! This move in frame of mind is significant on the grounds that, by being earnest and constructive, you've kept up your own capacity. Stunning, such control! You've accomplished another approach to breathe easier about your association with food!

A portion of the stress-related issues with emotional eating is our own evaluation of our appearance, our weight, and the advancement we have made in arriving at our weight objectives. The emotions encompassing these issues can prompt negative discernments about ourselves. Think of how you feel/felt at your heaviest weight. Keep in mind:

- What did your attire feel like?

- What is it like to stroll up five flights of stairs? Well, will you make it?

- Even without physical action, how was your breathing very still?

- Did you wheeze?

- What would you say it felt like to tie your shoes?

- Could you contact your toes?

- Could you see your feet?

- How did people look at you? Did anybody make remarks?

- Has your weight influenced your activity? Life? Family? Exercises with your family? Closeness?

- How much do you spend on food and liquor every day?

- How much weight have you gained over time? How does it feel to be of this size? Presently feel these feelings! Sit in them and accept the emotions. Pen them down and recollect.

Have you been there? Then you would understand better what it feels like! You can envision what arriving at your objective will mean. How is it going to be to slip into a smaller size of pants—feel absolutely great, thin and trim? Envision your skin is tight and sound. Envision your legs being more fit and conditioned than they have ever been! Picture yourself in a thinning swimsuit at your objective weight with a brilliant sparkle all over your body. Picture your body on the seashore and being agreeable in your skin. You can contact your toes, you can fold your knees up to your chest, and you feel incredible. You have the energy to save! You can complete five flights of stairs easily and still need to accomplish more! You don't wheeze any longer. You rest so refreshed and loaded with the vitality you ricochet up with a spring and a grin for the afternoon. You see, your objective is getting too enormous for you since you are conditioning your body and feel so fit. You are arranging your day's food, effortlessly, and fun. You have such extraordinary confidence and positive self-talk that you realize you can do anything you put your psyche to. You are resolved, and you have the entirety of your capacity! You are extraordinary! Furthermore, you have a sound body at your objective weight!

CHAPTER SIX
EMOTIONAL EATING AND CHALLENGING CIRCUMSTANCES

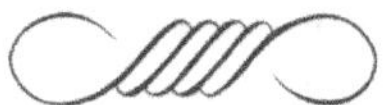

In life, we come across circumstances and individuals that can confuse us! Have you experienced a circumstance or a domain where you didn't feel good, however, needed to remain where you were? For instance, put yourself into this scene: a great friend welcomes you to a gathering. You show up and are making some great memories when your ex strolls in the entryway with their new date. Wow! The environment abruptly gets charged. You feel awkward and clumsy.

This circumstance with these specific individuals could send even the most secure individual into a portion of food or liquor free-for-all. Uplifted feelings and stress will make us "bargain" with the circumstance as well as can be expected, regularly adapting or soothing ourselves with food or potentially drink. The "fix" for our trouble may appear to be practically programmed; we need frantically to plan something to make us feel much improved. Be that as it may, over the long, all that we accomplish is that we've subverted our calorie admission for the afternoon. Contingent upon the degree of feelings and agony, the damage can keep going for quite a while. While the facts confirm that we have feelings related to cumbersome circumstances, we ought not to enable them to devastate our objectives and our arrangement for solid living.

Passionate responses are typical, and they alert us to our alternatives for activity. You can encounter the enthusiastic reaction, recognize that you have the feeling, and afterward ensure you manage it in a solid way. You can likewise recognize that in time, the misery that caused your enthusiastic reaction will scatter, and you will start to mend.

Similarly, as we wind up in moving circumstances with our relationship to food, there are additionally testing individuals that can push us over the edge. Maybe you know individuals who get resentful when you don't eat the entirety of a dinner they have arranged for you. Their reaction is to 'push' food on you, and your reaction might be to indulge. Another difficult individual is somebody who punches your catches or offends or focuses on you to the degree that you are disturbed to the point that you choose to adapt by eating or drinking. Food 'Pushers' can be steady, and you can create systems to manage them. You need to let them know courteously, "Forget about it," and not joke about this. If vital, you can include that you have been told to watch what you are eating for wellbeing reasons. Call your hosts ahead of time. Be open about saying that you have a lunch plan for the afternoon, and you know the dinner that they are offering doesn't accommodate your arrangement. You could offer to bring your own food, acknowledge their substitutions, or plan to land after supper. Plan your time there and have an out. Stand firm; you won't be compelled to eat what isn't in your arrangement.

Counsel your procedures in your journal before you go, have a positive psychological arrangement, and be solid. Keep in mind, by putting your own breathing apparatus first, you are better ready to think about yourself and afterward care for other people. The equivalent goes for the individuals throughout your life who continue pushing your catches. Attempt to constrain your time with them. If those individuals are jokesters, grin and giggle with them. Do whatever it takes not to pay attention to them as well. If they are hostile, considerately let them know along these lines, and afterward make an agile exit. Peruse your diary early and have an arrangement. Inquire as to whether you need to invest energy with these individuals. Be solid and don't give anybody a chance to destroy your day or your wellbeing! Try not to give anybody a chance to influence how you eat. Relax!

Once in a while, an assortment of components can meet up capriciously and upset our eating plan. We experience certain individuals in an unforeseen circumstance, and, all of a sudden, we're focused, and an enthusiastic eating or drinking scene is all of a sudden in our sights. You are presumably gesturing because you have thought of the individual, spot, feeling, and food that may consolidate to cause you trouble! Monitoring these difficulties and how they may emerge is extremely significant. For instance, would you be able to envision a circumstance that is typically fine, yet with the expansion of a difficult associate or the beginning of a dismal day, your reaction to food could turn into a debacle? Try not to leave it alone. Envision these mixes of variables; attempt to maintain a strategic distance from those circumstances, individuals, and negative self-talk until you have an arrangement!

LONGINGS AND IMPULSES

Having a longing and being eager to eat are altogether different things. A longing is that annoying feeling of needing a specific food or a specific taste in your mouth. Some of the time, our creative mind will stay at work past 40 hours to concentrate on that food, and afterward, we can wind up wanting that food throughout the day! Longings for food can develop whenever. Yearnings are not constantly negative—they can flag our body's lack of specific minerals, nutrients, or proteins.

They might be identified with our nourishing needs, or they may caution us to certain hormonal irregular characteristics, adrenal exhaustion, or even insulin obstruction.

All food yearnings, be that as it may, can turn into a negative in our general wellbeing when we react improperly to them. The outcome is that we harm our digestion, increment weight gain, and imperil our wellbeing. You ought to counsel a certified nutritionist or potentially your primary care physician if you have worries about longings and the impact they have on your digestion. What I need to talk about here are a few systems for adapting to and wiping out regular yearnings. There are two significant thoughts regarding desires.

In the first place, they don't have anything to do with self-control. Also, we have to focus on what foods we desire and how we react to them. Here are a few techniques to assist you with perceiving and managing food desires: Foods that have a solid flavor may make you want another food. For instance, tomato sauce, cream sauce, or zesty foods containing garlic may make you long for a portion of sweet food. This is because your sense of taste and tongue are loaded with taste receptors; the solid enhanced food may have a waiting taste, and you have to purify your sense of taste to get over it. Eating grapes, apples, watermelon, and cucumber can do this. You will be very shocked by the outcomes. Other non-food choices are to attempt a tongue scrubber to dispose of the taste, or brush your teeth or bite some gum. Some different longings are about texture. You may long for fresh or crunchy food; you may ache for delicate or smooth food sources.

If the surface of food is more important to you than the carbohydrate level, then you can choose cooking strategies that will give the ideal surface and still be a solid other option. For instance, if you want the smash of tortilla chips, which are high in starches, salt and fat, pick heated pita bread. Cut the round bread into reduced triangles and heat or flame broil for two or three minutes on a cookie sheet. This dries out the pita and makes it fresh—and it turns into a fantastic substitute. You could add a few flavors to modify the flavor, however, watch salty flavors, for example, garlic salt, onion salt, or flavoring salt. If you long for rich surfaces, give a portion of the new yogurts a shot. Peruse the marks for the sugar content; watch the fake sugars as well. A few yogurts have less fat. Plain yogurt can be utilized in cooking and in blend with crisp products of the soil. As the establishment for natural product smoothies, plain yogurt is unsurpassable.

Blending foods grown from the ground improves the yogurt normally as a result of the fructose or common sugars found in an organic product. Take a stab at solidifying natural products, for example, pineapple pieces, grapes, mandarins, and blueberries. Blended with yogurt, they are an awesome substitute for frozen yogurt. Eaten by themselves, these solidified natural products likewise will help scrub the sense of taste. A few people discover they have a craving for salt. If your eating regimen is excessively high in sodium or salt, it can influence your pulse, your cardiovascular condition (heart), just as influence your body's water maintenance and flow. If you, as of now, have difficulties in these territories, you ought to have direction from your doctor and a nutritionist. If it has been over a year since you had an audit of what foods and amounts of sodium are in your eating routine, you need a survey! Indeed you do! It is for your life! It is astute to know about foods high in sodium, regardless of whether you are solid.

Handled foods can be higher in sodium due to how these foods are made to give them a more extended time span of usability. Models are handled meats, canned veggies, canned soups, sauces, bundle seasonings, cheeses, prepackaged dinners, pickles, restored hams, canned fish, bacon, cold cuts, chips, wafers, and considerably more. Peruse the names and search for sodium in the fixings. There are some low sodium items available; make certain likewise to check those names. A few people long for counterfeit sugars. A portion of these are produced using modified amino acids—an adjusted amino corrosive is a protein building obstruct whose sub-atomic structure has been changed. The truth of the matter is, we have given sugar negative criticism! Sugar is OK with some restraint—when we don't revel in it!

If this sounds unnerving, it is. I am adversely affected by any counterfeit sugars, and, as a food instructor, I am frightful about what fake sugars are doing to the assortments of individuals who revel in them. Any fixing with 'ose' or 'ol' toward the finish of the word has a few characteristics of sugar. Peruse your fixings marks. Correspondingly, "palatable oil" items are healthfully bankrupt. I make some hard memories with those also. When we pick counterfeit anything, accept it as an image that we are altering our sustenance for the purpose of accomplishing a specific taste. Because artificial is regarded as safe, you truly need to consider this one.

Mindfulness is the way to managing desires and finding the starting points of them. We have to inquire as to whether we ache for specific foods, certain surfaces, or particular preferences. Controlling perilous desires might be as straightforward as utilizing distinctive planning or cooking systems, substituting various foods, or eating what we pine for with some restraint. If longings become overpowering, then you ought to consistently counsel a wellbeing professional.

TANGIBLE TRAPS: SMELL, TASTE, SURFACE, LOOK, RECOMMENDATION.

Before we even eat food, we are dependent upon an assortment of upgrades that can make us need food. We can smell food and see it and be enticed by it. We can envision the surface of specific foods—their crunchiness or their smoothness pulls in us. Only the memory of the flavor of food from the last time we ate, it tends to be a solid boost. Indeed, even another person discussing food can send us into emotions of want. I will always remember how, in the wake of directing around 16 individuals one day, I returned home needing shrimp and strawberries. Two of my customers had discussed those foods that day. It was an exceptionally odd proposal to hunger for them together, yet that was all it took for me to need shrimp and strawberries. I lived behind a pastry kitchen, and each morning, with the fragrance originating from that spot, I ached for doughnuts! I was nearly drooling as I got into my vehicle.

As a rule, when I drove away, the temptations passed; however, I will consistently recall the intensity of those fragrances. The smell of grilled meat does likewise for me. I always cherished how those things looked so heavenly, yet when I ate them, it wasn't on a par with I had envisioned. So I quit getting them. Presently, I can basically see them, recall my failure by the way they taste, and I don't have to eat them. The surface of certain foods—crunchy, smooth, or grainy—is sufficient to bait us into eating them. I used to appreciate a specific mousse yogurt because of its bubbly surface. The surface was so imperative to me that, if the yogurt mousse was knocked or dropped, so the air bubbles left it, it simply wasn't the equivalent, and I wasn't as keen on eating it. I feel a comparative dissatisfaction when I envision corn chips being delicate or stale. A few people like the texture more than they like the flavor of crunchy food. I love the smash of bread in a plate, garnished with mixed greens, however, put them in the ice chest, and they become unappealing—simply spongy bits of bread. Give your senses a chance to direct you to thoughts regarding food; however, know what it is— just a thought, not a proposal to hurriedly eat. Let the smell simply be that, a smell. Give the sight a chance to be only a decent view. Fulfill your craving for something sweet with new natural products. Solidified pineapple pieces work for me unfailingly. When you need food with crunch, attempt veggie sticks or make your very own prepared pita chips. Investigate different seasonings other than salt to enhance your foods. Most importantly, assess your desires inside the setting of your day's food plan. If you should yield to a hankering, settle on it a sound decision! Searching for a total tactile food experience? Have an orange. You cut into the strip with a blade and the juice showers softly on your lips, and you lick your lips and taste the sweet orange splash. Strip away all the skin and partition the natural product into the areas. Nibble into a piece and experience the crisp squeezed orange as it sprinkles your taste buds. It is so cold and sweet on your tongue.

Each piece is succulent to the point that it trickles down on your hand and onto your plate. Decent, isn't it! The demonstration of fulfilling your very own feeling of joy and surrendering to your food wants can compromise your day by day food plan. Do you live hazardously by eating what you see as taboo foods? You may laugh at this now, however, dive into the thought! As grown-ups, would we say we are carrying on what our folks or the grown-ups in our lives let us know was prohibited or incautious to devour?

Is it safe to say that we are silly? Or on the other hand, will I say incorrupt? What does it mean for us to eat or even revel in these foods? For instance, I cherished hot new pastry shop buns as a kid, yet was told, "No, you can't eat the entire sack!" Then as a grown-up, I enjoyed devouring an entire pack of those buns. Most adults wouldn't think about this a judicious or shrewd decision, yet I've done it! What's more, I realize that a significant number of my customers have done it or something comparative. Is it accurate to say that we are doing this because of resentment? Or on the other hand, since we are grown-ups, we can settle on these decisions if we decided to? Do you have confidence in self-satisfaction concerning food? Here's a critical inquiry that will offer you the response: "Okay, do this conduct freely before others?" What do you do? If you have a self-delight slip by? Here's a story to show what I did. At some point, I requested four cuts of a lemon poppy seed portion to bring home. In the pastry kitchen, I asked for a lot of napkins, demonstrating that the four cuts would be shared by a gathering of individuals.

The fact of the matter was that I was too humiliated even to consider admitting that I may eat two or three of these cuts in a single sitting—in private, obviously. Also, I did only that. The cuts were heavenly; I tasted each chomp! I understood I enjoyed three cuts and concluded that I would skip lunch to remain on track then have a light nibble before supper, and afterward have a light dinner. Do I suggest this as a decent habit? By no means! In any case, if a self-delight slip happens, simply fuse it into your day's food plan. Next time plan better: just have one piece and afterward quickly solidify the rest. Alter your lunch or the remainder of the day for food utilization—and proceed onward!

If I weren't happy enough with my choices to do this, I would not have gone to the café that sells the portion. I would not wait over the feature of treats; I would concentrate on my associates and our discussion. If my mates were a piece of my care group, I would say to them, "My plan is that by no means am I to leave with a few cuts of lemon poppy seed portion."

SELF-ABUSE AND FOOD

What do you consider when you eat? This is a different inquiry, aimed at the individuals who consider hurting themselves with food or abandoning food for long hours or days. This subject of self-misuse may be the place your self-talk should be more profound, and you don't know what is happening inside. Here are a few questions that might pop up if you are abusing your food intake:

- Are you indulging in being taken note of?

- Are you under-eating with the goal that somebody will take note?

- Are you attempting to pay back somebody?

- Do you sense that you don't have the right to be sound?

- Have you overeaten or gorged on foods so much that you have made yourself debilitated?

- Have you utilized food to make yourself wiped out deliberately?

- Are you binging because you feel more secure if you are not seen—particularly seen sexually?

I discovered that I was accomplishing something intuitively to hurt somebody in my past with the decisions I made for myself. In established truth, I was harming myself and destroying my life as a result of it. That was a major eye-opener! When I made sense of that one, I was stunned for a considerable length of time, then weeks, and at last for almost a year. After I was out of shock, I knew what I was doing, yet I continued abusing myself without really thinking. It was increasingly agonizing and disappointing to know about this harmful habit.

I looked for advice from an expert, chipped away at it like a vocation, and now I understand my inspirations and my decisions with the goal that I never again hurt myself. All is fine currently, yet would you be able to imagine what would have happened had I not made sense of it? It was because I was bold enough to be happy to confront my negative ideas behind abusing my body! So take courage; you can do this! If you believe you need some professional help with this region, you are settling on an insightful choice. I settled on that decision, and it was one of the most significant things I accomplished for myself. You can do it!

COMPULSIVE EATING

Compulsive eating is indulging in food and doing it without control, without having the option to stop. Compulsive eaters are not really mindful of what they are doing. This is more than simply eating a whole sack of hot new pastry shop buns in a periodic slip up. This sort of eating occurs all the time. If you feel that you are eating compulsively, you have in any event ventured out—advancing toward staying alert! That is incredible. The subsequent stage is making sense of why you take part in this conduct, what makes you do it, and afterward to assemble some action steps in a plan to stop your habitual eating. Sounds simple?

It tends to be if you are happy to go up against the conduct and find a way to dispose of it. If you accept that you have an issue with urgent eating, I suggest rounding out a food journal in a different note pad to understand what you are consuming. If you don't record everything, you are deceiving yourself! You have to deal with yourself first so you can be seen to others as a fit and capable person.

There are some critical questions to pose about compulsive eating, and they may require some intense reflection. Here are some primer inquiries to consider before you write:

- What do you feel when you eat compulsively?

- What is at the base of the why you eat along these lines? (To numb anything that is going on inside?)

- What feelings do you experience when you are eating habitually?

Look at your self-talk—there are heaps of signs there. You may feel humiliated to concede what you eat. However, you can see it outwardly of your body, right? You are eager to understand this, so you should ask yourself, "Why?" Look somewhere inside for what you are educating yourself regarding your habitual eating conduct. Take as much time as necessary and tune in to what you state to yourself.

MODERATION WITH YOUR CHEAT MEALS

Our aim for eating ought to be eating out of a requirement for energy, vitality, and nutrition. Who thinks about that any longer? Very few. There are sure non-food things that we consume that can fundamentally influence how we eat and what we eat. A few, when done without control, present dangers for the vast majority, including the danger of habit.

Specifically, I'm alluding to the use of liquor, medications, and smoking. Liquor is high in calories, it can numb our feelings and our choices, and it can make us not think about what we eat and why we eat. With regards to settling on a decision about hard versus delicate alcohol or wine versus hey balls, you just need to recollect every mixed drink that is high in calories.

There is an explanation that most diet experts allude to mixed beverages as "empty calories." They give little in the method for sustenance; however, it is nearly as high in calories as fat. Liquor is utilized by our bodies more quickly than fat or protein and is stored rapidly as fat — one drink averages more than 100 calories. In a night out, without control, you effectively could drink your day's energy needs in liquor! If you are overdoing the alcohol in your diet routine, you have to ask yourself why.

If you feel that you may be found napping at a get-together where you know alcohol will be served and don't have a plan before that time, then just don't go. That is genuinely outrageous, so here are a few procedures for keeping away from mixed beverages that I have prescribed to my customers: At parties or in the bar, have a low-calorie drink in your grasp consistently. Individuals will be more averse to offer you a beverage. If you have one in your hand or before you, tip the server or barkeep early and instruct them to give you pop or juice if you request an alcoholic drink. Plan ahead.

- Combine juice with the diet for the spritzer impact.

- Opt for juice or soft drink water rather than a drink.

- Have water with a lemon or lime.

- Have diet pop—however, with some restraint.

- Have a non-hard brew.

- Mix wine with a soft drink for a spritzer.

- Tell others you are on some medicine that you can't consolidate with liquor

MEDICATIONS

Regardless of whether it's a doctor prescribed tranquilizer or a sedative, drugs do practically what alcohol does from an enthusiastic level, however not from a caloric level. Medications can numb our feelings and our choices, and they can make us not mind what we eat or don't eat. Every physician endorsed sedative has adverse reactions. Check with your pharmacist as well as your doctor about the reactions of any medication you take. Street drugs are intended to have a major effect on our minds and our emotions. Time and again, individuals use medications to numb emotions or stop mental agony. Essentially, there is nothing of the sort as a "recreational drugs"— they're all dangerous and possibly fatal. You should know that both prescription and street drugs can be abused. As I educated you about the extreme use concerning alcohol, it would be ideal if you look for proficient assistance quickly if you are abusing or dependent on drugs.

SMOKING

Tobacco is one of the most addictive substances we can place in our bodies, and smoking is one of the most addictive practices all over the whole world. While I have compassion toward the individuals who have reliably attempted to stop smoking, my recommendation is to attempt over and over until you are fruitful. Nicotine is exceptionally addictive, and like different synthetic substances found in cigarettes, for example, cyanide, it is a toxic substance that, in large dosages, can kill. We, as a whole, know the dangers that smoking presents for our general wellbeing—lung malady, emphysema, organ harm, osteoporosis, and coronary illness—however, smoking likewise alters your metabolism. The sooner you quit smoking, the better. There are various projects and care groups that can help if you would like to stop. Staying smoke-free brings several advantages: more vitality, healthy metabolism, better appearance, and a better relationship with food.

MENTAL TRAPS

There are mental snares that we can fall into that influence our association with food. One of the most widely recognized is our mental appraisal of our own bodies. I think we are, for the most part, incredulous of our bodies sooner or later in our lives. When that occurs, our self-perception is most likely lopsided. The media, Hollywood, and the style, diet, and cosmetic industries have extraordinarily impacted our thoughts regarding the ideal body types. They have set an incomprehensibly elevated requirement of what comprises the "perfect" that hardly any of us can accomplish. Closer to home, loved ones can impact our self-perceptions through negative or positive remarks. The genuine inquiries are: are we are ceaselessly contrasting ourselves with that perfect, and are these practical objectives?

Stop comparing yourself with a body type that isn't yours. The human populace has various kinds of shapes and sizes—one isn't perfect over another. We are essentially unique due to race, hereditary qualities, condition, and culture. We, as a whole, have diverse body shapes, and we, as a whole, come in various sizes. The proportion somewhere in the range of stature and weight, bone structure, and bulk is diverse for each human. Go up to a mirror with a friend, stand facing the mirror, stand sideways into the mirror, and see these distinctions. Without being basic, value the distinctions. A positive or solid self-perception is a recognition that leaves you alright with your size and shape. A positive self-perception is crucial to your wellbeing and a sound mental frame of mind. A negative self-perception is likely a mutilated discernment dependent on poor correlations with others that leaves you loaded with disgrace and tension. This can prompt low self-esteem, depression, and eating disorders. Get yourself reintroduced to your body, and, if you don't as of now, acknowledge and love it! Truly. It's the single body you have—approach it with respect! It will treat you pleasantly right back!

CHAPTER SEVEN
STRATEGIES FOR ORGANIZING YOUR FOOD AT HOME

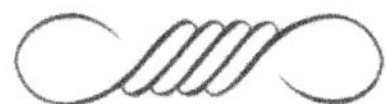

You can control your home food condition by devising a couple of straightforward systems—and now and then, this task involves effective planning and organization. When you are feeling incredible and inspired, here are a few techniques that may help food organization in your home:

- Only purchase the foods in small portions as you require.

- If you are buying more foods than you can use within a brief time, freeze it, share with other individuals, offer it to a food bank, part with it, or even toss it out. You may think it a loss to dispose of food, yet is it a big deal if massive food purchases are exchanged for excess weight gain on you? What is the cost, and will it be worth it? Is it safe to say that you are exchanging your excess food for your wellbeing, your relationship with yourself, your association with your loved ones, or your job?

- Place things that entice you, and you accept that you have to have close by in a zone hard to get to.

- When you are enticed by treats and bites, choose to permit yourself a humble serving and set the rest away. For instance, if potato chips or confections are an exceptional treat for you, partition some into a little bowl and, before you expend the treat, set the rest away in an inaccessible, difficult to reach shelf.

Distinguish most loved foods that push you into difficulty. It is important that you know about specific foods that you hunger for, gorge on, or eat wildly. Normally, individuals have issues or extraordinary difficulties with foods that fit into four classes:

- • Sweet

- • Salty

- • Fatty or Greasy

- • Crunchy

Put foods that are a test to you into one of these classifications. Maybe there is a typical gathering that overwhelms your preferences. You realize what foods are powerful and can jeopardize your eating methodologies. In time, you may change starting with one trying food class then onto the next. The progressions might be because of conditions, evolving hormones, or new anxieties brought about by individuals or circumstances. For me, a most loved food challenge could be as basic as setting off to the sales register at the nearby corner store and seeing the brownies in the pastry shop case by the clerk. The portion size of those brownies is crazy—estimating 4 x 5 inches! What's more, would I finish the entire set in one sitting? Truly—in around 15 seconds! Is there some other way? There totally is another approach to manage this issue, yet not at the time I am slobbering over the brownie remaining in line to pay for my gas. Around then, control isn't at the forefront of my thoughts or in my jargon.

Would you be able to relate? Supplant my preferred food— brownie—with one of your difficulties? Here are the means by which I may take a look at the brownie in an alternate way. Here are my three choices:

1. I genuinely ask myself and answer this question: "Is today a terrible day that I have to eat the entire 5" x 4" brownie? The appropriate response: YES! I was having a terrible day, and I need to eat the entire brownie in the vehicle—even before I leave the parking area. The exciting ride may have recently started. Will self-talk win? Perhaps, perhaps not!

2. If it is an awful day, being straightforward with myself, I will keep away from that difficult food by paying at the siphon where I can't see those beast brownies. Potentially, I can actualize some other technique that I have talked about in the section about enthusiastic eating, for example, making an interruption for this food propensity or desiring.

3. I will be in charge, buy the brownie, put it in a sack, request that the agent tape the pack shut. What's more, when I return home, I am going to cut it into a lot of 1 x 1-inch pieces and stop everything except one. Having given myself consent, I will eat that one brownie parcel without blame.

Can you see the distinction? In picking choice 1, I can hear myself say, "I am so furious at myself that I wolfed it down. I feel so remorseful! What's more, since I have blown this day, I should begin once again on Monday. I didn't taste it, what a waste! I am such a disappointment. I could very well too have an immense supper and dessert, and the remainder of the week is shot! I will eat a lot by the end of the week. I can't remain on track any longer."

Then I would be set to increase another 6 pounds in the following 4–5 days. Negative self-talk around testing foods has outcomes that are difficult to escape—and can be so foolish! In picking alternative 2 or 3,

I have recently finished a potential restraint debacle and kept to my arrangement for progress. I have decided to focus on my methodologies with the goal that I may appreciate the incidental treat and appreciate it by continuing everything with some restraint! I will appreciate each nibble of that brownie parcel, instead of wolfing down the first enormous piece, which would leave me sickened with myself.

Did I get away from the snare of negative self-talk and wrecking consequences? Indeed, by being eager to survey the circumstance with attention to my critical choices to abstain from falling into difficulty, and by picking positive self-talk. Is this as simple as it sounds? Most likely, not! What's more, I am certain that you and I will get loads of practice with similar difficulties! We presently realize that we must be careful around specific foods in specific circumstances. Awareness is simply the key to controlling and making sound meal choices. It's imperative to know about what your preferred foods are, because those food sources make you defenseless against binging or eating without control. Keeping in touch with them will carry you to another degree of self-disclosure. If you realize what foods are hazardous for you, you would then be able to pick procedures to assist you with managing them!

SHOPPING FOR FOOD: AN PLANNED ADVENTURE

When you are increasingly mindful, it isn't as simple to settle on thoughtless food choices. Alone in the supermarket walkways, you are your very own emotionally supportive network, and you should depend on yourself to settle on the right decisions. Some of the time, be that as it may, your negative self-talk—which is not your strong framework—kicks in. Where do you turn? Mindfulness is the way to shop for food. Monitoring your decisions offers you a chance to be responsible for your choices, to be eager to acknowledge duty regarding your choices.

Mindfulness gives you the capacity to settle on decisions without blame or lament but with trust in your feelings and simplicity in basic leadership. The outcome is that you have a superior association with yourself and with the food you buy since you have an arrangement.

Here are some essential tips to use on your next shopping for food adventure:

- A list of every one of your suppers and snacks for a bustling week. (Haul out plans ahead of time.)

- A look into your organizers to perceive what fixings you have close by and what you should buy.

- A basic food item list to guarantee you buy all that you need.

- A date to go shopping for food.

- A plan for water consumption. Carry a water bottle with you all over the place and top off it throughout the day!

Here are a few procedures to help your week by week food arranging: Plan your suppers early and make singular cooler dinners that are pre-partitioned, so you will realize what and the amount you are eating. For example, when you warm a meat and rice dish, simply plan to add new veggies or plates of mixed greens to finish your supper. If you are hurried, this is an incredible method to follow and keep away from inexpensive food.

- Plan your dinners as indicated by where you will be that day. Is there a microwave open? If not, make a point to get ready for progress. Have a feast that is chilled in your lunch pack; however, it is anything but difficult to eat. Have snacks that work with your timetable, including some that are anything but difficult to eat in a hurry.

- Make foods ahead of time, for example, broiled chicken that can be added to hot dishes, or slice up cold to place in plates of mixed greens, or slashed up and made into a chicken serving of mixed greens with a light dressing for a sandwich.

- Using extra-lean ground hamburger, make a dish of lasagna with light cheeses, crisp vegetables, and low-sodium seasonings. If you have scraps, cut the cooled lasagna into pre-parceled pieces for snacks and meals and rapidly freeze them.

- Make spaghetti sauce without any preparation, so you know precisely what you put into the sauce. Pre-partition cooked spaghetti and sauce into holders to use during the week. Freeze what you don't anticipate utilizing in the main couple of days.

- Precook some fish and rice dishes.

- Cut up vegetables for tidbits and put them into proportioned packs to rapidly get when you are in a hurry. Buy a protected lunch sack and load it up with the entirety of your day's food necessities, and you are composed for the afternoon!

- Perhaps later in the week, you can plan to get a serving of mixed greens in a hurry if you foresee that you'll be low on veggies. That is fine, particularly if you have the remainder of your suppers all arranged and prepared. Or on the other hand, dash by the supermarket after you have eaten and get some new organic products or veggies for the remainder of the week.

Arranging when and how to eat is as essential as arranging what to eat. When you eat, ensure you set aside the effort to sit down and taste your food. Our body takes 20 minutes to tell the cerebrum that we are full. If you eat in a short time and haven't yet gotten the sign that you've had adequate food, simply think what harm you would be able to do in the staying 15 minutes that you keep on eating! When you chew, put down your utensils until you have swallowed. Or then again, when you are eating finger food, assume a bite then position the thing on your plate until you are finished swallowing. Slow down. Think positive contemplations as you eat. You are nothing more than trouble for anybody if you arc vcxcd or furious with yourself. Think about your kids and the dietary patterns you are instructing them. Think about the future and how it could be more beneficial if you change a few things today! Relax!

CHAPTER EIGHT
STRATEGIES FOR PLANNING HOME MEALS.

Earlier in the book, I talked about emotional eating and the disorders associated with emotional eating. Go through those points, and you'll notice that it is so simple to have a kitchen loaded up with intentional and healthy decisions to assist you with keeping on track with your healthy diet program. As a part of my expert practice, I visited numerous homes. Because of what I have seen and what a large number of my customers have let me know, I accept that a great many people who have attacked their eating systems need to address revamping their kitchen—and I'm not looking at placing in new machines or counters. I mean, they have to accommodate what food they keep in their homes with how they store it and how they control it.

EFFECTIVE WAYS FOR PLANNING YOUR HOME MEALS

You can control your home food condition by devising a couple of basic procedures—and here and there, this undertaking involves association and arranging. When you are feeling extraordinary and inspired, here are a few procedures that may help food redesigns in your home:

- Only purchase the food in small portions as you need.

- If you purchase more food than you can use within a brief time, solidify it, share with other individuals, offer it to a food bank, part with it, or even toss it out. You may think about what a loss to dispose of food. However, is it a big deal if enormous food purchase is exchanged for excess weight in your body? At what expense? Is it accurate to say that you are exchanging your food abundances for your wellbeing, your association with yourself, your association with your loved ones, or with your activity?

- Place things that entice you, and you accept that you have to have close by in a territory hard to get to. For instance: If you have an ice chest, put the thing far away or put the thing high in a cabinet where it is hard to reach —Place enticing food in a storage room you don't utilize and see constantly.

- When treats and tidbits entice you, choose to permit yourself a humble serving and set the rest away. For instance, if potato chips or confections are a treat for you, partition some into a little bowl and, before you devour the treat, set it away in an inaccessible place. Have a list dependent on your arrangement for the whole week! Record it.

- Shop after you have eaten. When you are hungry, everything looks great, and you will perpetually fill your shopping basket with hasty purchases.

- Buy however much foods as could reasonably be expected to eat. The greater part of your fresh things is along the edge of the store, for example, milk and dairy, leafy foods, grains, and meats. A portion of the things in the passageways are hazardous because they contain handled food, snacks, high-fat, and fatty treats.

- Watch out for displays of specials or new foods that are, for the most part, bargains. These presentations are in your face deliberately, and organizations pay truckloads of money to be in your face!

- When it goes to those powerful specials in tempting displays or in food coupons—ask yourself, "Is it a deal if I don't have it on my list and it's not part of my program?"

- Know the areas where you are easily attracted to food. Write in your Journal and survey the segment on "Most loved foods that push me into excess weight gain," and audit your systems for keeping away from those difficult foods.

- Pick who you go to the supermarket to shop with. A few people who go with you can undermine your best expectations: kids who need sugary treats, family members who have various thoughts regarding what you ought to and shouldn't eat, and good-natured companions who may have an effect on your shopping.

- Read names if you are picking bundled or handled foods. (See what you should search for in the following segment on perusing food names.) As a savvy, key customer, state to yourself, "I will...":

- Plan ahead for your weekly food needs and make a composed basic food item list.

- Shop after you have eaten.

- Shop the dividers to buy new foods however much as could be expected.

- Read the names when you have to buy bundled or prepared foods.

- Stick to your list.

- • Leave the kids at home, if possible, so there is less impulse to purchase outside of your list.

- Abstain from going shopping for food with somebody who could attack your arrangement.

- Purchase just those things on your list and abstain from utilizing coupons since you have them for different things, not on your list.

- Avoid spur of the moment purchases and promoting ploys to make such buys.

- Shop with a help individual, or if you should shop alone, be sure you adhere to your list.

CAREFULLY READ FOOD LABELS

When you read food labels, you are searching for a lot of sugars, fats, fiber, or sodium in the list of fixings. Essentially, you have to know a couple more things about reading food names to guarantee that you're getting the entire picture. The first ingredient recorded is the most important arranged by weight; the last fixing recorded has a minimal sum in an amount in the specific item. Additives and flavorings should likewise be recorded.

Sugars: Names for sugar are glucose, sorbitol, sucrose, dextrose, lactose, xylitol, etc. Different types of sugars include corn sugar, unadulterated sweetener, darker sugar, crude sugar, mannitol, corn sugar, corn syrups, sorghum, molasses, and nectar. There are various distinctive fake sugars available today. New fake sugars are springing up in food items all the time. The best way to remain careful is to eat everything with restraint.

Fats: Components in many of the foods we eat are soaked in fats, including oils, grease, suet, shortening, and spread. Soaked fats are additionally found in meats, for example, hamburger, and other creature items, for example, egg yolks, spread, cheddar, sharp cream, and all milk aside from skim. Palm and coconut oils are likewise soaked fats. Unsaturated or polyunsaturated fats are found in fish and plant foods, for example, avocados, nuts, seeds, olives, and oils, for example, sunflower, soy, nut, and canola oils. Mono-saturated fats are olive oil and rapeseed oil. Omega 3 unsaturated fats are found in sleek fish, for example, salmon and mackerel.

Trans-fats, which means fluid vegetable oils that have been transformed into strong fats by hydrogenation, are found in margarine, many nibble foods, heated products, and seared food. The words hydrogenated or halfway hydrogenated methods trans-fats are in the food—generally prepared food sources. Fats are frequently used to make mayonnaise sauces, flavors, and plate of mixed greens dressings. Different names for fat are mono-glycerides, diglycerides, triglycerides, lecithin, lipids, egg yolk, and mayonnaise.

Salt: A mineral fundamentally made out of sodium chloride, salt, is basic for most life. It is one of the fundamental tastes and is utilized as a significant additive. Salt is found in fixings records for ocean salt, kelp, heating powder, preparing pop, monosodium glutamate, sodium saccharin, sodium nitrate, sodium propionate, and anything with sodium in its name. Sauces, flavors, plate of mixed greens dressings, onion salt, garlic salt, celery salt, canned tomato items, ketchup, bean stew sauces, grill sauces, Worcestershire sauce, cooking wines, escapades, miso, hydrolyzed vegetable protein, yeast, arranged mustards, soya sauce, tamarin, pickles, corned meat, handled items and cheeses can be high in sodium. A general rule is to constrain your admission of foods that contain more than one mg — sodium per calorie. Foods guaranteeing "low-salt" or "no-salt" on their marks are best—however, read the name to ensure the case is valid. Fiber: Diets are improved with fiber. Dietary fiber originates from plants and isn't processed in the intestinal tract yet might be used in the lower gut.

Various plants have various types of fiber: gelatin and gum (which are water solvent), and adhesive, cellulose, hemicellulose, and lignin (which are water-insoluble). Wellsprings of dietary strands are discovered distinctly in plant foods—for instance: entire wheat, entire grains, oat wheat, multi-grain, rye, oats, dark colored rice, wild rice, entire grain pasta, crisp foods grown from the ground, plates of mixed greens, beans, lentils, split peas, nuts, seeds, and dried products of the soil considerably more. They aid absorption and guarantee that the stomach and digestion tracts function admirably. In marking, the fiber substance of food is recorded in weight just as a level of the day by day admission esteem. Also, here's the last word on shopping for food: If you need somebody to buy staple goods for you since you feel that you are excessively occupied or accept that being in a market is unreasonably enticing for you at the present time—proceed.

Keep in mind this is about YOUR success, and success implies loving and taking care of yourself. When you are more certain about your capacity to the basic food item shop, return to your list of strategies that you feel are significant for you to pursue and go complete it.

FAMILY MEALS

Our general public is portrayed by busy people from every walk of life. We are occupied individuals in our business and in our private lives. Family life can be as entangled as it is occupied, as we attempt to be all over and everything for the remainder of our relatives. Our youngsters are the ones who will endure the most if they never realize what it feels like to have sound, formal dinners with discussion and family. Family suppers ought to be solid in sustenance—for the soul and mind just as the body. You can serve scrumptious dinners that are brisk, nutritious, and engaging for the whole family.

There are numerous sources to assist you with structuring and planning healthy family dinners: cookbooks, magazines, the web, and unique media programs. From these sources, you will find food organization and cooking methods that are lower in fat, sugar, and sodium. While there are great deals of pre-arranged sound foods at the supermarket that can be served rapidly for your benefit, there are many inexpensive food dinners you can make at home utilizing whole foods. For instance, look at certain plans in cookbooks for diabetics, low-fat cookbooks, or heart-savvy cookbooks for solid supper plans. Explore them all and most of all: plan, plan, plan!.

If being too occupied is your major challenge, there are a few procedures that can help conquer time-challenging weeks. For instance, be imaginative and amass freezer suppers on Sunday before the week begins. Have an assortment of dinners prepared for whatever state of mind strikes you and your family. Everybody could have something other than what's expected if they like. You can make cooler dinners that are sound and fun, as well. For all suppers, however, particularly family dinners, it is ideal to take a seat at the table to eat as opposed to eating in your vehicle or before the TV. The standard here is to slow down!

Set aside some effort to visit with the family, talk about the day, and put your fork or knife down if food is in your mouth. Bite your food as opposed to breathing in it! Appreciate each nibble and taste the food! If the family demands foods that you know are unmistakably not in your eating plan and you have a test with them, you may settle on a decision to remain in charge by eating your principle supper previously or after the family eats. While they eat, you can have a plate of mixed greens.

Along these lines, you are not enticed by their decisions are as yet at the table for discussion and participating in the family gathering. You realize what will work for you. Make an arrangement early. If you don't feel great getting ready family dinners, request support from your family for some assistance. You may be astounded what they think of it. The perfect, obviously, is to plan foods you would appreciate that are nutritious and good for your entire family. One father told me that he was not very good at arranging dinners and continued putting it off. He additionally said that his teenage girl was always delighted in preparing meals, so I proposed that he let his little girl plan the suppers for the week, and he could double-check them for taste and satisfaction. His food organizing challenge was understood.

Food preparation can be one of the absolute most noteworthy factors in making healthy meals. Be aware of food preparation descriptions, for example, deep-frying, coated or adding of fat/oil to cook. These techniques include a bigger number of calories and fat than is vital. Better strategies for planning healthy meals include grilling, baking, steaming, boiling, broiling, microwaving, barbecuing, roasting, poaching, braising, and stir-frying.

Here are a couple of tips to reduce the fat, sodium, and sugar in your cooking:

- Drain off the fat that collects during cooking.

- Refrigerate sauces, soups or stews, and flavors before serving so as to skim off the hardened fat that has ascended to the top. Warm them.

- In planning meats, cut back on excess as much at conceivable and expel the skin from poultry before cooking.

- When you pan sear, utilize a low-sodium stock instead of oil to cook meats and vegetables. To thicken sauces, use cornstarch or rice flour.

- In preparing, supplant fats with fruit purée or no-fat yogurt fitting for the formula.

- Reduce the measure of sugar or salt in a recipe.

- Reduce the measure of cheddar in the recipe (low-fat obviously).

- Avoid cooking your vegetable dishes with fat and salt or including fat and salt at the table.

- Use garlic, onions, peppers, or new herbs in your dishes.

- Add a dash of flavor to your dish; decrease the sugar and include vanilla or almond concentrates or cinnamon powder for the season.

Snacks are a significant piece of family dinners, whether they are eaten at home or while away. Organized and laid out in your kitchen, custom made snacks and tidbits have a few benefits.

When taken to class or work, they frequently free us from the stress of what we will have for lunch and questions regarding how to remain on our eating plan. Other than being savvy, pre-made snacks fend off us from enticing and normally less nutritious cheap food and eatery suppers. We know precisely what is in our pre-made snacks and can incorporate the best possible adjustments for ideal sustenance and good dieting. Assortment in lunch and snacks isn't an issue since we can bundle and convey hot and cold food sources. Scraps frequently make amazing snacks. Utilize a canteen for hot or cold foods; warm sacks and little cooler packs can guarantee freshness. Making snacks and bites at home takes effective planning.

Plan ahead for seven days of snacks and lunch that will cater to the entire family. Set a suitable time for collecting snacks sacks ahead of time—for certain families, the prior night functions work well, and for other people, the morning appears to be less difficult. I plan my lunch and snacks for my days off as well; then, when I'm getting things done, I realize I can adhere to my eating plan.

Put variety and nutrient-filled ingredients in every snack, keeping desserts, carbonated beverages, sodium, and fats to the base or disposing of them all together. If you need recommendations, ask your family, different guardians, or search for data on lunch proposals on the web. If you are enticed to nibble on the fixings as you set up the lunch meals, request that other relatives assist you with making them. If you are eating at home, pursue similar standards for all family dinners: sit together, take part in the discussion, put down your utensils between bites, chew completely, and turn off telephones, radios, and TV interruptions. Make the most of your time together over lunch!

CHAPTER NINE
HOW TO BURN FAT AUTOMATICALLY
AND FEEL FULLER ON LESS

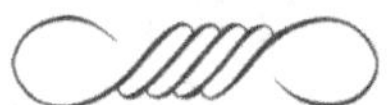

In this chapter, you're going to figure out how to reduce your size, become healthier, and feel full even when you're eating less food. Utilizing the simple and straightforward nutrition rules stated in this section, you'll effectively accomplish your ideal weight, and it won't appear as though you're on an eating regimen. In fact, you don't need to starve yourself or surrender your preferred foods. You'll likewise have no issue keeping up your new body shape since you're not going to do anything strange or extraordinary to achieve it.

Losing fat doesn't rely on fat grams, sugar grams, feast timing, food blends, macronutrient proportions, singular micronutrients, or any of a hundred other extraordinary diet program subjects. None of those things matters if you're eating excessively. At last, almost every weight reduction system returns full-cycle to whether it encourages you to keep up a calorie deficit. Remaining in a calorie shortage reliably, be that as it may, is a challenge on the grounds that many factors impact the amount you eat and number of calories you consume.

Energy balance is dynamic, which implies the measure of calories you require can change. Alongside thinking little of food utilization, neglecting to alter your calorie consumption when your vitality needs change is the most widely recognized reason for weight reduction levels. The central issue is, "What is the most effortless, proficient, and most beneficial approach to keep up that imperative caloric shortfall?" For my cash, I'll wager on what I call "high-low" food, a way to deal with food determination dependent on three significant standards:

1. Energy density, otherwise called calorie density, is the number of calories in a portion of food for every serving.

2. Nutrient density is the dietary benefit per serving (nutrients, minerals, phytonutrients, and fiber).

3. Satiety is defined by how full a portion of food or dinner makes you feel and how that influences the amount you eat. To boost fat loss while enhancing your wellbeing, you will likely pick foods that contain the most noteworthy supplement density, the highest satiety level, and the least calorie density.

Is a calorie, "Just a Calorie?" You might be thinking, "There's significantly more to nutrition than just calories, and a calorie isn't only a calorie!" That is the general purpose of eating nutrient-dense, normal foods. Clearly, 200 calories from pretzels and soft drinks won't give the equivalent dietary benefit or satiety as 200 calories of broccoli and salmon. Various foods can significantly influence your wellbeing, your hormones, and even your disposition, sharpness, and mental work.

Various kinds of foods can likewise have marginally various consequences for body structure at a similar gross caloric consumption. This can be clarified by the thermic impact of food, calories in stringy foods that aren't totally assimilated, and the impact of food on hormones and consequent craving. In any case, this doesn't negate the calorie law; it checks it. Representing every one of these components, when you take a look at the net outcome, you're left with precisely what the math directs: weight changes depend on calories in versus calories out. From a vitality balance perspective, a metabolizable calorie is only a calorie.

There's a major distinction between "don't count calories" and "calories don't count." Some diet regimen programs discourage calorie counting; they basically show you what to eat and what not to eat. The exceptional food blends or remarkable topic of the diet regimen is generally credited for the weight reduction. What they don't let you know is that their eating rules cause you to eat less consequently.

A DIFFERENT DEFINITION OF COUNTING CALORIES

At this point, you might be thinking, "God help us, not another calorie-counting program!" If so, take a deep breath. You won't need to check calories.

Truth be told, in case you're determined about not including anything, I won't demand it. I'll essentially request that you complete three things:

1. Recognize the calories-in versus calories-out equation.

2. Know about your bite sizes.

3. Increase or reduce your portions in light of your week by week results.

My definition of checking calories may not be what you think. Checking calories doesn't need to mean strolling around with a scratch pad or electronic gadget, recording each piece you eat consistently. Rather, you make a day by day menu plan as your eating objective for the afternoon. Utilizing this strategy, you possibly need to tally calories once when you make your menu.

This technique is proactive, not responsive. You record what you intend to eat first, then eat it, as opposed to eating first and afterward recording what you just ate. Consider it menu arranging as opposed to calorie checking. To counteract weariness and get a dietary variety, you can make various menus or make food substitutions from a similar class with comparable caloric qualities. Making your very own menus is simpler than you might suspect. Basically, pursue the ten Body Fat Solution food rules, and your menus will nearly make themselves.

CALORIES 101: ASCERTAIN YOUR DAILY MAINTENANCE CALORIES

One size doesn't fit all with regards to calories. It's senseless to endorse a similar measure of calories for everybody, particularly if it bumps people or dynamic and inactive individuals together. For instance, 1,500 calories daily may be ideal for most ladies to reduce fat; however, it could be semi-starvation for a gigantic and active man. The greater and increasingly dynamic you are, the more calories you have to have to keep up your weight. Keep in mind these focuses and that both can change. Likewise, remember that ladies are commonly littler than men, so ladies, for the most part, need around 600 to 800 fewer calories every day. Calorie needs likewise decline as you get more established. As indicated by exercise physiologists Victor Katch and Frank McArdle, the normal female between the ages of twenty-three and fifty has a calorie maintenance level of around 2,000 to 2,100 calories for each day and the normal male around 2,700 to 2,900 calories.

CALORIES 102: MAKE THE ALL-SIGNIFICANT CALORIE DEFICIT

To shed fat, you should make a caloric deficit. A caloric deficit, otherwise called negative energy balance, implies that the quantity of calories you devour is not exactly the number of calories you consume. You can make a shortage by diminishing your food admission, expanding your movement level, or both. If you require 2,800 calories for each day to keep up your weight and you eat 3,300 calories every day, you're in positive energy balance by 500 calories, and you'll put on weight.

If you eat 2,300 calories every day, you're in negative energy balance, and you'll get thinner. A caloric shortfall is a basic subtraction. To figure your optimal caloric admission for diminishing muscle to fat ratio, subtract 20–30 percent from your support level. 20% is viewed as a preservationist shortage, 30 percent a forceful shortfall. In case you're a normal male, and your support level is 2,800 calories for each day, then a 20 percent shortage is a 560-calorie decrease, which gives you an objective of 2,240 calories for every day. In case you're a normal female, and your upkeep level is 2,100 calories for each day, then a 20 percent shortage is 1,680 calories for each day.

It's commonly best to keep your calorie decrease preservationist from the outset. In case you're not getting the pace of fat loss you need, you can make a progressively forceful shortfall later by diminishing your calories a little further or expanding your movement. Overall, most ladies will decrease muscle to fat ratio adequately and securely on 1,400 to 1,800 calories for every day. Most men will accomplish healthy, safe, and effective fat reduction around 2,100 to 2,500 calories each day. Keep in mind that these are midpoints. If your body is huge and you're dynamic, utilize the upper end of these ranges. If your body is small in size or if you're inert, utilize the lower end of these ranges.

CALORIES 103: MODIFY YOUR CALORIE INTAKE OR EXERCISE OUTPUT ON THE BASIS OF YOUR RESULTS

There are numerous equations you can use to ascertain your calorie needs with accurate precision. In any case, don't be excessively worried about calorie calculations, since you'll need to modify your calories dependent on your week after week results in any case. All you need is a decent pattern. At last, it's progressively significant that you comprehend the 10,000-foot view of energy balance. Despite the number of calories you believe you're eating at the present time, if your body weight isn't changing, then you don't have a calorie shortfall. This implies one of three things:

1. You thought little of what number of calories you are eating.

2. You overestimated what number of calories you are consuming.

3. Both of the above-mentioned. Whatever the explanation, you have to make or restore a shortage by eating less or exercising more.

THE SELECTIVE REDUCTION OF CALORIES

There are two different ways to make a shortfall: increment your vitality use or decrease your food utilization. On the food decrease side, the following inquiry is, "Which food sources do you cut?" Do you basically eat somewhat less of everything? That would work, because any caloric deficiency will cause weight reduction. In any case, there's a superior way.

At that point, when a reduction in calories is called for, you specifically decrease the calorie-density basic sugars, dull carbs, and grains. That leaves the fundamental proteins, fats, and micronutrients from products of the soil. If the calories fall too low to even think about satisfying your vitality needs, you essentially include caloric counterbalance by somewhat expanding your lean protein and solid fats. In case you're an insightful reader, you may be thinking, "Hello, hold up a moment, aren't you making another low-carb diet in a mask?" Well, yes and no. Truly, on the grounds that we're expanding your caloric shortfall by diminishing certain carbs. No, because there are some significant contrasts in my methodology contrasted with "conventional" low-carb diets:

To start with, this diet plan isn't an outrageous low-carb diet. It's a moderate-carb sustenance program. Second, the measure of carbs you decrease isn't fixed; it's a variable dependent on your needs and inclinations. Third, the sort of carbs you wipe out directly from the beginning are the prepared carbs, refined sugars, and man-made carbs.

As a result, you additionally lessen normal starches and grains, which are calorie thick. There's no motivation to evacuate high-nutrient density foods like leafy foods. Fourth, the essential center isn't around carbs, yet where it ought to be — on the calories. Conventional low-carb slimming down mindset can sometimes lead to the misconception and judgment of alive and well and nutritious foods and makes carbs resemble the reason for heftiness. The reason for weight isn't carbs; it's an overabundance of calories, an abatement in physical activity, and every one of the components that lead to this vitality irregularity.

The Macronutrients:

Protein, Carbohydrates, and Fat Like calories, the correct admission of the three macronutrients—proteins, solid carbs, and fundamental fats—is basic. Be that as it may, if you essentially pursue the ten Body Fat Solution food runs, your macronutrient needs will be met, and you'll naturally be in the ballpark with every one of your numbers. What's most significant is to get the fundamentals first and locate a restorative macronutrient balance that keeps away from the boundaries. From that point, you can alter the arrangement to address your issues. Before we proceed onward to the ten principles, how about we quickly review the three macronutrients. The Power of "protein" originates from the Greek word proteos, which signifies "of first significance." This is fitting since, when you set up a feast, I need you to consider lean protein first.

Consider protein building material for the body on the grounds that the amino acids in protein are utilized as development material for almost every cell and tissue, including muscle. Protein is found in numerous foods, even vegetables, beans, vegetables, and grains. While this is significant for veggie lovers to know, when we allude to "lean proteins" in this program, we're alluding fundamentally to the lean wellsprings of complete proteins, ones that contain all the basic amino acids. Complete proteins incorporate chicken breast, turkey breast, lean red meat, fish, shellfish, egg whites, and low-or nonfat dairy items. Protein assumes some significant jobs in weight control. Slender protein encourages you to keep up your fit weight when your calories are confined. It additionally smothers your craving. Eating lean protein expands your digestion because of the thermic impact of food, which is how a lot of vitality you consume to process the food. Protein has a thermic impact of 30 percent. This implies, if you eat a lean protein food that has 100 calories, 30 of those calories are utilized to process the food, leaving just 70 calories of net vitality accessible. Sugars have a thermic impact of 10–15 percent, while dietary fat has the least thermic impact of just 3 percent.

CHAPTER TEN
PLANNING, ORGANIZING, AND IMPLEMENTING

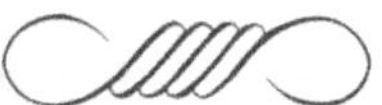

If we gave your fitness and health habits an unexpected assessment today, what might be the prognosis? Be sincere. Would your eating routine be a critical condition, in critical need of crisis treatment? Would your training program need a bit of fixing up to a great extent? Do you, at any point, have an organized training program? What about your lifestyle? Is your body enduring the impacts generally late nights, liquor use, or significant levels of stress?

Notwithstanding your current physical condition, the absolute quickest method to improve your outcomes is by planning and prioritizing. Your central goal is to recognize which regions throughout your life need prompt consideration and afterward sort out the entirety of your exercises around those needs.

By following the recipe, you'll learn in this chapter how you could go from a total stop to pedal to the metal and really show signs of improvement brings about less time. 80-20: The Magic Formula for Achieving More by Doing Less There's presumably no better method to set needs and increase your energy than observing the 80-20 rule.

It was first discovered in 1897 by Vilfredo Pareto, an Italian business analyst who saw a striking lopsidedness in the circulation of riches. He found that 20 percent of the populace had 80 percent of the cash and resources. In wellness, the 80-20 guideline is nonsensical. You may expect that all aspects of your preparation and food would have similar importance. Subsequently, you, as a rule, treat every viewpoint similarly. Be that as it may, the 80-20 principle applied to fitness and wellness says that 20 percent of your food, planning, and habits will create 80 percent of the adjustments in your body.

Understanding this guideline can be unpleasant from the outset since you'll understand that the vast majority of what you were doing each day created almost no outcomes. You may wind up feeling like the proverbial gerbil on the wheel—lots of action, yet going nowhere fast. Then again, it's a significant disclosure since it implies that it's completely conceivable to get more results because of doing less. When you see how to utilize this to further your potential benefit by actualizing the standard, it's a groundbreaking change in perspective. You understand that you don't need to perspire the little stuff, so in that sense, it's freeing. Your frame of mind turns out to be progressively loose, and the entire undertaking is less upsetting because you quit stressing over each modest detail.

Applying the 80-20 guideline is a procedure of recognizing needs and concentrating more on those and less on everything else. It's not time; it's action. It's the embodiment of working savvy. There are two different ways to apply the 80-20 standard:

1. Invest additional time and vitality on the imperative few (the 20 percent).

2. Invest less time and vitality on the unimportant many (the 80 percent). The million-dollar question is, how would you know the contrast between the significant needs and the paltry subtleties? What are the 20 percent of exercises that are creating most of your outcomes?

Finding and Eliminating Bottlenecks: Think of the way to your ideal weight and perfect body as a gigantic multilane expressway. Then envision there's something blocking at least one of the paths. As autos must converge to the other side to press through a restricted passageway, a gag point is made, making traffic back up for miles, hindering your movement time or, in any event, carrying you to a stand-still. Any individual who has ever been trapped in rush hour gridlock in Los Angeles or Chicago can identify with this since turnpike bottlenecks in those urban areas cause 25 to 27 million hours of delay each year. Unnecessary delays likewise happen in your fitness venture since at least one significant path of progress is blocked. Coaches regularly whine about their customers demolishing all their difficult work in the exercise center because, even that can't be expected to make up for a lousy eating routine. One change in your regular lifestyle routine, for example, lack of sleep, poor decisions in cafés, or end of the week gorging can demolish a whole seven day stretch of smart dieting.

A solitary restricting conviction, negative frame of mind, or enthusiastic issue can attack all that you do. Other basic limitations incorporate poor travel propensities, skipping breakfast, passionate eating, hitting the bottle hard, poor practice structure, wasteful practice projects, and irregularity in any part of your sustenance or preparing. Requirements can either be heavily influenced by you (inside) or out of your control (outer). For the most part, you'll find that the greatest requirements are interior. As Pogo stated, "We have met the enemy, and he is us." If you're not gaining ground toward your objective, there's quite often one significant requirement obstructing your way, and you quite often have authority over it. When you separate and get rid of it, your advancement begins to move through again at the most extreme conceivable speed. Your body's shape and size will begin changing so quickly it's practically alarming. A basic question or two can help flush with excursion the significant restricting imperative: What one snag is keeping down your advancement in each other territory? What one deadly defect has been keeping you from arriving at your objective? When you've bound the limitation, your need is to pour most of your vitality into settling that one major issue.

THE HIERARCHY OF NUTRITION

One of the ideal approaches to organizing is by utilizing the chain of command approach. Abraham Maslow's progressive system of necessities, a mental hypothesis of inspiration, was one of the most celebrated chains of command. Shown as a pyramid, basic physiological needs, for example, food, water, and rest framed the biggest part at the base, and regard or self-realization needs, for example, accomplishment and imagination, were the littler pieces stacked on top. As indicated by Maslow's chain of command, if the most fundamental life needs aren't satisfied, then they should become quick needs. Just when the basic endurance needs have been met can the higher needs be sought after. This pecking order idea is amazingly useful when you apply it to your preparation and sustenance. More than forty supplements are fundamental for your wellbeing, to give vitality, fabricate or fix body tissues, and perform different substantial capacities.

A caloric deficiency is a fundamental prerequisite for fat loss; however, outrageous and delayed starvation eats fewer carbs to reduce your metabolic rate. Caloric hardship additionally makes it hard to get the various basics. Food is fuel, and you need to top off the gas tank each day if you need to go anyplace. It is safe to say that you are getting enough fuel, basic amino acids. Protein is seemingly the most significant macronutrient when you're concentrating on fat loss. Protein causes you to clutch lean tissue while you're in a caloric deficiency, and it even smothers your hunger. Basic amino acids, which are the structure squares of protein, can't be made by your body, so you should get them from your food. Is it safe to say that you are eating a lean protein with every supper and meeting your day by day protein necessities? Fundamental unsaturated fats. Fundamental unsaturated fats are imperatively significant for cardiovascular wellbeing and various body capacities, including consuming fat. Like basic amino, the fundamental unsaturated fats can't be integrated into your body and should be gotten from your food. Is it true that you include solid fat sources, for example, salmon consistently? Fundamental nutrients and minerals. Nutrients and minerals are natural or inorganic mixes vital for the legitimate working of your body. They're basic because your body can't make them or can't make them in sufficient amounts, so you should get them from your food. Foods grown from the ground are among the most extravagant wellsprings of these micronutrients. Is it safe to say that you are eating them consistently? Water. Your body is, for the most part, water. Water is fundamental to the point that, without it, you'd pass on in merely days. Indeed, even mellow parchedness diminishes physical execution. Satisfactory water admission is likewise important to consume fat, ideally. Is it accurate to say that you are drinking enough water? These are the fundamentals that must frame the establishment of your pyramid. There are numerous minor subtleties that can take your sustenance to a more elevated level. In any case, if you understand you're inadequate in any of the basic pieces, that is the place your needs should go. Allude back to Chapter Six and the ten food rules to be certain your fundamental needs are met, to the exclusion of everything else. The Hierarchy of Training: The primary fundamental is that you are preparing. Any preparation is superior to no preparation. Numerous individuals go through a long time examining preparing methods, yet never begin. Numerous individuals, particularly ladies, are reluctant to lift loads. Yet, weight preparing is a higher priority than vigorous preparing. Weight preparing can give cardiovascular medical advantages, yet heart stimulating exercise can't give quality or solid advancement benefits. Your selection of activities ought to likewise be organized, utilizing a chain of command of significance. All activities are not made equivalent. Continuously make the compound free-weight activities, for example, squats, thrusts, deadlifts, lines, and presses your first need.

The workouts, for example, twists, triceps augmentations, and calf raises, are useful yet less significant, and accordingly, put rearward in the exercise. If you're at any point in a hurry and need to abbreviate your exercises, drop these detail practices first and consistently keep the significant developments. Most machines, except for certain workouts, take lower need than freeloads. If your lower body exercise comprises leg expansions, leg twists, inward thigh machine, and butt blaster machine, you have to take care of your needs. Start hunching down and deadlifting. You'll get progressively out of those two free weight practices than every one of the four of the machines joined. Cardio is lower on the activity chain of importance than weight preparing, yet significant in any case. The perfect program contains weight preparing and cardio preparing.

Cardio gives its very own one of a kind wellbeing and wellness advantages and expands your all-out calories consumed. Similarly, as with weight training, the kind of cardio ought to likewise be organized. Try not to pass judgment on a cardio exercise dependent on time alone. A twenty-to thirty-minute cardio exercise could consume the same number of calories as an hour-long exercise. The thing that matters is force. If you're healthy, fit, and have no orthopedic or therapeutic issues, then extraordinary cardio goes higher on the chain of importance, particularly if time proficiency is essential to you.

TRY NOT TO WASTE TIME

If 20 percent of your activities produce most of your outcomes, then by definition, 80 percent of your activities produce the minority of your outcomes and are generally insignificant. Worrying over details is the deadly problem in a large number of individuals' fat loss goals. For instance, we have Mike the Macronutrient Micromanager, who sweats over spreadsheets for a considerable length of time attempting to change the proportions of protein, carbs, and fat to the tenth of a rating point. Is it worth the issue? All things considered, take a look at it along these lines: If you're on a hunger diet that leaves you insufficient in protein, do you think it makes a difference whether your negligible calorie admission is adjusted impeccably to a 40-30-30 balance or whatever enchanted proportion you're attempting to hit? Then we have Annie, who is forty pounds overweight and needs to know whether she ought to eat natural products of the soil to assist her with getting thinner. Before I even begin to clarify any potential natural advantages, for example, dodging pesticides or getting more elevated levels of micronutrients, I ask her what number of foods grown from the ground she's eating now. I can't resist the urge to laugh when she reveals to me she isn't eating any vegetables whatsoever and just an incidental natural product. Yet, she has an issue kicking the day by day treat propensity. Wouldn't it bode well to cut the sugar and eat more foods grown from the ground before agonizing over natural versus conventional, or crisp versus solidified, or any of twelve different subtleties that don't make a difference if you're not eating any veggies? At long last, we have Pete the Pill Popper, who needs to recognize what fat killers to take—the whopper of every question and answer. If you become tied up with the cases in many promotions for diet pills, you'd leave away accepting you'd found the Holy Grail of weight reduction. Unexpectedly, in well-planned clinical research preliminaries, at any rate, 80 percent of enhancements publicized for weight reduction have never been demonstrated to work for people. Of the staying 20 percent, 80 percent of those items don't do what the ads guarantee they'll do. One broadly publicized fat-eliminator pill guaranteed that it would fix stomach fat and soften away 20 percent of your muscle to fat ratio in a quarter of a year. The examination recounted to an alternate story. A large portion of the investigations said it didn't work by any means. The other half said it worked; however, the outcomes were scarcely huge. One twofold blind, placebo-controlled clinical preliminary demonstrated just a single kilogram of weight reduction in a half year. A huge number of individuals surrender $240 for a six-month supply of an enhancement that delivered paltry advantages, which effectively may have been ascribed to something different, even the misleading impact.

Don't the Details Make a difference Too? A few people misconstrue the 80-20 principle to imply that nearly all that they're doing is useless. While that is not a long way from reality now and again, it's not so much exact. The 80 percent essentially speaks to bring down worth exercises. In case you're an aggressive competitor, propelled student, or refined calorie counter who has just aced every one of the basics and fundamentals, the subtleties matter. A great deal. Another significant achievement guideline is known as the triumphant edge hypothesis, which expresses that everything aides or damages; nothing is nonpartisan. This is particularly significant in sports, business, or aggressive undertakings, where the smallest edge tallies. Do subtleties make a difference? Approach an Olympic swimmer for whom the distinction between a gold and a silver award was one-hundredth of a second. Ask the sprinter who set forth and missed the decorations by a tenth of a second. If you're an expert competitor, then apparently unimportant subtleties, arranging, and execution are the distinction between leaving a mark on the world and being a spectator. Everything matters. Everything tallies. A little 100-calorie-per-day awkwardness in vitality—that is around four chocolate chips from the sweet snack at work—could make you fat if you kept it up for a long enough timeframe and everything else stayed equivalent. The 80-20 standard doesn't infer that subtleties don't make a difference. It says you don't stress over the subtleties until you've aced the fundamentals. As Goethe stated, "The things that issue the most should never be helpless before things that issue the least." Always Have a Plan—Never Wing It. Imagine strolling by a building site and soliciting one of the laborers, "Hello, what are you all building?" A specialist answers, "I have no clue." I wager you've never heard a wonder such as this, since beginning to manufacture something without an arrangement would be senseless. In any case, did you ever think it's just as senseless to go to a rec center, go shopping for food, or even take a seat during supper without an objective and composed outline for your sustenance and preparing? I once heard a statement from persuasive orator Jim Rohn that changed my reasoning for eternity. He stated, "Never start your day until you finish it." From the start, it seemed like a puzzle. How are you expected to complete your day before you start it? Then the light went on, and I understood that he was talking about arranging before acting. The sensible augmentations are, never start your week until you've completed it, never start your month until you've completed it, and never start your year until you've completed it. Activity without arranging is perhaps the greatest reason for disappointment. Arranging requires genuine ideas and exertion. It requires a peaceful, centered time with a pen and paper or PC, frequently with a mentor or accomplice. Proficiency specialists state that consistent time spent in arranging will spare you ten minutes in execution. When you apply this basic arranging idea to your sustenance, preparing, and way of life, the outcomes will stun you. Better results and increasingly productive utilization of time aren't the main benefits. Feeling ill-equipped or capricious makes tension and stress. That makes arranging and arrangement an amazing pressure reducer and certainty developer. Arranging and organizing around priorities start each day, week, month, and year on paper. Continuously work from a rundown, plan, or timetable. Compose a list of objectives, a list of day by day activity steps, an everyday plan, a week by week plan, a composed supper plan, a composed shopping list, and a composed preparing plan. Make need records, not plans for the day. Need records center around the imperative few. The plan for the day is generally jumbled with the minor many. The arranging procedure starts with an objective setting, since every one of your exercises must be sorted out around your high-need objectives and wanted a new way of life propensities. When your objectives are recorded as a hard copy, apply 80-20 reasoning. What is the one wellbeing, wellness, or body-weight objective that would have the greatest effect in your life? If you accomplished it in the following twelve weeks? Organize that objective by composing it on a card, conveying it with you wherever you go and perusing it regularly. Take a look at every one of the five Body Fat Solution standards—mental training, cardio training, quality training, food, and social help. In every one of these classes, what is the one most elevated need objective or activity step that will have the greatest effect in your life? Make your week after week calendar and everyday activity plan around these needs. Every day and Weekly Scheduling: Do you make meetings with your primary care physician? What about your dental specialist? Your bookkeeper? Your beautician? What about your life partner or noteworthy other—do you plan a period and a day for dates? (Neighborly tip: If you don't, leave visas are impending.) If you make arrangements for everything else in your life, for what reason would you leave your preparation for whatever pieces of time happen to be leftover every day? Prepare to have your mind blown. There never is whenever left finished. Strangely, your schedule will consistently top off each day except if you set needs and calendar squares of time for what's generally critical to you. You can begin the arranging procedure with only a pen and a clean sheet of paper. I prescribe putting resources into an arrangement book or time organizer. Planning every week ahead of time is simple since you, as of now, might suspect and arrange your life on a week by week premise. You'll additionally be setting body-weight and body composition objectives and outlining your advancement on a week after week premise, making seven days the ideal square of time for arranging your preparation and food. I propose composing your week after week preparing plan into your time organizer each Sunday evening for the up and coming week. Then each night before hitting the hay, survey your timetable and set everyday objectives and needs for the following day. Along these lines, your oblivious personality can assimilate and coordinate the data while you're dozing. You'll get down to business in the first part of the day with the center and course. At any rate, one of your day by day arrangements will be exercise. Record the specific time you'll be preparing, the activities or body parts you'll be working, and your objectives for the session. Be explicit. There's an enormous distinction between saying, "I'm getting down to business tomorrow," and saying, "Tomorrow at seven a.m. sharp at Gold's Gym, I'm preparing hip-predominant lower body, even push, level force, and lower abs, and I mean to break my own deadlift record."

THE COUNTDOWN METHOD

Another incredible arranging procedure is the "commencement schedule." I began utilizing this technique preceding my first weight training rivalry. It worked so well for me, I've utilized it from that point forward and have prescribed it to a large number of my customers who have additionally utilized it with colossal achievement. Utilizing a commencement, you'll get increasingly engaged and progressively persuaded as time passes as you see the cutoff time drawing nearer and closer. If you don't have looming cutoff times to give you a twinge in your stomach that shouts, "Make a move now or disaster will be imminent!" then you'll see it simpler to state to yourself, "I have a lot of time, so one cheat dinner or skipped exercise doesn't make a difference."

Then, when you understand you don't have time, all things considered, you freeze and participate in a last-minute scrambling practice or resort to outrageous strategies and risky solutions. Here's the means by which it works: get a divider or work area schedule—the sort that shows every week extending on a level plane over the page with an open square of room for every day—or make your very own eighty-four-day (twelve-week) graph on a PC in a word processor or spreadsheet. Circle the objective cutoff time or rivalry date on the schedule and imprint that as day zero. In each of the crates, start checking in reverse from the present day: T minus eighty-four days; T minus eighty-three days; T minus eighty-two days. This will program your oblivious personality to acquire you for an ideal arrival on your cutoff time date, similar to an F-14 on a plane carrying warship. Menu Planning: A composed menu might be the absolute most significant piece of your arrangement. The upside of working off a menu is that it's a proactive arranging system. Numerous individuals keep food journals or diaries, and I don't debilitate that at all since diaries are a fabulous device for training and responsibility. Nonetheless, journaling isn't a similar thing as working off a menu. With food diaries, you eat something and afterward record it. That is responsive. If you make a menu plan and then tail it, that is proactive. A menu plan is your eating objective for the afternoon. Beginning your day without a menu plan is an encouragement to a stray course at the smallest allurement or interruption. Working off a menu additionally implies that you don't need to include your calories consistently progressively. You possibly need to check your calories once when you make your menus. Then you essentially pursue the menu by gauging and estimating your food partitions. The perfect menu is one you make yourself utilizing a format and general standards of feast development, for example, the ten sustenance rules you learned in Chapter Six. You can make menus on a clear sheet of paper and include the calories by hand with a mini-computer, or you can utilize any of the business programming programs accessible available today. Spreadsheets, for example, Microsoft Excel, likewise work consummately for menu arranging and come previously introduced on numerous PCs. Sorting out Your Kitchen: Your following stage is to make a key arrangement for setting up your dinners, including how you will eat at home, at work, in eateries, and when voyaging. The best spot to begin is in your very own kitchen. I've seen coolers loaded up with so much garbage you'd need a GPS to explore your way through them. Kitchen pantries run a nearby second as the most jumbled spot in the home. There's most likely a great deal of stuff in your kitchen that isn't good for your new wellbeing and wellness objectives. Let it be known. Then start Operation Kitchen Clean Sweep. The greatest reason I hear is, "I would prefer not to squander anything." We put that one to rest in Chapter Four, so don't consider it. Toss it hard and fast. Because there's a large portion of a pack of potato chips in the pantry doesn't mean you ought to eat them and afterward start your program after the sack is done. If you're not going to drink sugary, fatty soft drinks any longer, then toss that two-liter cola bottle. I couldn't care less if you just got it and haven't split the seal. Pour it down the sink. It probably won't go to squander all things considered—it will likely wipe some rust off your funnels. If you have food stored in the storm cellar, carport, or some mystery hideaway, get those spots out. Dispose of all the messiness, all over the place. If all else fails, toss it out. When your kitchen is spotless, keep it clean. If the garbage's not there, you can't eat it. Kitchen Essentials: Next, ensure you have all the fundamental kitchen apparatuses, utensils, cookware, and holders you'll require. Notwithstanding the standard things found in each kitchen, like an icebox, broiler, and stovetop, here are a portion of the fundamentals I have in my kitchen: Optional things incorporate a blender and a George Foreman flame broil or some electric barbecue that can accelerate your planning time by cooking chicken breasts and other lean meats rapidly and in amount.

A rice cooker that serves as a vegetable steamer is a gift from heaven. Machines that enable you to cook in mass are a superb help. Office Clean Sweep: Once your house is all together; it's an ideal opportunity to get out of your office. Experience every one of your drawers and dispose of sweets, pretzels, chips, and other low-supplement, fatty] snacks. You'll be carrying solid tidbits to work starting now and into the foreseeable future. While you're grinding away, set up your workplace with little suggestions to keep you concentrated on your objectives.

Post rousing statements and photographs. Show your composed objectives conspicuously where you'll see them throughout the day. Shouldn't something be said about that associate seductress who drops off the doughnuts each morning? Advise her, "No, thank you," and ask her not to leave them anyplace in your sight, or you'll toss them out. If she leaves them in any case, hurl them and ensure she sees you do it. Keep in mind; individuals hate to squander "splendidly great food." I ensure she won't bring you doughnuts any longer. It has exactly the intended effect without fail—particularly If you dump them in the trash can directly over the pencil shavings and espresso beans. Arranging your workday likewise incorporates choosing what you will have for lunch. Try not to venture out from home toward the beginning of the day without knowing where you'll have lunch and what you'll be having.

If you figure you won't have a wide enough scope of alternatives to make a solid, low-calorie decision, then put together your lunch. No reasons. The equivalent goes for your midmorning and mid-afternoon snacks.

CHAPTER ELEVEN
ARRANGING TRIPS TO THE SUPERMARKET

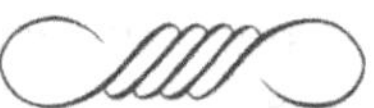

Dietitians gauge that 40 percent of store purchases are made on motivation. Now and then, you'll need to examine food marks at the store to settle on the better decision between two things, yet the entirety of your significant purchasing choices ought to be made ahead of time. Follow my shopping tips below, and you'll turn out each time with low-calorie, high food that draws you nearer to your objectives. Ensure you shop from a list.

Shopping records are anything but difficult to make by utilizing everyday menu designs and including the provisions required for seven days of menus. When you have your list, stay with it. As indicated by New York University sustenance teacher Marion Nestle, 70 percent of customers carry records into the grocery store; however, just around 10 percent stick to them.

- Try not to shop when hungry. I'm certain you've heard this counsel previously, yet do you heed to it?

- Never shop on an unfilled stomach.

- Be aware of your physical and emotional state, also.

- In case you're worn out or upset, you're bound to snatch low quality food on motivation.

- Shop rapidly. Did you realize that general stores play downtempo music to impact you to shop all the more gradually? It's valid. If you wait longer, you purchase more. Rather, with a list close by, perceive how quick you can hurdle through the store. It helps if you shop during off-top hours when there are no groups and shorter lines.

- Do the greater part of your shopping in the aisles of the store. 80% of the foods you'll need to eat all the time can be found on the outskirts of the store: natural products, vegetables, servings of mixed greens, potatoes, yams, lean meats, fish, fish, dairy items, and eggs. Be careful with food item promoting. In each square inch of the store, you're being advertised to always. Food organizations pay for prime areas on the racks.

- Watch out for craving animating colors, for example, red, orange, and yellow are utilized to cause you to notice foods. Adhere to your arrangement and don't be taken in by promoting, including wellbeing and weight reduction claims. Eat generally foods with one fixing and no name. 80% of the foods you eat every day will come without a mark (think products of the soil).

- If they have a mark, they'll normally have just a single fixing, as on account of lean meats, fish, eggs, or antiquated cereal.

- Become a specialist at checking the names.

- Prior to eating anything in a crate, can, or bundle, read the mark cautiously.

- Reduce the quantity of white flour or any refined sugars; for example, sucrose or high-fructose corn syrup, are high on the list.

- Do likewise if the fixings incorporate trans-unsaturated fats or synthetic substances with names you can't articulate. Additionally, observe the calories, serving size, and fiber sum. Watch for name escape clauses. As indicated by food naming laws, if there's not exactly a large portion of a gram of fat, the mark can say "fat-free." If there are less than five calories for every serving, the name can say "zero calories." Food organizations exploit these escape clauses by contracting their serving sizes. For instance, a run of the mill nonstick cooking shower will say "calorie-free" on the name, yet cooking splash is 100 percent oil. How would they pull off it? The serving size is a 33% of-a-second shower. Oppose drive buys at the register. Indeed, even as you're looking, regardless, you're being showcased too. Pretty much every checkout path has treats and soft drink inside arm's lengths.

- Shop for food supplies on the web. A study distributed in the International Journal of Behavioral Nutrition and Physical Activity found that individuals on fat loss programs who requested their staple goods utilizing on the web conveyance administrations bought 28 percent less calorie-thick foods than individuals who shopped in the grocery store.

ANTICIPATING RESTAURANT EATING

If there's one huge error that is bound to disrupt your program, it's making awful decisions at cafés. In many investigations, eating every now and again in eateries corresponds to the higher muscle to fat ratio. Everything bodes well when you take a look at how things have changed in the previous few years. In 1955, Americans burned through 19 percent of their food spending plan on dinners arranged outside the home. Today that number has dramatically increased to 41 percent.

The quantity of individuals now overweight has dramatically

increased with it. Stoutness has significantly increased. As indicated by the U.S. Branch of Agriculture, $222 billion is gone through consistently at cafés and $118 billion of that at drive-thru eateries. The huge issue: unhealthy dinners, to a limited extent, because of expanding segment sizes. Numerous ordinary café suppers contain 1,000 calories or more in principle course alone. If you incorporate a tidbit and treat, that could include at least 1,000. One cut of cheesecake can have 700 calories. Cheddar nachos or seared mozzarella sticks have around 800 calories, the "ordinary" servings that is. As indicated by a report in Men's Health magazine, the most noticeably awful nachos checked in at 2,740 calories. A run of the mill steakhouse prime rib or porterhouse could without much of a stretch fall in the 1,200-to 1,500-calorie extend. Suppose you had hors d'oeuvres, fries, sweet, and beverages with that. The National Restaurant Association reports that the normal individual eats out 4.2 times each week. With that recurrence, if you picked any of these "calorie bombs" each time you ate out, it would totally undermine each nutritious handcrafted supper you ate and all that you did in the rec center throughout the entire week.

Obviously, I understand that telling individuals they can't eat in cafés won't make me extremely well known, so my progressively moderate idea is essentially to downplay eatery eating. One of the qualities I've found in most of the lean individuals is that they like to keep tighter command over their wholesome admission by making their very own large portion suppers. If the national normal is four café dinners for every week and you don't need a normal individual's body, then don't do what normal individuals do. Do what lean individuals do. Keep eating at the cafe a few times each week and settle on the correct decisions when you're there. Notwithstanding how regularly you feast out, you need to instruct yourself about the healthy benefit of eatery food and have an arrangement in advance.

- Start with low-calorie plates of mixed greens rather than fatty hors d'oeuvres.

- Stay away from broiled foods, for example, French fries, onion rings, and calamari.

- Inquire if you don't know how something is readied, particularly about additional sauces, oil, spread, or other shrouded calories.

- Look into menus and calorie data on the web and settle on a sound decision ahead of time.

- If you don't have the foggiest idea of what number of calories are in a dish, don't eat it.

- Pick broiled chicken or fish for lean protein. Pick lean sirloins or filets and get nine-to twelve-ounce cuts or littler.

- Request steamed vegetables as side dishes.

- Request dry heated potatoes, sweet potatoes, or darker rice as sides or part of the primary course.

- Request crisp natural product for dessert.

- Split a customary sweet with a friend.

- Try not to clean your plate—take a doggie pack home with you.

- Eat until you are 80 percent full.

- Never stuff yourself.

- Try not to eat at buffets.

ARRANGING YOUR WEEKENDS

Unless your Saturdays and Sundays follow a similar schedule to what you pursue on weekdays, it's imperative to design your ends of the week ahead of time, particularly your dinners. A study led at Washington University and distributed in the diary Obesity found that adjustments in timetable, dinners, and way of life practices on ends of the week were sufficient to cause weight increase or hinder weight reduction for the whole week. Numerous individuals can't understand why they're not getting results when it appears as though they invest a lot of exertion throughout the entire week.

The appropriate response is that two days of extravagance can fix five days of work. Making arrangements for Holidays, Birthdays, and Special Occasions Planning is likewise instrumental for exploring your way through occasions, birthday events, parties, and other unique events. I accept that these are events where it's superbly suitable to unwind and appreciate the food, family, and fun that are a piece of these unique occasions. Be that as it may, this doesn't mean overeating or tossing all alert to the breeze. Stay away from all-or-none reasoning. You don't need to pick between getting a charge out of the special seasons or remaining lean and solid—you can pick both.

Occasions and other get-togethers can undoubtedly be worked into your 10 percent consistency rule. Be that as it may, when you focus on 90 percent consistency, respect your guarantee to yourself. A typical example, particularly every November and December, is the "I'll start when" mentality. For reasons unknown, three occasions—Thanksgiving, Christmas, and New Year's—some way or another convert into about a month and a half of relentless dietary destruction. It's imperative to place this in a legitimate viewpoint. It's extremely just three days you need to manage.

Truth be told, it's just a couple of suppers. Appreciate the occasion food with some restraint. The remainder of the period it's preparation and nutritious eating, not surprisingly. If you discover yourself saying, "I'll start when I move beyond the special seasons," be cautious, since that sort of reasoning typically reaches out a long ways past January 1, and you'll generally be hoping to begin when conditions are perfect. They never are. Making arrangements for Vacations and Travel: Because you're voyaging doesn't mean you can't pursue your ordinary food and preparing routine. You invest a lot of energy arranging the flight, the vehicle rental, the lodging, and different subtleties of your excursion; why not prepare and food?

Here's the absolute most dominant method I've utilized for health and wellness: each time I travel, I set an objective to return home as fit as when I left. Here are the means by which to do it:

- Get lodging with a kitchen. Numerous inn networks offer rooms with a full kitchen. Or attempt transient loft or condominium rentals. Search the Internet, and you might be amazed at the sort of cabin accessible and now and then at preferable costs over inns.

- Go food shopping following checking in. Subsequent to checking in, make a straight shot to the neighborhood supermarket, shopping list close by. Any place you are on the planet, if you have a kitchen and a well-loaded icebox, your supper arranging and food readiness is very little, not quite the same as when you're home.

- Check the neighborhood eatery menus ahead of time. When you travel, almost certainly, you'll have more café suppers than expected. Utilize all the eatery arranging techniques you adapted before and consistently ponder what you'll eat each time you eat out.

- Prepare various types of foods and pack healthy snacks for drives, flights, and day trips. For long flights and drives, nothing beats convenient dinners and tidbits that you can take with you. You can figure out how to make a variety of compact foods, including various kinds of cereal flapjacks, solid burgers, and sound sandwiches. Traveling, flying, or driving is never a reason for poor eating.

- Work out your exercise plan in advance. Continue utilizing your time organizer or timetable book when you're away from home. Continuously work from a composed arrangement.

- Pick your training area ahead of time. You can do bodyweight practices directly in your lodging. If you like, utilize the Internet to find a rec center before your outing. Bring ahead of time and inquire as to whether there is day by day or week after week rates. Inquire as to whether your inn has an exercise center or an alliance with a nearby fitness center.

If you use an exercise center in your neighborhood, check whether they are associated with different clubs around the nation. Make physical diversion part of your sightseeing plans. On one ongoing excursion, I spent a whole day climbing on the slopes of a wonderful national park. On another, I leased a bicycle and rode for miles along a beach. I've additionally seen other individuals, a significant number of them unfit, tooling around outside on those high-quality bikes. Which would you pick?

THE SUREFIRE WAY TO IMPLEMENT NEW HABITS AND LIFESTYLE CHANGES

There's no chance to get around it—to handle an issue like a muscle to fat ratio, which has such a large number of causes, you should make changes in each aspect of your life. You need to eat better, train reliably, deal with your feelings, change your reasoning, get the help you need, and set up everything together into a solid way of life. In any case, there's extraordinary power in organizing and focusing on the absolute most significant errand at some random time.

Numerous individuals attempt to do excessively, too early. The amazingly roused sorts may pull it off, yet the vast majority who make a plunge and roll out clearing improvements at the same time only dissipate their center, diffuse their endeavors, and end up with a lower achievement rate over the long haul. Another propensity, as a rule, takes around twenty-one sequential days to shape. If you center on each essential objective or conduct change in turn, while keeping everything else in a holding design, you can shape seventeen new propensities in a year.

With this methodology, one year from now, you will be such a changed individual, you'll need a telescope to think back to where you began. Locate your greatest restricting imperative, adhere to the 80-20 principle, and utilize the progressive system to deal with picking the most sensible spots to begin. Every individual has one of a kind qualities and shortcomings, so you'll need to painstakingly pick which territories you need to organize and concentrate on first. Here's one case of how the initial six habit changes may play out.

1. Hit the sack at ten to eleven p.m. sharp, so you get seven to eight hours of value rest.

2. Take up yoga, contemplation, or unwinding activities to help lessen pressure.

3. Start having breakfast each day, which you may have skipped regularly. Attempt regular oats, blueberries, and an egg-white scramble with one entire omega-3 egg.

4. Exchange the leg "conditioning" practices you were accomplishing for weight squats and deadlifts.

5. Quit drinking liquor or lessen to one to two beverages a few times per week.

6. Quit drinking pop and change to water or unsweetened green tea as your essential refreshments.

CHAPTER TWELVE
EATING OUT: STRATEGIES FOR DEALING WITH EMOTIONAL EATING OUTSIDE YOUR HOME

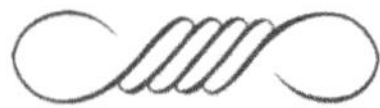

With our fast-paced ways of life, I think individuals now and then eat out more than they eat at home. Eatery and inexpensive food eateries, buffet meals, get-togethers, occasion meals, huge family social occasions, and excursion dinners can become uncommon difficulties for the greater part of us. Why? There are numerous reasons. When we eat out, we see that since we are not responsible for fixings, arrangement, or in small sizes, "feasting out" signifies "getting out" or deserting our food plan. We may get confounded or feel vanquished by the number of decisions we should make when we eat away from home. Lastly, we may make presumptions about what is fitting conduct when we're eating out or even give ourselves authorization to binge.

A few people have not many challenges with eating out, yet they may battle with eating plans at home. Still, other individuals find that they are in charge when they eat at home, yet a gathering or eating out can be shocking for their eating plans.

Regularly, we don't recollect every one of the things that work for us in a period of tumult, when feelings are running high or when our quick paced world stretches us as far as possible. Know about one's self-talk at that time. What are you letting yourself know? Is it accurate to say that you are looking into effective techniques or feeling despair on account of negative considerations? Decide to compose what works in the diary, utilize the diary, and keep mindful and change your self-talk. Work on that self-talk and alter territories of concern. Take 20 seconds to allude to the fitting segment—particularly this segment on eating out—and be set up for all outcomes with the goal that you can stay in charge and be fruitful.

Have an arrangement all set in your mind before you break the flow from your home meal plan. More than once, we have said, "To hell with the arrangement, I'll simply begin once again on Monday." It isn't an alternative—and it is anything but a sensible methodology. You can deal with every one of your difficulties through mindfulness and arranging! In North America, the cafe experience is frequently appraised on the measure of food in singular servings. The pattern has been that the normal client will gripe whenever served a sensible portion, by all accounts dependent on the nature of the food, but on the amount of food on individual plates. You have to prepare when you eat out in eateries. When placing an order, request a smaller part or a half-portion. Lots of eateries will readily do this. If the eatery doesn't agree, request a "take out" compartment to accompany your dinner.

This gives you the chance of passing judgment on your own part size and putting what you won't eat in the holder to bring home. Do this before you dive into the supper, and you will find that you most likely have enough in your holder for another dinner!

The reward: You won't be enticed to binge. A few eateries will guarantee that they don't have littler divides as a choice. However, they will furnish a plate with less food on it—in spite of the fact that they will charge you the maximum. This is really a sensible choice. If you eat the bigger feast, what is the genuine cost you are paying regarding feelings, blame, fault, or disgrace? Is it justified, despite all the trouble to forfeit smart dieting, trouble with your association with food, and to endanger your associations with the ones you love?

Here is a list of systems I have discovered supportive when advising individuals about eating out concerns and difficulties:

- Call the café early and have the menu faxed to you with the goal that you can choose what to arrange early that accommodates your eating plan.

- Pre-order your food to guarantee achievement if you are truly not certain about your capacity to arrange astutely before other individuals.

- Ask your host if it is OK to arrange first, so you are not enticed by what others are requesting.

- When you request, ask how things are readied. Inquire as to whether your request can be broiled or poached rather than fried.

- Order broiled veggies with your supper rather than pasta or pureed potatoes with sauce.

- Be cognizant with regards to requesting food with flavors, cream sauces, or sauces when all is said and done. Request them as an afterthought, so you can control the sum you expend. Simply dunk your fork into the sauce for enhancing as you take a nibble of food.

- Be mindful of requesting food that accompanies serving of mixed greens dressings, nuts, high sodium meats, cheeses, bread 3D squares, nacho platters, olives, and guacamole. Request serving of mixed greens dressings as an afterthought—

dunk your fork in them for enhancing as opposed to pouring them on your plate of mixed greens.

- Offer to part a supper with a friend if it is suitable. Approach your server to bring another side plate with the goal that you can partition the dinner into two segments. Cafés are frequently glad.

- Ask the server beforehand to carry your plate when you are finished.

- When you are finished eating, place your knife and fork on your plate. Treat your plate like a clock: place the knife and fork together with handles at 5 o'clock, indicating 10 o'clock. Push the plate only a couple of inches from you with your thumbs on the edge of the plate to flag you are finished. If you have been utilizing a paper napkin, place it over your plate. (Legitimate behavior implies that you would not do this with fabric napkins; they ought to just be set on the table close to your plate.) These are signals to your server that you are done with your supper.

- • If you decide not to eat the full segments you have been served, inquire as to whether you can have the rest of it to go.

FAST FOOD

Normally, fast-food eateries serve foods that are high in fat, sugar, sodium, and starches. Late drifts in good dieting have incited some fast-food chains to make some solid decisions. Anyway, those things are not as well known, in some cases, sit on the rack for broadened timeframes, some of the time turn sour, and very regularly are immediately supplanted in the menu. Fast food ordinarily keeps to things that are prevalent and sell reliably, for example, high-fat substance burgers, fries, and carbonated refreshments stacked with sugar.

Fast food eateries have additionally experienced esteem in the amount of their food. "Super-sized" suppers can be twofold or even triple the segments of fat, sugar, and sodium that we regularly devour in a whole day! If you decide to go to a fast-food eatery, plan to go to one where you will use sound judgment. One methodology is to arrange a children's feast to exploit the littler size; give the toy to the children. Look on the web and become more acquainted with a few fast food menus, so you know the rates and dietary benefits of their things and can make sense of what will work best for you early — that way, you are set up with a strategy.

Think about all the squandered vitality related to decision making and the squandered vitality if you don't settle on informed choices. The outcomes in your self-talk could be: blame, thrashing on yourself, disgrace, and emotions of loss of control. These emotions could ruin the entire occasion, in addition to influencing your determination to keep up your good dieting arrangement. Relax! Eating fast food is unavoidable—so why not make it pleasant and keen! Settle on shrewd decisions. Select fast food suppers that will fit into your day by day eating plan and keep to your objectives.

This might be simpler than it sounds if you recall thoughts regarding balance. For instance, envision that you enable yourself to have one little request of fries with a broiled chicken burger, mayo as an afterthought, with juice or water to drink. Gradually eat each fry in turn, tasting each nibble, appreciating the supper. Understand that you don't need to complete the fries, realizing you are content with just having 6–8 pieces. Settle on a choice that the remainder of the fries are not worth going short on different foods later in the day. Acknowledge that, although a couple are delicious, they are oily and too salty to even think about eating the whole bit. You realize that eating every one of them may give you an annoyed stomach, and you choose it's not justified, despite any potential benefits to eating them all. Poise implies you decide to be content as you pursue your arrangement and feel glad for yourself. You've put your breathing device on first: you are dealing with yourself and breathing simpler about your association with food.

Well-Being: "It will be awful! I don't have the foggiest idea of what to request to keep on my arrangement!" That is the way it will be. That is the thing that you have let yourself know, in this way you will make it so. Instead, you may state, "I will set myself up early, find out about my decisions, and settle on the best choice for my well-being." That is the thing that you will probably do.

BUFFETS

The scandalous buffet is regularly charged as "Everything YOU CAN EAT!" as though this were the objective of buffet feasting. Some dread the buffet table; some adore it! Regardless of which side you are on, the visual effect of the buffet spread is sometimes overwhelming. The primary thought that strikes a chord concerning decisions was— what decisions are to be made, yet what are the best worth choices. A few people need to get their cash's value. Typically, the last decision to be made is, "Is the thing that on this buffet table solid and does it fit into my eating plan?" Buffets sensibly connect with us in a great deal of self-talk because there is such a significant number of decisions to be made about such a large number of enticing dishes.

Self-talk may be very surprising for every individual, except it regularly comes as a test to our feeling of decency. It doesn't need to be. If you are vexed about the value contrasted with the amount of food you intend to devour, who truly pays? It is safe to say that you are practical or sharp? Examine what is happening in your mind. Be progressively mindful of what you are informing yourself regarding food. Again and again, we have negative self-talk! Consider this. I did when I directed individuals. I would believe that it has cost a few people—in one year alone—3300 dollars to shed 45 pounds. I needed to inquire as to whether they were going to pass up being affected by their negative discussion about their association with food.

They had a decision to make. Is it safe to say they would get every piece of significant worth from an eatery or buffet supper by devouring as much as they could, or would they say they would connect an incentive to the nature of their feasting out? I would regularly transcend their protests and legitimizations by soliciting, "Shouldn't something be said about the cost of your well-being?" If buffets alarm you, don't go to one until you are alright with picking the correct foods and eating as indicated by your eating plan. Cost is extra; accept that you are paying for the experience, not the amount you can eat.

Here are a few methodologies for eating out at a buffet:

- If it is a cooperative choice to go to a buffet, and you are awkward with that decision, inquire as to whether anybody minds heading someplace else. If you feel bolstered, disclose that to the individuals in your gathering.

- Ask if you could meet them at the eatery after they eat. Or state that you are tied up to that point, and you will seek an espresso after.

- If you wind up heading off to the smorgasbord café, request a menu as opposed to picking the smorgasbord alternative. Feel certain of this great decision and maintain a strategic distance from the buffet table.

- Ask to be situated far away from the smorgasbord. If the smorgasbord is in somebody's home, sit far away from the smorgasbord table.

- If you decide to participate in the smorgasbord, study the spread for savvy decisions and furthermore for thoughts that will advance your prosperity. Adhere to your arrangement.

- Tell yourself that the foods on a smorgasbord table consistently look obviously superior to the taste. In reality, this is likely obvious because the foods are set up in enormous amounts and kept warm or cold for quite a long time as opposed to being readied new for singular plates.

- Choose a littler plate if you can. If a littler plate isn't accessible, then remain inside the inward ring of the supper plate and don't put any food past that edge.

- Have a little soup to begin or an enormous serving of mixed greens.

- Have only a spot of what you might want to attempt. When you place the food on your plate, orchestrate it with the goal that foods don't contact one another.

- Take your time. Plunk down and make the most of your food. Taste each bite; appreciate the organization.

- Have an organic product for dessert.

- Share a sugary pastry. If you should, however, have only a couple of nibbles. Appreciate them. Enjoy the flavors. Enable yourself to have the taste without overindulging.

- When you are finished eating, place your knife and fork on the plate and cover your plate with your paper napkin. Move the plate away from you two or three inches. This flags you are done eating and a server can expel your plate.

- Resist the compulsion to return to the table for quite a long time.

Be straightforward with yourself about your eating design and be in charge. Relax!

GET-TOGETHERS

In many societies, numerous get-togethers are associated with foods. In your home, at work, and around your companions, you may feel responsible for your food. However, get-togethers may show an entire diverse arrangement of difficulties for you. Weddings, organization feasts, mixed drink parties, potlucks, retirement festivities, leaving parties, political meetings, craftsmanship opening gatherings, and church picnics are only a couple of instances of get-togethers that frequently serve food. The greatest test is that the food is generally free! My most exceedingly terrible time is "free" food at a gathering, meeting, or at another person's home.

As I examine the food table, I consider new plans, new food thoughts, food sources I don't typically have close by or don't ordinarily eat because they are on my "dangerous foods" list. Like such a significant number of individuals, when I'm in this circumstance, my first thought is that I should top off with free food. I am mindful that, in my school years, this demeanor helped me to increase 15 additional pounds. This is such a notable marvel in new undergrads in Canada and the States that it is regularly alluded to as the "Green bean Fifteen"! I presently realize that "getting my fill" appeared in my midriff! Presently, as a grown-up, I am mindful that at a get-together, I can decide to have one taste of a food and be fulfilled. I have figured out how to move my spotlight and rather focus on the event, the individuals, and the social parts of the occasion as opposed to the food.

Here are some more methodologies that can assist you with concentrating on the occasion and not the food:

- Plan your day when you realize you will go out later. Pack your lunch and snacks prior in the day. Else you will be eager to such an extent that you will try too hard when you get to the occasion.

- Compensate for an event that you realize will be focused on food: plan additional activity and equal out your everyday food admission.

- Ask what will be served, so you realize how to prepare it in time.

- Plan to eat with some restraint and alter your bits as need be. Pick solid foods.

- If you should have a sweet pastry, select one that is your least favorite, so you do not eat a lot of it.

- Ask your host or leader if you may carry a dish to the occasion—make it something that you can fit into your eating plan.

- Do you have a helpful individual with you? Tell that individual early about any food or eating difficulties you hope to experience. Discussion the help you need.

- Show up to the occasion later to maintain a strategic distance from the tidbits. Eat before you go.

- Pre-divide your plate with foods that fit your arrangement and just eat what is on your plate to abstain from picking.

- Focus on the non-food themes and on different visitors.

- Keep a solid beverage in your grasp consistently; make it a full or half-full glass to guarantee nobody inquires as to whether you need a beverage.

- Keep a handbag, or a plate, cutlery, and a napkin in the other hand to shield you from snacking at the food or topping off your plate.

- Keep the discussion going as you avoid the table or the treats.

- Help the hosts by taking empty plates or cups the kitchen to abstain from being enticed to snack at the food contributions.

Here are some close to home instances of procedures I use. As you probably are aware, I love chocolate brownies. However, if they have nuts in them, I am less inclined to eat them and enjoy them. Along these lines, if I have brownies on my very own occasion, I purchase ones with nuts in them. At Halloween, I get the chocolate bars that simply don't taste great to me, so I avoid them. A choice is to plan the get-together to occur at your home. Have a lot of sound options on the menu. Maybe you could get ready just what you know you need to remain on track as opposed to having enticing foods on the menu that are not a piece of your arrangement. Plan to serve a few foods that you enable yourself to eat, so you don't feel denied.

If planning an occasion at your home is excessively unpleasant or is an over the top allurement with food planning, propose that another person have the occasion. Thoroughly consider it—what will be better for you? If you do have the occasion at your home, do you trust you can control things better? Make sense of this. Have an arrangement in any case. Here are some self-disclosure journaling questions that may assist you with seeing progressively about your association with food at get-togethers.

HOLIDAYS AND FAMILY FESTIVITIES

Holidays can be a challenge for us all. There is one holiday for each month in America—and maybe more if we incorporate strict and ethnic occasions. For some families, occasions, for example, weddings, commemorations, birthday events, and reunions are events celebrated with food. Thus, with regards to eating out, at any rate once per month, we have the chance to be tested in the good dieting division. Where do we start? You have to tune in to your positive self-talk, know, prepare, have techniques set up and inhale each day—or you could be in a tough situation. Possibly you sense that you are now in a tough situation. It's OK—take it each day in turn, and you can deal with these events. Your packed food schedule didn't occur without any forethought. Be caring to yourself and work through this diary; keep it with you and use it! Take the entirety of your systems for eating out and apply them to holiday and family festivities too.

Plan ahead and choose what you will do together, not to try too hard. On the event, ensure you have a sample of everything if you wish. Simply don't surpass your everyday food consumption plan. Maybe you have a most loved occasion or family food. Appreciate it, however, balance it inside your day or choose to practice more to redress. Discover some help, focus on partition size, tune in to your self-talk, and change it if essential. Hold returning to mindfulness and your systems. Remind yourself about your objectives, why you need to be sound.

GET-AWAYS

Being away from home resembles eating out three times each day, so survey your techniques in this part, "Why You Eat." When you are on an excursion, utilize a meal plan that ensures you remain a similar weight or keep up your weight. Be savvy, healthy, be sound, and be effective! How and what would you be able to design? Here are some explicit get-away techniques to increase the ones we have just secured:

- Plan ahead and find out about the foods that are in your movement region.

- Be safe with foods! Counsel your nearby trip specialist and your well-being facility about risky foods in underdeveloped nations.

- On the street, bring a cooler and fill it with healthy food and snacks–organic product, squeeze, and hacked up veggies.

- When in an inn or motel, approach early for a kitchenette; inquire as to whether your room has a microwave and cooler.

- At your goal, go to prescribed nearby food markets for sound tidbits and feast fixings.

- Ask if the kitchen in your inn, motel, or resort highlights solid menu options.

- Eat with some restraint

EMOTIONALLY SUPPORTIVE NETWORKS: GETTING ENOUGH AIR

Having individuals who bolster you is significant with regard to your weight, the executives, and dealing with yourself. This emotionally supportive network gives positive consolation while simultaneously keeping you responsible. Here are a couple of general thoughts regarding how emotionally supportive networks work. Individuals in your care group ask how they can best help you in the challenges you face with eating and food. Bolster individuals don't chasten you or treat you gravely when you have had an awful food experience; rather, they tune in, offer proposals, and ask how they can help you later.

At different occasions, you may require your care partners to be firmer with you than on different occasions. Be clear with them ahead of time that you depend on them to help you in specific manners and not in others—speak with them and reveal to them what you need. Together, you and your care partners can have any kind of effect. Try not to control your helpful individuals. They are there for you. I realize it can happen because I have done it—I've controlled somebody who was attempting to help me so as to get what I needed temporarily. Luckily, it didn't work since I could have endangered my objectives to practice good eating habits.

Monitor what works for you. Every individual has an alternate approach, and every individual has various needs. Some like help to be conveyed delicately, however solidly; others acknowledge productive encounters, inspirational talk, and fervor. Still, others favor severe support. You choose what you need right now and be adaptable enough to transform it as your needs change.

SUPPORT FROM HOME

Specifically, our home support depends on the individuals who live with us and are generally acquainted with our needs and difficulties. If your emotionally supportive network is comprised of relatives or individuals who live with you and are not exactly alluring, it is imperative to chat with these individuals. Tell them how glad it would make you if you had somebody on your side to help you. If you have individuals who need to be on your help group, but are really are out to attack your prosperity, you might need to constrain your time with those individuals until you feel less enticed to bargain your arrangement and increasingly enabled to stay with it.

Maybe you live without anyone else. Who else could give home help? A few thoughts for help individuals who don't live with you but who know about your home life may be a nearby family member, a companion or colleague, a parent or kin, your neighbor, a rec center accomplice, your fitness coach or weight reduction advocate, or your chiropractor or specialist.

Here are a couple of ways your home emotionally supportive network can work successfully:

- When you are enticed to have foods that are not part of your program, food sources that you have distinguished as being hazardous, or if you figure you may start to gorge on food, your help people will be aware of those perils and inquire as to whether they can do or say whatever would assist you with moving beyond this scene. For instance, they may help with an interruption system to assist you with forgetting about food.

- When you feel enticed by foods, converse with your helpful individual immediately and request that the person help you. Try not to anticipate that that individual should think about what you are thinking or police everything you might do.

- Ask your help individuals to move high-hazard foods to a zone you are ignorant of or that is difficult for you to reach.

- Suggest that your care partners do not eat high-calorie foods before you, or if nothing else inquire as to whether it OK to eat before you.

- Support individuals ought to be urged to inquire as to whether you need some rousing consolation to deal with your eating program. Maybe they could help you to remember your objective to eat good food, deal with your weight, and not feel caught or worried about your food decisions.

SUPPORT AT WORK

Do you have an emotionally supportive network at work? If you invest a great deal of energy at work, you will require support there similarly as you need at home. If you feel great doing as such, request that individuals at work assist in bolstering your good dieting objectives. Work can be a hazardous situation if there are colleagues or individuals in your work environment who are not on a similar wavelength as you in attempting to practice good eating habits.

Some colleagues or companions will need you to eat as they do with the goal that they don't feel so terrible about what food and well-being decisions they are making. If so, enroll some collaborators to help you. Likely, they will perceive these as difficulties for themselves, and you may find that you will shape a common bolster group. With mindfulness, eagerness, procedures, positive self-talk, and a decent, emotionally supportive network, this could be your key to progress!

At work, your help individual or group is there for you. Like your help individuals at home, these supporters don't chasten you or hate you when you have had a terrible involvement in food. Rather they ask how they can support you. They get you persuaded, keep you propelled, and cheer you on if that is the thing that you need. They remind you how significant your objectives are.

When you are going to eat something that isn't in the arrangement and is unfortunate, speaks with your help individuals: request that they help you, don't simply accept it's their accountability to comprehend what is happening in your mind. Your help individual would then be able to assist you with maintaining a strategic distance from the circumstance. Maybe they will help with one of your interruptions to get you away from food. Perhaps they will help by moving high-chance foods to a territory out of your sight and reach. Your work bolsters individual or group will be delicate to eating high-hazard foods before you. They can investigate with you a few inspirations to keep to your arrangement and objectives to be successful.

If your emotionally supportive network at work is not exactly alluring, maybe it is essential to converse with them. Tell them how glad it would make you if you had somebody on your side to help you. If you have an emotionally supportive network that is out to attack the entirety of your prosperity, you might need to constrain your time with those individuals until you feel progressively good about being around them in circumstances where enticing foods are being served. Keep occupied with work and ventures until you feel increasingly sure about this.

If there are no genuine help applicants in your work environment, attempt other people who could bolster you where you work. Is there somebody that you believe works near your office? Is there somebody that you constantly see during noon? When you do discover some help in your workplace, monitor what works for you. Every individual has an alternate approach, and every individual has various needs. You choose what you need and change it to fit.

Here are a few methodologies that you and your work environment support group can do together to help one another:

- Keep occupied with your work. It is imperative to keep centered and abstain from pondering food.

- Plan your snacks with your breaks; bring solid snacks and snacks from home.

- Always eat from your work area.

- Drink water during the day and have your water bottle full.

- Resist the impulse to keep desserts and snacks on or in your work area.

- Get up and stroll around if you are situated throughout the day!

- Challenge the workplace to choose progressively nutritious tidbits and suppers.

- Switch to more advantageous choices for office birthday, move, or retirement festivities—for instance, attempt a natural product flan as opposed to a chunk cake with thick icing.

- Ask if the sound tidbits can be placed in one organizer and less nutritious bites sorted out in another cabinet that you won't go into.

- Get the workplace roused to begin strolling at noon.

- Encourage others to pursue your propensity for taking the stairs as opposed to the lift.

If your working environment doesn't present specific difficulties—that is incredible—however, imagine a scenario in which you move to a new position in an alternate office or even to an alternate organization. You could wind up in an alternate working environment dynamic later. I suggest that, regardless, you answer the inquiries beneath in this diary, move a portion of those plans to your Journal, and afterward occasionally, particularly if your work environment changes, survey what is essential to you and what works. You may decide to impart a portion of these plans to your work environment, or if you have framed a shared help group, you may jump at the chance to examine a portion of these thoughts together.

If they feel that it is sheltered to do as such, a few people will converse with the individual who is persistently pushing food and clarify that this conduct might be hazardous for others attempting to control their food consumption. To evade that individual, you can eat in an alternate zone, make outside lunch arrangements, or get things done outside the workplace. If an experience is unavoidable, consistently be lovely to the food pusher. For instance, when I wound up in an office with an individual who was continually pushing food on others, I kept my plate loaded with solid food sources and pleasantly stated, "Not this time—I have something as of now."

Much the same as the systems you use at home, interruption strategies can be essential to assist you with enticing or testing foods and food circumstances at work. Contingent upon your particular work, you may have the option to fit a portion of these interruptions into your workday. Here are five classifications that may support you:

1. Things that should be possible rapidly during work:

    - Take a restroom break. Enjoy your reprieve early and appreciate the nibble you arranged.

    - If you are responsible for reusing and need to clear the little containers, do it now.

    - If you have to go to verify the mail or drop something in another office, do it now.

2. Busy exercises during work—things that will absolutely remove your psyche from food or occupy a ton of time:

    - Engage in any venture that requires close scrupulousness.

    - Set a motivation for your next gathering or review the minutes from the last gathering.

    - Work on your yearly report.

    - Contact customers.

3. Things you can do on breaks at work:

- • Go for a walk.

- • Walk the stairs.

-

- • Run a task.

- • Balance your checkbook.

4. Things that are unwinding during breaks:

- • Take a breather outside.

- • Go into the meeting room if it's empty and unwind.

- • File your nails.

- • Go to your vehicle for a rest and have somebody call you in a short time after your break is finished.

5. Things you can do with others or with others around you:

- • Plan the workplace softball match-up.

- • Plan the staff BBQ.

- • Organize the following office philanthropy occasion.

- • Start an office book club, sports lottery, or class arrangement.

When you have a challenge with food and eating at work, choose which classification will fit into your work routine. Select one of the exercises to finish, and if you need more interruption, then proceed with choosing another action. You may find that you can consider just a couple of interruption classifications in view of the sort of work that you do. Maybe your classifications are, for the most part, fit to exercises that you can do during snacks or breaks. That is fine—simply record pragmatic interruption techniques that fit you and your work environment. If you telecommute, you will have some extraordinary interruption thoughts from those you would have in an increasingly traditional office circumstance. Whatever your work environment, if food and food circumstances are a test, be set up to plan your very own interruption classifications. This strategy works! You will occupy yourself from considering food so you can continue ahead with your work—and conceivably proceed onward to greater and better things.

COMPANIONS AND SUPPORT

Companions can be an extraordinary help—or they can be an issue. A few companions can be exceptionally strong, while different companions can need you to remain unfortunate, so they have somebody to be undesirable with. Try not to confuse support with compassion. Try not to believe that, by sharing food, you are getting support; you could wind up becoming involved with another person's pity party. That isn't the target. If you get great help from companions and are a decent help to other people, you would be shocked how well you will do. I comprehend there will be days that you won't give or get impeccable help; however, quiet yourself at the time and consider your self-talk. Gain power by utilizing your Distraction Techniques. Remind yourself why it is imperative to be solid. Get support from companions and, thus, be a mentor and an incredible model! If your emotionally supportive network is not exactly attractive, maybe it is significant in any event to converse with your companions and let them realize how glad it would make you if you had somebody on your side to help you in arriving at your objectives. If you feel that your companions may unknowingly or incidentally damage the entirety of your endeavors to control your food admission, you might need to constrain your time with them until you feel progressively great around circumstances where you might be enticed to surrender your program. Try not to control companions' help. They are there for you. More than family or work connections, companions might be the most powerless to our controls on the grounds that, out of kinship, they need to satisfy us and not feel they have over-ventured the limits of good kinship. There are uncommon difficulties in requesting that companions bolster you—be delicate and know about them! Yet, additionally, know about the endowment of a companion's help; it might be the most valuable blessing you claim or can give. Do you and companions consistently assemble around food? When you are with companions, keep occupied with exercises and activities that don't include food until you feel progressively sure of remaining in charge. Plan getting together after supper or for espresso. Make the most of your kinships, yet additionally, recall the agony related to eating undesirably as opposed to breathing simpler about your association with food. Keep your fellowships invigorating and steady!

IN CONCLUSION

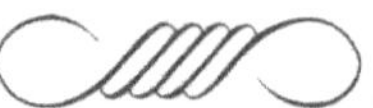

Here are a couple of definite instances of techniques and indications to support you on your voyage to a healthy wellbeing while successfully managing emotional eating:

- Unless you have a lot of weight to lose and you can't traverse with the dress you have, hold on to purchase smaller attire until you arrive at your objective.

- Alter some exemplary pieces you effectively possess until you accomplish your objective weight, or relying upon how a lot of weight you intend to lose, purchase just a couple of outfits to endure this progress time until you arrive at your objective.

- Get free of your bigger apparel. Give the garments or put them in a recycled shop or transfer store. Get a portion of your garments there too—you may locate some awesome outfits there while you change to your objective weight!

- For inspiration, experience your wardrobe and compose your garments from the biggest size to the littlest size. Mess around with your storeroom as you progress through the sizes from enormous to little. Make certain vestments small objectives.

- Hang outfits that you are practically prepared to fit into before your room entryway, so you physically need to stroll past them in the first part of the day and night. These "objective outfits" will help you to remember what you are doing.

- Write notes containing positive self-talk and certifiable articulations. Stick them everywhere throughout the house to remind yourself about your objectives. Compose your objectives on the notes too.

- Wear marginally more tightly fitting garments to remind you all the time that you have to eat better to quit being awkward. Indeed, even go to the extraordinary of putting on a somewhat tight swimming outfit under your apparel for the day to keep you propelled. When you get too agreeable is the point at which you are bound to eat inaccurately. This is works, however!

- Picture yourself 5 or 10 pounds lighter—or 20 pounds lighter! Go to the supermarket and buy a 5, 10, or 20-pound pack of potatoes and put them in a knapsack. If your back will permit it, convey this potato-filled pack around for a day. Feel the help by the day's end when you remove that rucksack. See what shedding those pounds can feel like? Pounds not lost distinctly to be found once more—you've freed yourself of those pounds for good!

- Visualize yourself in your ideal weight. What will your body feel like at that point? Your body will feel extraordinary. Indeed, even 10 pounds has an effect. Thus, eating great and doing activities will make you feel much improved. If you are keeping up your objective weight. Imagine your feeling of success as an individual who can smile at your relationship with food.

Motivation, amazing thoughts, positive energy, and a general feeling of well-being are the prizes of utilizing the Strategies and techniques delineated in this book. You just have to envision yourself at your objective weight and realize that you are the creator of your own success story. By what means will your apparel fit? What will it feel like to settle on healthy food choices? How empowering is it to feel that you are not just settling on savvy decisions with regards to food and eating, yet that these are your decisions! Don't give up! Don't relent! I will be cheering and rooting for you!

EMOTIONAL EATING

How To Develop Healthy And Guilt-Free

Eating Habits

INTRODUCTION

A good number of us have a general, rationale feeling of what to eat and when—there is no lack of ideas regarding this matter. However, there is regularly a distinction between what we know and what we do. We may have the facts; however, making choices must involve our emotions. Numerous individuals who battle with emotional struggles likewise struggles with an eating disorder. Emotional eating is a well-known term used to describe eating that is affected by emotions, both positive and negative. Emotions may influence different parts of your diet, including your inspiration to eat, your food choices, where and with whom you eat, and the speed at which you eat. Emotions incite most overeating as opposed to physical hunger. People who battle with obesity will generally eat in light of how they feel.

Be that as it may, individuals who eat for emotional reasons are not frequently overweight. Individuals of any size may attempt to get away from an emotional encounter by engrossing themselves with eating or by fixating on their shape and weight. Here are a few instances of what emotional eating may present as:

- Snacking when you don't feel physically hungry or when you are full

- Feeling an exceptional longing for a specific type of food

- Not feeling satisfied in the wake of eating satisfactory measures of healthy meals

- Restlessly picking more foods/snacks while your mouth is full

- Feeling emotionally calmed while eating

- Eating during or following a distressing encounter

- Numbing your feelings with specific foods

- Eating alone to maintain a strategic distance from others seeing you.

People who eat for emotional reasons frequently eat trying to self-alleviate or to find short-term relief from emotional trauma. A few people eat certain kinds of foods as a psychological approach to adapt to pressure. Emotional eating is identified with emotions of deficiency or inadequacy. Feelings may appear to be serious to the point that we believe we have to cope with them by getting away with choice meals, or we may feel we need other means to cope with emotional stress.

Consider your experience over the years. Do you experience valid or long-lasting relief while eating? Or on the other hand, is the relief temporary or halfway at the best-case scenario? Similarly, when we impulsively sit in front of the TV, drink liquor, or shop, we may wish to escape through eating. In later sections of this book, I will discuss some tried and tested methods to adapt to stress. In this book, you will figure out how to understand and deal with your emotions with the aim of feeling less averse to or overwhelmed by your feelings. These important tips will guide you into having perfect control over your eating habits as well as your emotions. However, you must take time to understand the problems before understanding how to pick the best solution that will work for you. Allow me the privilege to walk you down the path of guilt-free, emotion-free healthy eating habits!

CHAPTER ONE
UNDERSTANDING EATING DISORDERS

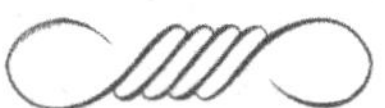

Emotional eating isn't a particular eating disorder worth losing your peace of mind over; however, emotional eating happens in eating disorders. Emotional eating is related to obesity, binge eating, and bulimia. You might or might not have an eating disorder, yet every now and then, I will refer to eating disorders to delineate the manners in which emotions influence eating disorder conditions.

To begin, I'll quickly explain how the Diagnostic and Statistical Manual of Mental Disorders—Fourth Edition (DSM-IV-TR) explains eating disorders. Anorexia includes over-evaluation of shape and weight. Individuals who battle with anorexia characterize their self-esteem to a great extent based on their weight. In this disorder, people keep an unusually low body weight (under 85 percent of average weight). To meet the criteria for anorexia, a lady must lose her menstrual period because of her dietary limitations.

Bulimia correspondingly involves an over-evaluation of one's shape and weight and inflexible struggles to control one's body size. Individuals who battle with bulimia intermittently "binge eat" or eat an enormous amount of food and experience loss of control at the same time. Notwithstanding binge-eating, individuals with bulimia participate in certain compensatory practices, or endeavors to "make up" for unnecessary caloric intake, by limiting their food consumption, intentionally inducing nausea, over-exercising, or abusing laxatives. Eating disorder not generally indicated (NOS) is the most widely recognized eating disorder. This classification depicts an eating issue of clinical seriousness that doesn't meet the criteria for anorexia or bulimia. For instance, a lady who is a heavy, however, ends up unreasonably engrossed with worries about her shape may meet the criteria for eating issue NOS. A man who is engrossed with his shape and restricts his food intake, but doesn't weigh under 85 percent of the normal human weight, would correspondingly get the eating disorder NOS diagnosis.

One type of eating disorder NOS is binge-eating disorder. Binge-eating disorder portrays intermittent binge-eating without extreme intentional efforts to control weight, and this issue regularly corresponds with obesity—however, it can likewise happen in individuals who are of average weight.

In contrast to anorexia or bulimia, which overwhelmingly influences women and young ladies, around 33% of individuals who binge-eat are males. We should pause for a minute to separate objective binges from subjective binges. An objective binge portrays devouring a considerable amount of food, joined by a sense of loss of control. An individual may consume a large number of calories in a sitting in an objective binge. An emotional binge includes feeling or thinking you ate excessively.

If you indulge yourself on Thanksgiving, this would be an emotional binge; if you ate what is normal on such a unique occasion, however, despite everything, you would have an inclination that you indulged yourself. Recognizing objective binges from subjective ones can assist us with starting to move away from seeing our practices in supreme terms or participating in pondering those practices. Feeling or thinking you ate an excess contrasts from losing control and quickly devouring unreasonable calories. Most eating disorders share specific center highlights, and numerous individuals who meet the criteria for one eating disorder wind up meeting the criteria for another eating disorder sooner or later. For instance, somebody who battles with anorexia may, in the long run, get a diagnosis of bulimia. For the most part, individuals who struggle with eating disorders over-evaluate their shape and weight and are strongly engrossed in fruitless attempts to manage their size. Binge eating likewise is prevalent among various diagnoses of eating disorders. Thoughtfully, this makes a lot of sense. If you characterize yourself by your weight, you may decide to restrict your meals, and limiting regular food intake brings about overeating, as your body's cells begin to feel denied of the required nutrients and energy to function. After a diet routine, individuals tend to indulge in foods and snacks they craved during the diet period. Individuals regularly likewise binge in light of negative states of mind or after having a stressful day.

EATING AND EMOTIONS

Individuals may either increase or decrease their eating rates because of stress. For instance, a few people experience an increase in craving when they feel discouraged while others experience a reduction. Restricting foods might be an approach to oversee feelings, as may binging. You may wind up reveling when you feel stressed out to calm yourself, and afterward placing yourself on harsh eating regimens trying to control your weight and your emotions. Psychologists conjecture that trouble in managing your emotions is the major issue behind both binge eating and bulimia. Binge-eating and different types of an unhealthy diet are regularly observed as social endeavors to impact, change, or control excruciating emotional states. Individuals who don't have an idea of how to manage feelings, either positive or negative, may depend on binge-eating, as well as cleansing, as an approach to oversee feelings. Anorexia is correspondingly determined by efforts to maintain a strategic distance from feeling any form of emotion. In particular, decreased awareness of emotions can happen in individuals with bulimia, and emotional shirking is normal for individuals who battle with anorexia. Emotions may influence eating in increasingly unobtrusive manners that don't enroll clinically. For instance, how many of us have plunged into a plate of cupcakes after a breakup or lost business deal? There is nothing amiss with appreciating good food during an unpleasant time; however, consistently relying upon food to deal with our emotions sends us the negative message "You can't adapt." Plus, what does a cupcake do to respect your emotions or to explain what matters to you? Research has shown that trouble recognizing and getting feelings, just as issues in controlling them, impacts gorging more than sexual orientation, food limitation, or exaggerating shape and weight do. At the point when individuals experience intense emotions or experience difficulty recognizing what their feelings are, they may feel they can't adapt to their emotions and may then attempt to keep away from the uneasiness by diverting themselves with food. You may see that you bounce from feeling any extreme emotions to eating, accordingly losing touch with your feelings. This may feel like a relief from the outset, yet it brings about your passing up on the chance to encounter the inclination for what it is (this is something you can work on doing effectively, as we will see in subsequent chapters). It is a must that we will encounter awkward emotions and reliably keep away from them, restraining our capacity to live with both wisdom and freedom. Specific individuals are all the more emotionally helpless, encountering feelings more strongly and feeling feelings for a more extended time than others.

If you are emotionally helpless and were brought up in a situation where you were not instructed how to adapt to emotions—or more awful, were rebuffed for showing your feelings—you may have figured out how to control emotions with food. When you experience a feeling and eat accordingly, you may encounter a normal feeling, just as different feelings that emerge because of emotional eating. Eating to numb your emotions doesn't completely assuage your emotions; instead, it only includes increasing mental (and caloric) weight to the experience. Likewise, if you eat because of your emotions, you may frequently neglect to value the message the emotions will teach you. Prominently, outrage and sadness are particularly identified with eating disorders; numerous individuals likewise see they will, in general, eat when upbeat, desolate, or restless.

Eating fried chicken may at first appear to be calming, yet overindulging in comfort foods when your emotions are unbalanced can give you significant emotional information, which will inevitably lead to disgrace and confusion. Food may likewise be utilized to increase the force of emotion. We may, for instance, use food to add to the standard experience of satisfaction, endeavoring to take our happiness up a notch.

Shirley, one of my clients, battled with an extraordinary bout of emotional trauma for a year. After a blend of intellectual, psychological treatment, and prescription meds, her state of mind improved, and she started to savor food. She depicted eating as relearning joy. At first, Shirley cherished exploring new wines and cheeses. In the long run, she chugged wines and ate cheeses, looking for an interminable divine understanding of what she tasted. Shirley had gone excessively far. A hyper insatiability exchanged for the straightforward delight of eating. The momentary advantages of turning into a cheese expert and an informal sommelier were presently being refuted by uneasiness and low self-esteem around her increasing weight.

CHAPTER TWO
ACCEPTING THE IDEA OF ACCEPTANCE

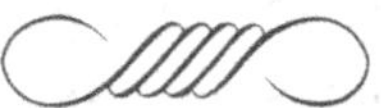

What is genuinely behind emotional eating? It is our reluctance to accept, or sit with, our feelings. However, when we eat for emotional reasons, we never really rid ourselves of our feelings. Or maybe, going into and tolerating our feelings is the entryway to opportunity and happiness, just as help from the cycle of emotional eating. However, this can be difficult to hear. Indeed, even my most charitable clients shiver when I state "accept" with regards to emotions and eating. Who wants to acknowledge difficult emotions or pain or acknowledge a burden that feels inadmissible? It can feel like I'm encouraging you to throw in the towel.

I submissively propose this procedure; a deep new worldview is a way into a new perspective and kinder association with food. Diets, food plans, blending and coordinating, enhancing, and denying may briefly help. Tolerating, minute to minute, is a long-term solution. A long way from being agonizing, acceptance is a type of graciousness: you recognize your facts and where you are at this time of your life. Will your weight go down as your psyche extends? Perhaps. Will your suffering decrease and become bearable? Truly. As you read further in this book, acceptance won't block change; rather, acceptance goes with change. Battling your body brings stagnation. Acknowledgment brings the flow into the best things life has to offer.

WHY DO WE HAVE EMOTIONS?

How about we step back for a minute and think about the various emotions we experience. Feelings give us a list of valuable information about our lives. The base of "feeling" is "motere," from the Latin for "to move." Emotions rapidly create changes in our mind and spinal cord to start an action—our conduct is frequently firmly attached to the feeling. An emotion is a precise signal that promotes survival instinct. Emotions spur our behavior, furnish us with significant information, and enable us to communicate with others in ways they will understand. How about we deliberate on two regular emotions and their functions. For example, say your partner becomes friends with an astoundingly alluring associate at your office, and you experience envy. Why? This emotion (envy) flags a risk, motivating us to plan ahead because our relationship may be in danger. At the point when we feel jealous, we are given information that our relationship is valuable and might be at risk. Our jealous disposition conveys our uneasiness to our partner; along these lines, envy guides us toward securing the relationship. If we eat to smother this feeling or to divert ourselves from it, we can't realize what the feeling is letting us know, and we can't respond in a fitting way, for example, communicating our emotions to our partner. Also, what is the incentive to feel cheerful? Bliss propels us to keep seeking after an action or esteemed bearing. The inclination gives data on what makes a difference to us. Satisfaction likewise conveys data to people around us, solidifying fundamental social securities. Would a friend be as excited to welcome you to a birthday dinner if you looked hopeless on the last occasion she hosted?

UNDERSTANDING ACCEPTANCE

Have you, at any point, eaten to cope with feeling fat? Time after time, individuals need to shed pounds and get baffled and somewhat frustrated when their weight reduction goals appear to go slower than expected. The process of weight reduction has become more like an ailment treatment than an experience to seek after. One may contend that obesity is a genuine medical condition, or eating for emotional reasons as opposed to hunger prompts, which may be hazardous. At the same time, would we energize an individual with disappointment to accomplish better psychological wellness by harping on how low his temperament is?

Or would we urge him to acknowledge his disposition—not in the soul of giving up on consistently improving, yet imaginatively and eagerly looking for unique arrangements? The idea of this continuous voyage requires continually coming back to an acceptance of self and mishaps and new challenges. The beginning of "acceptance" is the Latin for "to take." This is fitting because the best way to lessen the suffering is by taking the pain till you devise a means to living above the pain.

The fundamental equations are:

Pain = Pain

Pain + Non-acceptance = Suffering

Acceptance isn't abdication. It doesn't incorporate enjoying or approving the pain process. Yet, if "acceptance" is making you tingle, you may supplant it with a term like "extensiveness." Acceptance is deliberately receiving an open, nonjudgmental, responsive position, in any event, when faced with a challenge. This incorporates tolerating our feelings, contemplations, sensations, body shape, and reality, all in all, similarly for what it's worth at this time.

Non-acceptance—battling reality or our feelings—constrains our mindfulness and expands our struggles. Envision clutching one part of a scarf as I clutch the opposite end. If the scarf symbolizes your weight, what is your relationship with it? It is safe to say that we are loose as we hold the scarf together, or is there strain—would we say we are pulling in inverse ways? For a minute, consider the physical and emotional experience associated with a tug-of-war. It hoards our attention and vitality. Is it justified, despite all the trouble?

What is the other option? We could relinquish the fight, dropping the pull and opening our hands to receiving more energy. If we are eager to take an interest just in circumstances that give us great vibes, what will our life about? When we are reluctant to acknowledge our existence, we radically reduce our available options. That being stated, we can decide how to meet and acknowledge circumstances.

Acceptance, in a sense, is about empathy and dignity, not masochism. It is mind-boggling and dynamic—a continuous arrangement of decisions that relate our musings and activities to our profound qualities. Qualities depict what profoundly matters to you or what you need your life to represent. You may decide to acknowledge participating in a difficult relationship with a friend or family member if doing so identifies with your estimation of supporting your friends and family ("I will visit Mom at Christmas and assist her with getting out the loft"), while additionally doing what you have to do to in the administration of your benefit of securing and thinking about yourself ("I'll remain at a lodging, so I have my own place to go to if things start getting harsh").

If you can acknowledge the reality of a circumstance, instead of trusting or fantasizing things will, by one way or another, be different this time, you can take actions that respect the two sets of qualities. Correspondingly, you may acknowledge both your present shape and the emotional and social responsibilities required to transform it. You may acknowledge your emotions and, at the same time, change how you react to them. You don't need to acknowledge steady yearning and self-inflicted pains. Frequently, when we experience pain, we tend to get furious with others, accusing ourselves or responding indiscreetly. When our feelings trap us, it very well may be a test to back off and see whether our emotions are situated truly and whether our actions are serving our well-being and our qualities. Acceptance involves perceiving reality for what it's worth, non-judgmentally understanding the reasons for this reality, and drawing in with it instead of battling against it. Acceptance implies powerful seeking practices instead of stalling out in decisions with respect to what is "correct" or "wrong," "reasonable," or "out of line."

RADICAL ACCEPTANCE

Radical Acceptance is a functioning procedure involving being available to the experience of what is at every minute. "Acceptance without duty is a shallow triumph, and responsibility isn't practical without acceptance." Acceptance is mental and social, including tolerating with both our brain and our activities; tolerating our world altogether—the main extremely viable type of acceptance is called radical acceptance. It is hard to acknowledge what is at the time altogether; be that as it may, just incompletely tolerating our world won't support our torment. Envision that you "acknowledge" your relative. However, when you see her, you unremittingly consider how terrible she is as an individual. What does this kind of acceptance achieve? You may mentally acknowledge her; however, despite everything, you feel tense and pushed when she's near, and you can scarcely remain to address her. If you unapologetically accept your present weight or shape, you are neither scowling when you look in the mirror nor surrendering to failing to address it. Acceptance implies seeing without judgment. This doesn't mean you are not permitted to have an idea like "I can't stand how I look"— it just means you can see it when you have it ("that is an idea"). This naming can enable you to have and see the idea without joining misery or disgrace to it. You don't stifle the idea, and you don't harp on it—you watch it come, and you watch it go. For this situation, you've made a conclusion, yet you didn't pass judgment—you simply saw it—and this dulls its sting and may likewise enable you to take a look at the substance of the making a decision about the idea. As you may envision, this is a training that nobody ever gets flawlessly—we are human—however, once you start doing it, it's consistently there and accessible for you to use as you are capable. Imagine yourself, once more, before the mirror. Acceptance additionally includes moving toward the circumstance with both an exacting and a non-literal stance of ability—maybe truly loosening up your neck and shoulders, smoothing your brow, and unfurling your arms as you look in the mirror. This can assist you with seeing the idea, "I can't stand how I look" without becoming tied up with it. There is an input circle between our physical stance and our cerebrum; once more, so as to push toward acceptance, it is essential to do as such with both personality and body. If your brain accepts something while your body tenses, flagging dismissal, would you say you are drastically tolerating your existence? The accompanying action will give you practice in seeing the connection between your body and your mind with regards to acceptance.

CHAPTER THREE
EXERCISE PROGRAMS AND DIETS
WORKING TOGETHER

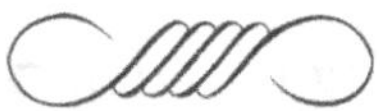

Throughout the years, I have remained friends with a considerable lot of my clients. It would astound you how, every now and again, they slip into the discussion some remark about being fat or humiliated or overweight. I recall one customer who had not physically met with me since she had recovered the weight she'd lost; she would just interface via telephone or by email. Goodness, we both felt like disappointments for various reasons. She felt she'd neglected to keep up her weight reduction, and I felt that I hadn't adequately met her mentoring needs. It was agonizing for the two of us.

This is the reason I composed this book: to decrease the pain in our relationship with food. Much of the time, the main question individuals ask me is, "Which program or diet functions admirably with results showing within a few weeks?" The appropriate response is straightforward. Journaling your experience is something that you can use related to any food or exercise program, and it will improve your goals. Regardless of what program you are following, since it is sound, it will work; please go for it and break the bad habits. Today, there is a variety of phenomenal programs and diets accessible to suit the necessities and desires for nearly everybody. They change contingent upon the individual and the particular needs of the person. Before

"

beginning any food or exercise program, it is basic that you check with your doctor or your local wellbeing authority. If you have any wellbeing concerns, you should counsel with your primary care physician to guarantee which sustenance or exercise program is for you. You can likewise counsel your locale wellbeing authority; inquire as to whether they offer any programs in food direction or advising. A few programs do all the arranging and thinking and cooking for you. That sort of controlled diet is the thing that a few people need. In these programs, feast arranging and sustenance preparing come later in the program as the customers quit utilizing the readied menu and prepare dinners for themselves.

Different programs require a more elevated level of customer inclusion from the earliest starting point, figuring out how to design and prepare suppers. Still, other diet programs use a blend of thoughts and methods with fluctuating degrees of dinner arranging and food preparing. As far as I can tell, regardless of what a program offers, there is only enough accentuation on the upkeep part of the program. While customers accomplish transient satisfaction through weight reduction or legitimate conditioning for their body, an excessive number of individuals think they have every one of the appropriate responses and leave the program with practically zero help. The outcome: their weight immediately rebounds. I know; I have seen it too often. There is an inquisitive incongruity here. Indeed, they do have every one of the appropriate responses. However, memory can be short, and old propensities can crawl back. Procedures and systems for program support can gradually start to bomb as memory blurs. Is it safe to say that we are impeccable? No. Would we be able to get ourselves before things go sideways with our weight? Totally! Breathing devices, as a self-disclosure instrument, encourages us to remember the strategies we have learned and to incorporate them to the point where they supplant old habits.

OBJECTIVE SETTING: WHAT'S IN IT FOR YOU?

All through my counseling profession, when I have moved toward the subject of objectives and defining objectives, customers have over and over made statements like, "I can't envision what arriving at an objective will resemble. I can't see past my stomach, don't worry about it the promising finish to the present course of action." Some objectives are only too far away for individuals to envision. Since you are getting into the swing of things, how about we get into the point. It is fantastic to have objectives—a guide of what we need to accomplish.

Here are a couple of tips for fruitful objective defining:

Make the objectives achievable. Maybe characterize transient objectives for the present—until you can see that famous promising finish to the present course of action. Why? I have seen many customers define an enormous objective for themselves, such as being a sure weight for their wedding.

What's more, when the wedding has gone back and forth, so wants to keep endeavoring to keep up that weight. To maintain a strategic distance from untimely deserting of an objective, ensure that, when you are drawing near to achieving one objective, you set another one for the prompt future. While you're grinding away, set an objective for the removed future also. Record your goals. Update your diary as you arrive at an objective or need to change your objective.

- Goals don't need to be about a specific number or accomplishing a particular weight. They can be close to home objectives.

- Reduce your waistline with the goal that you can tie your shoes on the top to bowing from your midsection as opposed to holding your leg to the side!

- Be comfortable in your present belt and not have it hit your sides.

- Have the jeans that are too short, really get some length to them—bafflingly! (As individuals lose or put on weight, the trouser legs don't abbreviate or extend. Individuals simply round them out increasingly, taking up more texture, so apparently, the jeans are shorter. When you get in shape, the texture isn't taken up to such an extent, and evidently, the jeans get longer.)

- Adjust your belt one step littler.

- Snore less.

- Get into the next smaller dress size.

CHAPTER FOUR
WHAT'S FOOD DOING FOR YOU?

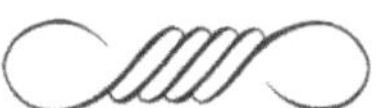

WHY WE EAT

The reasons we ought to eat are for sustenance and for fuel; in any case, we eat for numerous different reasons. We eat as a result of what our way of life lets us know is correct and appropriate behavior, and on account of exercises and thought patterns we learned in youth. We eat to fulfill social desires, without really thinking, because of feelings, for comfort, and to fulfill longings. We eat because we are enticed by the smell, taste, surface, look, and inviting nature of the served food. We eat to satisfy our creative mind, for self-satisfaction or discipline, and from impulse. Our essential purpose behind eating ought to be that we are hungry, having arranged our fuel admission to help with the exercises for the afternoon. This is rarely the situation.

In the last decades, our general public has changed significantly concerning action. Regardless of whether it is physical or mental movement, life in our bustling society here and there implies appropriate sustenance is impossible. We are attempting to pack such a great amount into our days that physical exercise goes as a second thought. The outcome? If our admission of food is more noteworthy and higher in calories and fat substance than would generally be appropriate, and our physical movement is lower or even non-existent, the main path for our waistline to go is out! The changing occasions influence all ages. In numerous parts of the nation, our kids have physical training as a choice in their schools as opposed to a compulsory course. Cooperation in sports appears to drop off in adulthood with the essential game movement a ride in a golf truck or sitting in the stands.

Since we have such a quick-paced way of life today, innovators are attempting to make everything simpler to achieve, so we are even less physical in what we do. At work, leaving our work area becomes restrictive with our connections to PCs; the time of the remote-controlled everything keeps us on the lounge chair for everything from tuning hardware to diminishing the lights to opening the window ornaments. However, for every one of the machines of comfort, we're accomplishing more while we take care of solid life-decisions less. These bustling components change the purpose behind "why you eat" and the decisions you make.

If you proceed on this hamster wheel, you will wear out. So take a DEEP breath and set aside some effort for you! Arranging your day around your exercises, your food prerequisites, and offsetting those components with time to rest is basic. Equalization! This is significant for your association with others also. You have to inhale effectively!

What's more, that takes us back to the genuine explanation of "why we eat"— it is for food, fuel, and rest—all to advance the parity of our real needs with the goal that we can live healthily. When your body appreciates balance, you appreciate life—and the others in your life. This is putting on your own breathing apparatus first! We should investigate a portion of the thoughts you have about offsetting your existence with your food, your eating, your exercises, and your rest times. Generally, when we have balance in our lives, we discover time to accomplish different things that we like doing.

SOCIAL DESIRES—HOW WE EAT

The various lessons from our social roots regularly form our relationship with food. Previously, the desires encompassing food utilization were more characterized than they are today. Individuals from various societies have different standards concerning food utilization. Where you are brought up on the planet, what religion you practice, can affect social thoughts, for example, the right blends of specific foods, the animals and plants that might be utilized for food, the significance of the individuals you share your table with, feasting with suitable refreshments, social graces, who eats first, sharing food, which foods might be eaten with the hands and when utensils are fitting. Social standards and desires assume a tremendous job by the way you characterize your relationship with food.

Numerous concepts and sayings began years ago, at various times and in various circumstances. When we hear these thoughts, we have to ask where they originated from and what was happening at the time. Was there a war? Was there a lack of any food? Did individuals need to shroud food to endure? Were there eight kids, and the best way to get a significant piece was to stack up your plate or you didn't get any food whatsoever? As children, we heard:

- Clean your plate.

- Don't squander food.

- Bread and spread with each meal.

- Pasta and potatoes with each meal.

- There are starving youngsters on the planet, so you need to eat the entirety of your food.

- Always finish with a sweet treat.

- You won't leave the table until you have completed your supper.

How about we address the value that you wind up paying for overeating?

Clearly, your wellbeing is endangered! What does it take to change this conduct? Abruptly, you may end up in a wellbeing emergency that will push you from 'I need to change how I eat' to 'I need to change how I eat!' Imagine a scenario where you were in the emergency clinic and not ready to deal with yourself or your children or your family or your pets. Or then again surprisingly more dreadful, if a wellbeing emergency would end your life? What cost would you say you will pay? You choose. Again, it's about what you realized in adolescence and have brought into adulthood as self-talk. What are you educating yourself regarding food that you learned as a kid, and how might you modify those thoughts?

COMFORT FOOD

Do you recollect what pacified you as a kid around food and eating? I remember how I would sneak treats off of grandmother's table when she was beating the batter before cutting the treats. I can nearly smell the bowl of chicken noodle soup that my mother or grandmother offered me to help with a cold or an irritated stomach. There were times when my father took me for a dessert to keep me at ease while thinking about a soccer match that my group lost. Did you sneak turkey cuttings off the platter at the special seasons as I did when my grandpa was cutting the feathered creature? I remember how I would sneak some pie crust off mother's counter when she wasn't looking as she prepared the mixture to make a pie. The smell of turkey and stuffing makes me remember my home. The smell of crusty fruit-filled treat makes me feel all warm inside, similar to a kid at grandma's—sheltered and warm.

Do you have fond memories that associate food with comfort? These are normal emotions. Food gives us joy and satisfies our hunger. It is essential to understand what your result is concerning food. Maybe you never thought of it that way. Once more, dive profoundly into your self-talk related to your relationship with food. When we speak about comfort food, what we truly mean is the food we eat to make us feel better when we feel pitiful or something has turned out badly in the day. It is food that will comfort us.

That is what our folks, grandparents, and grown-ups in our general public frequently thought when we were troubled: "How can I make you feel good? What about ice cream or chicken noodle soup...or hot cocoa?" Their consideration regarding us frequently came as food. Temporary comfort may originate from eating choice food; however, when we eat comfort foods in excess amounts or more every now and again, then our sound association with food decays and the blame and the negative cycle resumes. Mindful of the undesirable food decisions you've made and the sum you ate can prompt negative self-talk. You become disappointed over your inability to be fruitful with food. That is the point at which you start to deal with yourself, making statements like: "I'll simply begin once again on Monday...or next week...or one month from now." Eating solace food typically just sets aside a short effort to gain power. What amount of harm would you be able to do at this time?

GET-TOGETHERS

In the present fast-paced society, the expression "work hard, play harder" is by all accounts the standard. It is difficult to imagine a get-together without food and refreshments. The food business, from supermarkets to cafés, is intended to advertise food sources for each get-together from religious events to retirement parties, from Superbowls to chapel picnics, from private evening gatherings to Charity banquets. A major social event without food? Unimaginable, you would say, it isn't? Food and eating are customs fitted to get-togethers in our lives.

We hope to be properly fed when we play hard. In numerous societies, enormous and little get-togethers are not only defined by eating but by an excess availability of various food choices. Get-togethers are an opportunity to consider the types of food we are eating. It's an opportunity to consider our limits and our breathing space around the food that accompanies the occasion. It's an opportunity to set ourselves up to be aware of what decisions we can and should make about food.

Get-togethers are a major test for me! I frequently contemplate internally: "Free food...yummy. New plans and top choices I don't ordinarily have! Treats!" I get all energized—for a couple of seconds—then I return to strategies and boundaries that I have built for myself. I'll have just a sample of only one top pick, request the formula, and keep the social parts of the occasion as my core interest. I keep my hands full so that I won't be enticed to snack at the food.

Now and again, I have a mint before I stroll in the entryway, which will demoralize me from examining different foods. Or on the other hand, I eat before I go for any gathering, brush and floss my teeth, so I don't feel like I have to eat. I remind myself that the food does not deserve the struggle and pain to get the weight off or to feel wild. I remind myself how it feels to be in outfits that are my ideal size. I recollect the minute I put them on, and I feel like a million!

Almost immediately, distressing happens directly before the get-together that could factor into your choices. This is the point at which you will require your journal to help you to remember the motivations to remain on track and not let a person or thing influence your weight and your choices.

FOOD HABITS

A dietary pattern is something that we have become acquainted with doing, potentially out of routine or maybe even unwittingly. We routinely eat a few foods without a great deal of thought since it is simply programmed conduct. What is a food habit? It might be continually having potatoes with steak.

Or on the other hand, routinely eating bacon with your eggs or frozen yogurt with your cake. Without really thinking, you may consequently be adding salt to every one of your foods. These habits must be broken in a systemic way, not by forcing it or starving yourself. As they say, easy always does it!

FOOD REWARDS

Once I was in a dress store. I caught two individuals saying to one another that they merited a treat. Then they kept examining the sugary frozen yogurt and baked good treat that they got ready for themselves, portraying the foreseen food in such detail and with such eagerness that I hoped to check whether they were drooling. I was nearly drooling myself simply tuning in to them. Rewards don't need to be a sugary treat; it could be going out for supper and requesting what you wouldn't ordinarily request and afterward overindulging in that food too. We can treat ourselves every so often, however making food a reward is certifiably not a healthy habit. We have to concoct new thoughts regarding prizes and treats for ourselves. One of the genuine outcomes of utilizing food as a reward is that we can pass along with this negative behavior pattern to our youngsters.

SHOULDN'T SOMETHING BE SAID ABOUT YOUR METABOLISM?

In every one of the years that I trained individuals, I have always stumbled into many who didn't eat throughout the day—some of the time, holding up until 8 PM to have their first meal of the day. When individuals hold up until night to eat, they are upsetting their metabolism. They are either not eating enough regularly, or they may be compensating for it in a couple of days at the end of the week, or they are indulging each night because, before dinnertime, they are starving! Think about what befalls good judgment of your actions that occur when you are extremely hungry? It departs for good. You eat a great deal at the same time—and you feel qualified to eat anything you desire!

In this state, you are probably not going to settle on solid decisions. This is the most accurate explanation of why diet programs reliably caution individuals not to go shopping for food when they are hungry. The propensity is to purchase out the store and fill your truck with a ton of junk food and poor decisions since all food looks great! Would you be able to relate to that? So what job does your digestion play in why you eat? Think about your digestion as a fire in your body. If you put some fuel and paper on the ashes, a fire will start. If you continue including fuel and some littler logs, you will keep your fire consuming all through the entire day. During the night, or at whatever point you quit eating for a more extended timeframe, your body goes into a smaller than expected quick, and your digestion and processing will back off until you eat again in the first part of the day. That is the point at which you "break the fast" from the evening of not eating, hence what we call "breakfast."

So the sooner you eat at the beginning of the day, the more extended your digestion will work. The quicker your digestion begins toward the beginning of the day, the more productively you will utilize the food you have eaten to fuel your body. Your morning feast starts your digestion. In any case, it is essential to eat things that won't slow your digestion. A major heavy breakfast may not be shrewd. Rather, consider breakfast foods that you discover simple to process. All things considered, our assimilation needs to restart for the afternoon, so settle on decisions, for example, juice, yogurt, natural product, toast, and bubbled egg—foods that are gentler on the stomach.

If you don't eat your first supper until some other time in the day, that is the point at which your digestion will begin once more. Returning to my fire relationship, if you put on a major gigantic log—a major feast once per day by day's end—it will seethe and simply stay there. When leaving your food utilization until the day's end, two things can occur: you can be hungry to such an extent that you indulge, or you are enticed to devour all your everyday calories at one sitting. If you don't utilize that food vitality immediately, it gets put away as fat. Also, your digestion isn't working at its ideal. If you just eat once per day, your body will go into "fasting" mode, closing down for the evening and the daytime. Food is fuel for your body. You need great fuel, conveyed consistently, for your cerebrum to work appropriately. If you just eat once per day, either your body trusts you are fasting or shuts down, or your body trusts it is in starvation mode, and all food gets put away as fat. Tinkering with standard eating times undermines the manner in which the body should work. Eating 5–6 snacks or small meals a few times each day props up your metabolism.

If you are not acclimated with eating this regularly during the day, go gradually as you change your feast propensities. Ease into eating meals a few times during the day with the goal that you don't feel like you have tried too hard when you do eat. Cut back on your segments; space your dinners and snacks close to 3 hours apart. Much the same as those little bits of wood on the fire, littler measures of food eaten 2–3 hours apart keep your digestion working perfectly—and it starts toward the start of your day with that very significant dinner we call breakfast.

Don't overdo it; even a bit of dry toast in the first part of the day is superior to nothing. Later toward the beginning of the day, when you are more in a hurry, some wheat wafers with nutty spread would be a smart thought.

Here's an example day of what eating 5–6 little dinners and bites may resemble: Breakfast Whole wheat toast with jam.

- Snack: Whole-wheat wafers with some nutty spread.

- Lunch: Grilled chicken in a small plate of mixed greens with a balsamic vinegar dressing and a side of new natural product cuts.

- Snack: Yogurt with cut almonds and raisins.

- Dinner: Roast hamburger with pasta presented with a steamed veggie and an organic product cup.

- Snack: Celery sticks with light cheddar and an apple. (Note that I haven't put sums adjacent to the food things in this model.

Individuals will have distinctive vitality needs relying upon their movement, age, body type, sex, digestion, and wellbeing concerns). Notice I have put a protein—in this model, nutty spread, chicken, yogurt, nuts, hamburger, and cheddar—with pretty much every dinner. The explanation is because we digest sugars—organic products, vegetables, slices of bread, wafers, raisins, pasta, and so on first; then, we digest protein. We digest fats last; in this model, fats are a portion of the nutty spread, a plate of mixed greens dressing, a few sauces, margarine, meat fat, cheddar, and yogurt. By having a sugar with a protein, you get a transient vitality stretch and afterward have enough protein to last a couple of hours until the following dinner or bite. Plan out a day like what I have done above and report it in your journal.

Here's a recommendation: Set up a layout for your day like the one I have given you above and afterward swap out the foods every day. For instance, where I composed Lunch – Grilled chicken on a nursery plate of mixed greens with a balsamic vinegar dressing and a side of new organic product cuts, you can supplant the barbecued chicken with cuts of turkey or ground prepared hamburger for a taco serving of mixed greens or the meat with cheddar. You may supplant a nursery serving of mixed greens with cucumbers and tomatoes. You could substitute a light Italian dressing or a light cream for the balsamic vinegar. You get the image! You have the format for what you are eating; simply change the foods. This is only a proposal of how to begin; sooner or later, you will think of some more plans to have a fair day. (Bits will rely upon you as an individual and will consider the stage you are at in your weight program or wellbeing concerns. You can check with your food control, your eating regimen program, your exercise center, your locale wellbeing authority, your physician, or a neighborhood nutritionist for a progressively point by point rule.)

It is a great idea to have some gentle appetite signs just before you are expected to eat; this discloses to you that your digestion is working. Everybody is unique, yet some regular appetite signs are:

- Stomach protesting

- Cold nose, hands, and feet

- Slight crabbiness

- Slower response to things

- Decreased capacity to focus

- Drink water in the middle of dinners and bites - Water tops you off, yet water is significant for all parts of your body.

Water, water, water!

Much the same as the oxygen (O2) in your body, water (H2O) is fundamental for your organs, blood, skin, electrolytes, balance, and a large portion of all for consuming fat! Inhale, exhale, and relax! Slow down when you eat. It takes about 20 minutes for your stomach to tell your mind that you are full. What amount would you be able to eat in 20 minutes- in 5 minutes? The appropriate response is a ton! How to back off? Put your fork or spoon down when you are chewing. In the wake of gulping, get your utensils again and continue eating. Drink water between significant meal times. Take as much time as necessary chewing, savoring the taste your food, enjoy the different flavors and textures, and appreciate what you are eating—one piece after another.

CHAPTER FIVE
WHAT'S EATING YOU?

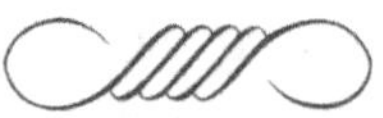

Knowing the various purposes for what you eat and what food is accomplishing for you was the subject of the last chapter. In this chapter, I will explore a portion of the reasons you eat. Recognize that what you eat might be pushed outside your ability to control by an assortment of variables. Beyond giving nutrition and fuel to your body, food is additionally associated with cultural, social, and social thoughts. Your food habits might be not quite the same as what your body and digestion require for ideal wellbeing.

Individuals are dependent upon passionate changes, testing circumstances, individuals, and conditions that make them go to food. For an assortment of reasons, yearnings and habitual practices may lose our control around eating. These elements—uniquely or in a blend—are genuine difficulties that can add to wild eating, which has nothing to do with fulfilling hunger or giving sustenance and vitality to our bodies. This piece of your self-revelation adventure might be especially uncovering, which is the reason I request that you give specific consideration to journaling your bits of knowledge and afterward moving your positive systems and ways to write a journal. Deep emotions encompass a significant number of our states of mind: stress, outrage, weakness, hunger, fatigue, pity, uneasiness, expectation, fervor, sadness, and delight. We, as a whole, encounter incredible emotions that can trigger passionate eating. What I mean by emotional eating is described by an out-of-control eating occasion that is utilized to battle, solace, or veil feelings that challenge our feeling of prosperity.

Put simply, emotional eating is bolstering your emotions, not your stomach. When you eat to fulfill something more than hunger, you are occupied with numbing pain or stress. A part of these behaviors can get neurotic—delivering such dietary issues as anorexia and bulimia—however, that isn't my core interest. Or maybe, how about we investigate a portion of the regular causes that a great many people involved in emotional eating. Feelings produce various responses in individuals; however, stress is, by all accounts, the most well-known factor in a poor diet. Stress can be communicated in an assortment of feelings and result in many harmful practices around food. Emotional eating can turn into your greatest test and even damage your weight reduction endeavors, so you must become mindful of what you are eating, yet additionally, why you are eating.

When you can perceive what is going on with your feelings and relate that to your conduct, you can modify what you are doing and defeat eating to fulfill awkward emotions. We all resort to eating for emotional reasons, yet when this turns into a primary focal point of our lives, which is the point at which the issue starts—we experience torment, battles, disappointment, and at last, weight gain. I had personal difficulties with enthusiastic eating: not minding what I ate when I got furious, irate, or tragic, eating out of weariness or dawdling. I ate when I was focused. Mindfulness and making an arrangement helped me escape the enthusiastic eating trench. I accept these two systems can help you as well, so relax! How about we take a shot at an arrangement!

When I have feelings that could lead me to eat wildly, I actualize the accompanying:

- Plan ahead for shopping for sound dinners.

- Plan to make additional foods early that can be solidified.

- Plan bites that have some assortment.

- Check my self-talk and alter it to be certain.

- Use my interruption systems to keep occupied.

- Eat little suppers and nibble 5–6 times each day.

- Slow down as I eat.

- Drink heaps of water, water, water!

Give myself the permission to have a few treats in minimal amounts and afterward change my day by day food admission: practice control as opposed to end.

EMOTIONAL DISTRACTION TECHNIQUE

Feelings can be strong to such an extent that we truly couldn't care less about our sound objectives any longer. It is essential to have an arrangement set up for when this occurs, so have your journal on you consistently. We don't create these feelings; they simply happen at the most awkward occasions. Any occasion can be ruined with a feeling that pushes you over the edge; outrageous feelings can drive you to settle on undesirable food decisions. What you need is something to remove your psyche from the feelings or worry until you can quiet down and settle on great food choices. Figuring out how to control your responses to profoundly charged emotions—regardless of whether it's satisfaction, pity, or weariness—and joining that control with a balance in your eating motivations will assist you with staying away from enthusiastic eating. During times when feelings brief you to eat or even gorge, ask yourself, "What is my motivation for needing to eat healthily?" This will help keep you spurred. Various programs offer an assortment of methodologies for turning away passionate eating. The system that has been effective for my customers has been an interruption strategy. The emotional distraction method starts with mindfulness. In the first place, list the classes of distractions that could keep you from emotional eating. Also, record exercises that relate to the classification that you think would help with diverting you from indulging as a reaction to enthusiastic pressure. Attempt to think of 4 to 5 great exercises for every classification that you would really take part in. Remember that, if the movement isn't appealing to you, what is the probability that you will expand your passionate eating? Keep it genuine for you!

Examples of classes of distractions:

6. Things that should be rapidly done at any time or place.

7. Your emergency distraction (which thoroughly removes your brain from food).

8. Things I can do while dressed up.

9. Things that are calming and relaxing.

10. Things I can do with others or with others present. A few instances of something that should be possible rapidly any place are:

- • Get the vehicle washed

- • Call a companion

- • Organize your day-clock or equalization the checkbook

- • Make game plans for a forthcoming occasion

- • Book a hair arrangement

- • Document your self-talk in your Journal

- A few instances of an emergency movement done any place would be:

- • Begin an art venture

- • Call your help person(s)

- • Organize a family carport deal

- • Repot your houseplants

- • Plan your youngster's birthday party

- • Go to the rec center

- • Get a nail treatment

- • Attend a game

This distraction process works a good number of times. When you have emotional difficulty, you choose which classification you need right then and there. Select one of the exercises in the classification that fits the condition and do that action. If you need more interruption, then select another action from that class. (Simply figure the amount you will achieve in your life when you are not doing enthusiastic eating!) Distraction methods remove your brain from food and grant you to jump on to greater and better things.

This urges you to settle on better choices and to like having that power. It additionally works you to inhale effectively in your relationship with food since you deliberately consider the circumstance. Knowing about your self-talk concerning your feelings can help you adjust self-talk if it is negative and settle on a savvy decision by maintaining a strategic distance from food or giving yourself authorization for control. You finish with power over your food admission and with an arrangement for the afternoon.

The following stage is to move your interruption classes into your Journal. Leave space to record new interruptions as thoughts arise for you. Take your Journal with you consistently, because we don't design these triggers, and the interruption arrangements you need will be readily available. That way, you remain on track, paying little mind to the time or spot. If you are finding that passionate eating is a major test right now, here is a progressively serious strategy for expanding your mindfulness and utilizing interruption methods. I consider it the envelope strategy and have thought that it was extremely successful.

Allude to the classifications you have distinguished and list everyone on the face of an envelope. Take bits of paper that will fit into the envelopes and record one interruption movement for each bit of paper. Spot that interruption action in the class envelope that compares with the movement. Convey these envelopes with you to assist you with traversing enthusiastic eating occasions; this is likely the most significant time that these interruptions work for you. I have utilized this envelope strategy with an assortment of individual difficulties. It works!

In the long run, you will move from the envelopes to your Journal. What's more, inevitably, you will do a diverting action; consequently, when an enthusiastic eating occasion comes around. You realize that you have the envelopes or your Journal to direct you—composed by you for you—helping you breathe easier about your association with food! Even better, place an additional duplicate in the ice chest or pantries to help keep you on track!

Home alone—that is presumably where we do the most harm to our eating plans and ourselves. When we are without anyone else's input, and in our very own homes, we give ourselves the authorization to eat any way. I know this as a matter of fact; when I have occupied with gorging, it has been in my home away from other observers. I felt truly senseless because I was acting like a child, avoiding everybody. It is miserable when individuals feel constrained to consume food hungrily. However, it occurs and is so harming to our self-esteem and to our prosperity.

What's more, a while later? The blame, shame, misery, and self-avocation that shows up in our self-talk isn't exceptionally beautiful, is it? Maybe, with our quick paced ways of life, we gorge significantly more in the protection of our own vehicles. Inexpensive food adds to the issue, yet it's not exclusively the fault for undermining our best eating goals. For instance, after grabbing some staple goods, we're frequently alone, and in the security of our vehicles, we enjoy eating anything we desire.

BINGE EATING IS THE ISSUE.

Binge-eating can prompt bulimia nervosa, a dietary problem for which there is no single recognizable reason. Gloom, eating less junk food, poor adapting aptitudes, and even hereditary qualities might be involved in gorging. Described by mystery and quick eating to the point of being awkwardly full, gorge eaters eat alone and regularly when they aren't ravenous. Regret and shame make bulimics cleanse their assortments of undesirable food by spewing or by utilizing intestinal medicines. If you are a gorge eater, what are you letting yourself know? "It doesn't make a difference any longer—I am a disappointment when it comes to food." If you state this, then it will work out.

If binging gets ceaseless in your life and you presume or have been informed that you have this dietary issue, you should look for help from a social insurance supplier: a specialist, analyst, or a doctor. There are numerous medications for bulimia nervosa. I encourage you to discover them. If you do have a passionate eating scene—since it will occur as it happens to us all—you can deal with it emotionally if you take some time, analyze the circumstance, and excuse yourself for settling on a poor food decision. It is essential to the point that when you understand that you committed a genuine error, or even basically decided to eat food to assist you with getting over awful or serious emotions, you should be sensible and take a look at your self-talk related with that occasion.

Hear what you are saying to yourself and change your affirmation if it is negative. Recognize to yourself that you settled on the choice to have that food and that you will alter your day by day food admission to be on track with your vitality needs. Say to yourself, "This isn't actually how I had arranged my day, yet I will change things for whenever and gain from this experience." Every opportunity that a test comes up, record it in your diary. Also, proceed onward. One scene is no major ordeal; it's a hindrance, much the same as we experience all through life! This move in frame of mind is significant on the grounds that, by being earnest and constructive, you've kept up your own capacity. Stunning, such control! You've accomplished another approach to breathe easier about your association with food!

A portion of the stress-related issues with emotional eating is our own evaluation of our appearance, our weight, and the advancement we have made in arriving at our weight objectives. The emotions encompassing these issues can prompt negative discernments about ourselves. Think of how you feel/felt at your heaviest weight. Keep in mind:

- What did your attire feel like?

- What is it like to stroll up five flights of stairs? Well, will you make it?

- Even without physical action, how was your breathing very still?

- Did you wheeze?

- What would you say it felt like to tie your shoes?

- Could you contact your toes?

- Could you see your feet?

- How did people look at you? Did anybody make remarks?

- Has your weight influenced your activity? Life? Family? Exercises with your family? Closeness?

- How much do you spend on food and liquor every day?

- How much weight have you gained over time? How does it feel to be of this size? Presently feel these feelings! Sit in them and accept the emotions. Pen them down and recollect.

Have you been there? Then you would understand better what it feels like! You can envision what arriving at your objective will mean. How is it going to be to slip into a smaller size of pants—feel absolutely great, thin and trim? Envision your skin is tight and sound. Envision your legs being more fit and conditioned than they have ever been! Picture yourself in a thinning swimsuit at your objective weight with a brilliant sparkle all over your body. Picture your body on the seashore and being agreeable in your skin. You can contact your toes, you can fold your knees up to your chest, and you feel incredible. You have the energy to save! You can complete five flights of stairs easily and still need to accomplish more! You don't wheeze any longer. You rest so refreshed and loaded with the vitality you ricochet up with a spring and a grin for the afternoon. You see, your objective is getting too enormous for you since you are conditioning your body and feel so fit. You are arranging your day's food, effortlessly, and fun. You have such extraordinary confidence and positive self-talk that you realize you can do anything you put your psyche to. You are resolved, and you have the entirety of your capacity! You are extraordinary! Furthermore, you have a sound body at your objective weight!

CHAPTER SIX
EMOTIONAL EATING AND CHALLENGING CIRCUMSTANCES

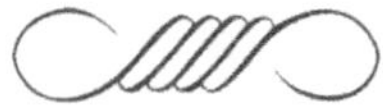

In life, we come across circumstances and individuals that can confuse us! Have you experienced a circumstance or a domain where you didn't feel good, however, needed to remain where you were? For instance, put yourself into this scene: a great friend welcomes you to a gathering. You show up and are making some great memories when your ex strolls in the entryway with their new date. Wow! The environment abruptly gets charged. You feel awkward and clumsy.

This circumstance with these specific individuals could send even the most secure individual into a portion of food or liquor free-for-all. Uplifted feelings and stress will make us "bargain" with the circumstance as well as can be expected, regularly adapting or soothing ourselves with food or potentially drink. The "fix" for our trouble may appear to be practically programmed; we need frantically to plan something to make us feel much improved. Be that as it may, over the long, all that we accomplish is that we've subverted our calorie admission for the afternoon. Contingent upon the degree of feelings and agony, the damage can keep going for quite a while. While the facts confirm that we have feelings related to cumbersome circumstances, we ought not to enable them to devastate our objectives and our arrangement for solid living.

Passionate responses are typical, and they alert us to our alternatives for activity. You can encounter the enthusiastic reaction, recognize that you have the feeling, and afterward ensure you manage it in a solid way. You can likewise recognize that in time, the misery that caused your enthusiastic reaction will scatter, and you will start to mend.

Similarly, as we wind up in moving circumstances with our relationship to food, there are additionally testing individuals that can push us over the edge. Maybe you know individuals who get resentful when you don't eat the entirety of a dinner they have arranged for you. Their reaction is to 'push' food on you, and your reaction might be to indulge. Another difficult individual is somebody who punches your catches or offends or focuses on you to the degree that you are disturbed to the point that you choose to adapt by eating or drinking. Food 'Pushers' can be steady, and you can create systems to manage them. You need to let them know courteously, "Forget about it," and not joke about this. If vital, you can include that you have been told to watch what you are eating for wellbeing reasons. Call your hosts ahead of time. Be open about saying that you have a lunch plan for the afternoon, and you know the dinner that they are offering doesn't accommodate your arrangement. You could offer to bring your own food, acknowledge their substitutions, or plan to land after supper. Plan your time there and have an out. Stand firm; you won't be compelled to eat what isn't in your arrangement.

Counsel your procedures in your journal before you go, have a positive psychological arrangement, and be solid. Keep in mind, by putting your own breathing apparatus first, you are better ready to think about yourself and afterward care for other people. The equivalent goes for the individuals throughout your life who continue pushing your catches. Attempt to constrain your time with them. If those individuals are jokesters, grin and giggle with them. Do whatever it takes not to pay attention to them as well. If they are hostile, considerately let them know along these lines, and afterward make an agile exit. Peruse your diary early and have an arrangement. Inquire as to whether you need to invest energy with these individuals. Be solid and don't give anybody a chance to destroy your day or your wellbeing! Try not to give anybody a chance to influence how you eat. Relax!

Once in a while, an assortment of components can meet up capriciously and upset our eating plan. We experience certain individuals in an unforeseen circumstance, and, all of a sudden, we're focused, and an enthusiastic eating or drinking scene is all of a sudden in our sights. You are presumably gesturing because you have thought of the individual, spot, feeling, and food that may consolidate to cause you trouble! Monitoring these difficulties and how they may emerge is extremely significant. For instance, would you be able to envision a circumstance that is typically fine, yet with the expansion of a difficult associate or the beginning of a dismal day, your reaction to food could turn into a debacle? Try not to leave it alone. Envision these mixes of variables; attempt to maintain a strategic distance from those circumstances, individuals, and negative self-talk until you have an arrangement!

LONGINGS AND IMPULSES

Having a longing and being eager to eat are altogether different things. A longing is that annoying feeling of needing a specific food or a specific taste in your mouth. Some of the time, our creative mind will stay at work past 40 hours to concentrate on that food, and afterward, we can wind up wanting that food throughout the day! Longings for food can develop whenever. Yearnings are not constantly negative— they can flag our body's lack of specific minerals, nutrients, or proteins.

They might be identified with our nourishing needs, or they may caution us to certain hormonal irregular characteristics, adrenal exhaustion, or even insulin obstruction.

All food yearnings, be that as it may, can turn into a negative in our general wellbeing when we react improperly to them. The outcome is that we harm our digestion, increment weight gain, and imperil our wellbeing. You ought to counsel a certified nutritionist or potentially your primary care physician if you have worries about longings and the impact they have on your digestion. What I need to talk about here are a few systems for adapting to and wiping out regular yearnings. There are two significant thoughts regarding desires.

In the first place, they don't have anything to do with self-control. Also, we have to focus on what foods we desire and how we react to them. Here are a few techniques to assist you with perceiving and managing food desires: Foods that have a solid flavor may make you want another food. For instance, tomato sauce, cream sauce, or zesty foods containing garlic may make you long for a portion of sweet food. This is because your sense of taste and tongue are loaded with taste receptors; the solid enhanced food may have a waiting taste, and you have to purify your sense of taste to get over it. Eating grapes, apples, watermelon, and cucumber can do this. You will be very shocked by the outcomes. Other non-food choices are to attempt a tongue scrubber to dispose of the taste, or brush your teeth or bite some gum. Some different longings are about texture. You may long for fresh or crunchy food; you may ache for delicate or smooth food sources.

If the surface of food is more important to you than the carbohydrate level, then you can choose cooking strategies that will give the ideal surface and still be a solid other option. For instance, if you want the smash of tortilla chips, which are high in starches, salt and fat, pick heated pita bread. Cut the round bread into reduced triangles and heat or flame broil for two or three minutes on a cookie sheet. This dries out the pita and makes it fresh—and it turns into a fantastic substitute. You could add a few flavors to modify the flavor, however, watch salty flavors, for example, garlic salt, onion salt, or flavoring salt. If you long for rich surfaces, give a portion of the new yogurts a shot. Peruse the marks for the sugar content; watch the fake sugars as well. A few yogurts have less fat. Plain yogurt can be utilized in cooking and in blend with crisp products of the soil. As the establishment for natural product smoothies, plain yogurt is unsurpassable.

Blending foods grown from the ground improves the yogurt normally as a result of the fructose or common sugars found in an organic product. Take a stab at solidifying natural products, for example, pineapple pieces, grapes, mandarins, and blueberries. Blended with yogurt, they are an awesome substitute for frozen yogurt. Eaten by themselves, these solidified natural products likewise will help scrub the sense of taste. A few people discover they have a craving for salt. If your eating regimen is excessively high in sodium or salt, it can influence your pulse, your cardiovascular condition (heart), just as influence your body's water maintenance and flow. If you, as of now, have difficulties in these territories, you ought to have direction from your doctor and a nutritionist. If it has been over a year since you had an audit of what foods and amounts of sodium are in your eating routine, you need a survey! Indeed you do! It is for your life! It is astute to know about foods high in sodium, regardless of whether you are solid.

Handled foods can be higher in sodium due to how these foods are made to give them a more extended time span of usability. Models are handled meats, canned veggies, canned soups, sauces, bundle seasonings, cheeses, prepackaged dinners, pickles, restored hams, canned fish, bacon, cold cuts, chips, wafers, and considerably more. Peruse the names and search for sodium in the fixings. There are some low sodium items available; make certain likewise to check those names. A few people long for counterfeit sugars. A portion of these are produced using modified amino acids—an adjusted amino corrosive is a protein building obstruct whose sub-atomic structure has been changed. The truth of the matter is, we have given sugar negative criticism! Sugar is OK with some restraint—when we don't revel in it!

If this sounds unnerving, it is. I am adversely affected by any counterfeit sugars, and, as a food instructor, I am frightful about what fake sugars are doing to the assortments of individuals who revel in them. Any fixing with 'ose' or 'ol' toward the finish of the word has a few characteristics of sugar. Peruse your fixings marks. Correspondingly, "palatable oil" items are healthfully bankrupt. I make some hard memories with those also. When we pick counterfeit anything, accept it as an image that we are altering our sustenance for the purpose of accomplishing a specific taste. Because artificial is regarded as safe, you truly need to consider this one.

Mindfulness is the way to managing desires and finding the starting points of them. We have to inquire as to whether we ache for specific foods, certain surfaces, or particular preferences. Controlling perilous desires might be as straightforward as utilizing distinctive planning or cooking systems, substituting various foods, or eating what we pine for with some restraint. If longings become overpowering, then you ought to consistently counsel a wellbeing professional.

TANGIBLE TRAPS: SMELL, TASTE, SURFACE, LOOK, RECOMMENDATION.

Before we even eat food, we are dependent upon an assortment of upgrades that can make us need food. We can smell food and see it and be enticed by it. We can envision the surface of specific foods—their crunchiness or their smoothness pulls in us. Only the memory of the flavor of food from the last time we ate, it tends to be a solid boost. Indeed, even another person discussing food can send us into emotions of want. I will always remember how, in the wake of directing around 16 individuals one day, I returned home needing shrimp and strawberries. Two of my customers had discussed those foods that day. It was an exceptionally odd proposal to hunger for them together, yet that was all it took for me to need shrimp and strawberries. I lived behind a pastry kitchen, and each morning, with the fragrance originating from that spot, I ached for doughnuts! I was nearly drooling as I got into my vehicle.

As a rule, when I drove away, the temptations passed; however, I will consistently recall the intensity of those fragrances. The smell of grilled meat does likewise for me. I always cherished how those things looked so heavenly, yet when I ate them, it wasn't on a par with I had envisioned. So I quit getting them. Presently, I can basically see them, recall my failure by the way they taste, and I don't have to eat them. The surface of certain foods—crunchy, smooth, or grainy—is sufficient to bait us into eating them. I used to appreciate a specific mousse yogurt because of its bubbly surface. The surface was so imperative to me that, if the yogurt mousse was knocked or dropped, so the air bubbles left it, it simply wasn't the equivalent, and I wasn't as keen on eating it. I feel a comparative dissatisfaction when I envision corn chips being delicate or stale. A few people like the texture more than they like the flavor of crunchy food. I love the smash of bread in a plate, garnished with mixed greens, however, put them in the ice chest, and they become unappealing—simply spongy bits of bread. Give your senses a chance to direct you to thoughts regarding food; however, know what it is— just a thought, not a proposal to hurriedly eat. Let the smell simply be that, a smell. Give the sight a chance to be only a decent view. Fulfill your craving for something sweet with new natural products. Solidified pineapple pieces work for me unfailingly. When you need food with crunch, attempt veggie sticks or make your very own prepared pita chips. Investigate different seasonings other than salt to enhance your foods. Most importantly, assess your desires inside the setting of your day's food plan. If you should yield to a hankering, settle on it a sound decision! Searching for a total tactile food experience? Have an orange. You cut into the strip with a blade and the juice showers softly on your lips, and you lick your lips and taste the sweet orange splash. Strip away all the skin and partition the natural product into the areas. Nibble into a piece and experience the crisp squeezed orange as it sprinkles your taste buds. It is so cold and sweet on your tongue.

Each piece is succulent to the point that it trickles down on your hand and onto your plate. Decent, isn't it! The demonstration of fulfilling your very own feeling of joy and surrendering to your food wants can compromise your day by day food plan. Do you live hazardously by eating what you see as taboo foods? You may laugh at this now, however, dive into the thought! As grown-ups, would we say we are carrying on what our folks or the grown-ups in our lives let us know was prohibited or incautious to devour?

Is it safe to say that we are silly? Or on the other hand, will I say incorrupt? What does it mean for us to eat or even revel in these foods? For instance, I cherished hot new pastry shop buns as a kid, yet was told, "No, you can't eat the entire sack!" Then as a grown-up, I enjoyed devouring an entire pack of those buns. Most adults wouldn't think about this a judicious or shrewd decision, yet I've done it! What's more, I realize that a significant number of my customers have done it or something comparative. Is it accurate to say that we are doing this because of resentment? Or on the other hand, since we are grown-ups, we can settle on these decisions if we decided to? Do you have confidence in self-satisfaction concerning food? Here's a critical inquiry that will offer you the response: "Okay, do this conduct freely before others?" What do you do? If you have a self-delight slip by? Here's a story to show what I did. At some point, I requested four cuts of a lemon poppy seed portion to bring home. In the pastry kitchen, I asked for a lot of napkins, demonstrating that the four cuts would be shared by a gathering of individuals.

The fact of the matter was that I was too humiliated even to consider admitting that I may eat two or three of these cuts in a single sitting—in private, obviously. Also, I did only that. The cuts were heavenly; I tasted each chomp! I understood I enjoyed three cuts and concluded that I would skip lunch to remain on track then have a light nibble before supper, and afterward have a light dinner. Do I suggest this as a decent habit? By no means! In any case, if a self-delight slip happens, simply fuse it into your day's food plan. Next time plan better: just have one piece and afterward quickly solidify the rest. Alter your lunch or the remainder of the day for food utilization—and proceed onward!

If I weren't happy enough with my choices to do this, I would not have gone to the café that sells the portion. I would not wait over the feature of treats; I would concentrate on my associates and our discussion. If my mates were a piece of my care group, I would say to them, "My plan is that by no means am I to leave with a few cuts of lemon poppy seed portion."

SELF-ABUSE AND FOOD

What do you consider when you eat? This is a different inquiry, aimed at the individuals who consider hurting themselves with food or abandoning food for long hours or days. This subject of self-misuse may be the place your self-talk should be more profound, and you don't know what is happening inside. Here are a few questions that might pop up if you are abusing your food intake:

- Are you indulging in being taken note of?

- Are you under-eating with the goal that somebody will take note?

- Are you attempting to pay back somebody?

- Do you sense that you don't have the right to be sound?

- Have you overeaten or gorged on foods so much that you have made yourself debilitated?

- Have you utilized food to make yourself wiped out deliberately?

- Are you binging because you feel more secure if you are not seen—particularly seen sexually?

I discovered that I was accomplishing something intuitively to hurt somebody in my past with the decisions I made for myself. In established truth, I was harming myself and destroying my life as a result of it. That was a major eye-opener! When I made sense of that one, I was stunned for a considerable length of time, then weeks, and at last for almost a year. After I was out of shock, I knew what I was doing, yet I continued abusing myself without really thinking. It was increasingly agonizing and disappointing to know about this harmful habit.

I looked for advice from an expert, chipped away at it like a vocation, and now I understand my inspirations and my decisions with the goal that I never again hurt myself. All is fine currently, yet would you be able to imagine what would have happened had I not made sense of it? It was because I was bold enough to be happy to confront my negative ideas behind abusing my body! So take courage; you can do this! If you believe you need some professional help with this region, you are settling on an insightful choice. I settled on that decision, and it was one of the most significant things I accomplished for myself. You can do it!

COMPULSIVE EATING

Compulsive eating is indulging in food and doing it without control, without having the option to stop. Compulsive eaters are not really mindful of what they are doing. This is more than simply eating a whole sack of hot new pastry shop buns in a periodic slip up. This sort of eating occurs all the time. If you feel that you are eating compulsively, you have in any event ventured out—advancing toward staying alert! That is incredible. The subsequent stage is making sense of why you take part in this conduct, what makes you do it, and afterward to assemble some action steps in a plan to stop your habitual eating. Sounds simple?

It tends to be if you are happy to go up against the conduct and find a way to dispose of it. If you accept that you have an issue with urgent eating, I suggest rounding out a food journal in a different note pad to understand what you are consuming. If you don't record everything, you are deceiving yourself! You have to deal with yourself first so you can be seen to others as a fit and capable person.

There are some critical questions to pose about compulsive eating, and they may require some intense reflection. Here are some primer inquiries to consider before you write:

- What do you feel when you eat compulsively?

- What is at the base of the why you eat along these lines? (To numb anything that is going on inside?)

- What feelings do you experience when you are eating

habitually?

Look at your self-talk—there are heaps of signs there. You may feel humiliated to concede what you eat. However, you can see it outwardly of your body, right? You are eager to understand this, so you should ask yourself, "Why?" Look somewhere inside for what you are educating yourself regarding your habitual eating conduct. Take as much time as necessary and tune in to what you state to yourself.

MODERATION WITH YOUR CHEAT MEALS

Our aim for eating ought to be eating out of a requirement for energy, vitality, and nutrition. Who thinks about that any longer? Very few. There are sure non-food things that we consume that can fundamentally influence how we eat and what we eat. A few, when done without control, present dangers for the vast majority, including the danger of habit.

Specifically, I'm alluding to the use of liquor, medications, and smoking. Liquor is high in calories, it can numb our feelings and our choices, and it can make us not think about what we eat and why we eat. With regards to settling on a decision about hard versus delicate alcohol or wine versus hey balls, you just need to recollect every mixed drink that is high in calories.

There is an explanation that most diet experts allude to mixed beverages as "empty calories." They give little in the method for sustenance; however, it is nearly as high in calories as fat. Liquor is utilized by our bodies more quickly than fat or protein and is stored rapidly as fat — one drink averages more than 100 calories. In a night out, without control, you effectively could drink your day's energy needs in liquor! If you are overdoing the alcohol in your diet routine, you have to ask yourself why.

If you feel that you may be found napping at a get-together where you know alcohol will be served and don't have a plan before that time, then just don't go. That is genuinely outrageous, so here are a few procedures for keeping away from mixed beverages that I have prescribed to my customers: At parties or in the bar, have a low-calorie drink in your grasp consistently. Individuals will be more averse to offer you a beverage. If you have one in your hand or before you, tip the server or barkeep early and instruct them to give you pop or juice if you request an alcoholic drink. Plan ahead.

- Combine juice with the diet for the spritzer impact.

- Opt for juice or soft drink water rather than a drink.

- Have water with a lemon or lime.

- Have diet pop—however, with some restraint.

- Have a non-hard brew.

- Mix wine with a soft drink for a spritzer.

- Tell others you are on some medicine that you can't consolidate with liquor

MEDICATIONS

Regardless of whether it's a doctor prescribed tranquilizer or a sedative, drugs do practically what alcohol does from an enthusiastic level, however not from a caloric level. Medications can numb our feelings and our choices, and they can make us not mind what we eat or don't eat. Every physician endorsed sedative has adverse reactions. Check with your pharmacist as well as your doctor about the reactions of any medication you take. Street drugs are intended to have a major effect on our minds and our emotions. Time and again, individuals use medications to numb emotions or stop mental agony. Essentially, there is nothing of the sort as a "recreational drugs"— they're all dangerous and possibly fatal. You should know that both prescription and street drugs can be abused. As I educated you about the extreme use concerning alcohol, it would be ideal if you look for proficient assistance quickly if you are abusing or dependent on drugs.

SMOKING

Tobacco is one of the most addictive substances we can place in our bodies, and smoking is one of the most addictive practices all over the whole world. While I have compassion toward the individuals who have reliably attempted to stop smoking, my recommendation is to attempt over and over until you are fruitful. Nicotine is exceptionally addictive, and like different synthetic substances found in cigarettes, for example, cyanide, it is a toxic substance that, in large dosages, can kill. We, as a whole, know the dangers that smoking presents for our general wellbeing—lung malady, emphysema, organ harm, osteoporosis, and coronary illness—however, smoking likewise alters your metabolism. The sooner you quit smoking, the better. There are various projects and care groups that can help if you would like to stop. Staying smoke-free brings several advantages: more vitality, healthy metabolism, better appearance, and a better relationship with food.

MENTAL TRAPS

There are mental snares that we can fall into that influence our association with food. One of the most widely recognized is our mental appraisal of our own bodies. I think we are, for the most part, incredulous of our bodies sooner or later in our lives. When that occurs, our self-perception is most likely lopsided. The media, Hollywood, and the style, diet, and cosmetic industries have extraordinarily impacted our thoughts regarding the ideal body types. They have set an incomprehensibly elevated requirement of what comprises the "perfect" that hardly any of us can accomplish. Closer to home, loved ones can impact our self-perceptions through negative or positive remarks. The genuine inquiries are: are we are ceaselessly contrasting ourselves with that perfect, and are these practical objectives?

Stop comparing yourself with a body type that isn't yours. The human populace has various kinds of shapes and sizes—one isn't perfect over another. We are essentially unique due to race, hereditary qualities, condition, and culture. We, as a whole, have diverse body shapes, and we, as a whole, come in various sizes. The proportion somewhere in the range of stature and weight, bone structure, and bulk is diverse for each human. Go up to a mirror with a friend, stand facing the mirror, stand sideways into the mirror, and see these distinctions. Without being basic, value the distinctions. A positive or solid self-perception is a recognition that leaves you alright with your size and shape. A positive self-perception is crucial to your wellbeing and a sound mental frame of mind. A negative self-perception is likely a mutilated discernment dependent on poor correlations with others that leaves you loaded with disgrace and tension. This can prompt low self-esteem, depression, and eating disorders. Get yourself reintroduced to your body, and, if you don't as of now, acknowledge and love it! Truly. It's the single body you have—approach it with respect! It will treat you pleasantly right back!

CHAPTER SEVEN
STRATEGIES FOR ORGANIZING YOUR FOOD AT HOME

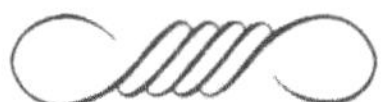

You can control your home food condition by devising a couple of straightforward systems—and now and then, this task involves effective planning and organization. When you are feeling incredible and inspired, here are a few techniques that may help food organization in your home:

- Only purchase the foods in small portions as you require.

- If you are buying more foods than you can use within a brief time, freeze it, share with other individuals, offer it to a food bank, part with it, or even toss it out. You may think it a loss to dispose of food, yet is it a big deal if massive food purchases are exchanged for excess weight gain on you? What is the cost, and will it be worth it? Is it safe to say that you are exchanging your excess food for your wellbeing, your relationship with yourself, your association with your loved ones, or your job?

- Place things that entice you, and you accept that you have to have close by in a zone hard to get to.

- When you are enticed by treats and bites, choose to permit yourself a humble serving and set the rest away. For instance, if potato chips or confections are an exceptional treat for you, partition some into a little bowl and, before you expend the treat, set the rest away in an inaccessible, difficult to reach shelf.

Distinguish most loved foods that push you into difficulty. It is important that you know about specific foods that you hunger for, gorge on, or eat wildly. Normally, individuals have issues or extraordinary difficulties with foods that fit into four classes:

- • Sweet

- • Salty

- • Fatty or Greasy

- • Crunchy

Put foods that are a test to you into one of these classifications. Maybe there is a typical gathering that overwhelms your preferences. You realize what foods are powerful and can jeopardize your eating methodologies. In time, you may change starting with one trying food class then onto the next. The progressions might be because of conditions, evolving hormones, or new anxieties brought about by individuals or circumstances. For me, a most loved food challenge could be as basic as setting off to the sales register at the nearby corner store and seeing the brownies in the pastry shop case by the clerk. The portion size of those brownies is crazy—estimating 4 x 5 inches! What's more, would I finish the entire set in one sitting? Truly—in around 15 seconds! Is there some other way? There totally is another approach to manage this issue, yet not at the time I am slobbering over the brownie remaining in line to pay for my gas. Around then, control isn't at the forefront of my thoughts or in my jargon.

Would you be able to relate? Supplant my preferred food—brownie—with one of your difficulties? Here are the means by which I may take a look at the brownie in an alternate way. Here are my three choices:

1. I genuinely ask myself and answer this question: "Is today a terrible day that I have to eat the entire 5" x 4" brownie? The appropriate response: YES! I was having a terrible day, and I need to eat the entire brownie in the vehicle—even before I leave the parking area. The exciting ride may have recently started. Will self-talk win? Perhaps, perhaps not!

2. If it is an awful day, being straightforward with myself, I will keep away from that difficult food by paying at the siphon where I can't see those beast brownies. Potentially, I can actualize some other technique that I have talked about in the section about enthusiastic eating, for example, making an interruption for this food propensity or desiring.

3. I will be in charge, buy the brownie, put it in a sack, request that the agent tape the pack shut. What's more, when I return home, I am going to cut it into a lot of 1 x 1-inch pieces and stop everything except one. Having given myself consent, I will eat that one brownie parcel without blame.

Can you see the distinction? In picking choice 1, I can hear myself say, "I am so furious at myself that I wolfed it down. I feel so remorseful! What's more, since I have blown this day, I should begin once again on Monday. I didn't taste it, what a waste! I am such a disappointment. I could very well too have an immense supper and dessert, and the remainder of the week is shot! I will eat a lot by the end of the week. I can't remain on track any longer."

Then I would be set to increase another 6 pounds in the following 4–5 days. Negative self-talk around testing foods has outcomes that are difficult to escape—and can be so foolish! In picking alternative 2 or 3,

I have recently finished a potential restraint debacle and kept to my arrangement for progress. I have decided to focus on my methodologies with the goal that I may appreciate the incidental treat and appreciate it by continuing everything with some restraint! I will appreciate each nibble of that brownie parcel, instead of wolfing down the first enormous piece, which would leave me sickened with myself.

Did I get away from the snare of negative self-talk and wrecking consequences? Indeed, by being eager to survey the circumstance with attention to my critical choices to abstain from falling into difficulty, and by picking positive self-talk. Is this as simple as it sounds? Most likely, not! What's more, I am certain that you and I will get loads of practice with similar difficulties! We presently realize that we must be careful around specific foods in specific circumstances. Awareness is simply the key to controlling and making sound meal choices. It's imperative to know about what your preferred foods are, because those food sources make you defenseless against binging or eating without control. Keeping in touch with them will carry you to another degree of self-disclosure. If you realize what foods are hazardous for you, you would then be able to pick procedures to assist you with managing them!

SHOPPING FOR FOOD: AN PLANNED ADVENTURE

When you are increasingly mindful, it isn't as simple to settle on thoughtless food choices. Alone in the supermarket walkways, you are your very own emotionally supportive network, and you should depend on yourself to settle on the right decisions. Some of the time, be that as it may, your negative self-talk—which is not your strong framework—kicks in. Where do you turn? Mindfulness is the way to shop for food. Monitoring your decisions offers you a chance to be responsible for your choices, to be eager to acknowledge duty regarding your choices.

Mindfulness gives you the capacity to settle on decisions without blame or lament but with trust in your feelings and simplicity in basic leadership. The outcome is that you have a superior association with yourself and with the food you buy since you have an arrangement.

Here are some essential tips to use on your next shopping for food adventure:

- A list of every one of your suppers and snacks for a bustling week. (Haul out plans ahead of time.)

- A look into your organizers to perceive what fixings you have close by and what you should buy.

- A basic food item list to guarantee you buy all that you need.

- A date to go shopping for food.

- A plan for water consumption. Carry a water bottle with you all over the place and top off it throughout the day!

Here are a few procedures to help your week by week food arranging: Plan your suppers early and make singular cooler dinners that are pre-partitioned, so you will realize what and the amount you are eating. For example, when you warm a meat and rice dish, simply plan to add new veggies or plates of mixed greens to finish your supper. If you are hurried, this is an incredible method to follow and keep away from inexpensive food.

- Plan your dinners as indicated by where you will be that day. Is there a microwave open? If not, make a point to get ready for progress. Have a feast that is chilled in your lunch pack; however, it is anything but difficult to eat. Have snacks that work with your timetable, including some that are anything but difficult to eat in a hurry.

- Make foods ahead of time, for example, broiled chicken that can be added to hot dishes, or slice up cold to place in plates of mixed greens, or slashed up and made into a chicken serving of mixed greens with a light dressing for a sandwich.

- Using extra-lean ground hamburger, make a dish of lasagna with light cheeses, crisp vegetables, and low-sodium seasonings. If you have scraps, cut the cooled lasagna into pre-parceled pieces for snacks and meals and rapidly freeze them.

- Make spaghetti sauce without any preparation, so you know precisely what you put into the sauce. Pre-partition cooked spaghetti and sauce into holders to use during the week. Freeze what you don't anticipate utilizing in the main couple of days.

- Precook some fish and rice dishes.

- Cut up vegetables for tidbits and put them into proportioned packs to rapidly get when you are in a hurry. Buy a protected lunch sack and load it up with the entirety of your day's food necessities, and you are composed for the afternoon!

- Perhaps later in the week, you can plan to get a serving of mixed greens in a hurry if you foresee that you'll be low on veggies. That is fine, particularly if you have the remainder of your suppers all arranged and prepared. Or on the other hand, dash by the supermarket after you have eaten and get some new organic products or veggies for the remainder of the week.

Arranging when and how to eat is as essential as arranging what to eat. When you eat, ensure you set aside the effort to sit down and taste your food. Our body takes 20 minutes to tell the cerebrum that we are full. If you eat in a short time and haven't yet gotten the sign that you've had adequate food, simply think what harm you would be able to do in the staying 15 minutes that you keep on eating! When you chew, put down your utensils until you have swallowed. Or then again, when you are eating finger food, assume a bite then position the thing on your plate until you are finished swallowing. Slow down. Think positive contemplations as you eat. You are nothing more than trouble for anybody if you are vexed or furious with yourself. Think about your kids and the dietary patterns you are instructing them. Think about the future and how it could be more beneficial if you change a few things today! Relax!

CHAPTER EIGHT
STRATEGIES FOR PLANNING HOME MEALS.

Earlier in the book, I talked about emotional eating and the disorders associated with emotional eating. Go through those points, and you'll notice that it is so simple to have a kitchen loaded up with intentional and healthy decisions to assist you with keeping on track with your healthy diet program. As a part of my expert practice, I visited numerous homes. Because of what I have seen and what a large number of my customers have let me know, I accept that a great many people who have attacked their eating systems need to address revamping their kitchen—and I'm not looking at placing in new machines or counters. I mean, they have to accommodate what food they keep in their homes with how they store it and how they control it.

EFFECTIVE WAYS FOR PLANNING YOUR HOME MEALS

You can control your home food condition by devising a couple of basic procedures—and here and there, this undertaking involves association and arranging. When you are feeling extraordinary and inspired, here are a few procedures that may help food redesigns in your home:

- Only purchase the food in small portions as you need.

- If you purchase more food than you can use within a brief time, solidify it, share with other individuals, offer it to a food bank, part with it, or even toss it out. You may think about what a loss to dispose of food. However, is it a big deal if enormous food purchase is exchanged for excess weight in your body? At what expense? Is it accurate to say that you are exchanging your food abundances for your wellbeing, your association with yourself, your association with your loved ones, or with your activity?

- Place things that entice you, and you accept that you have to have close by in a territory hard to get to. For instance: If you have an ice chest, put the thing far away or put the thing high in a cabinet where it is hard to reach —Place enticing food in a storage room you don't utilize and see constantly.

- When treats and tidbits entice you, choose to permit yourself a humble serving and set the rest away. For instance, if potato chips or confections are a treat for you, partition some into a little bowl and, before you devour the treat, set it away in an inaccessible place. Have a list dependent on your arrangement for the whole week! Record it.

- Shop after you have eaten. When you are hungry, everything looks great, and you will perpetually fill your shopping basket with hasty purchases.

- Buy however much foods as could reasonably be expected to eat. The greater part of your fresh things is along the edge of the store, for example, milk and dairy, leafy foods, grains, and meats. A portion of the things in the passageways are hazardous because they contain handled food, snacks, high-fat, and fatty treats.

- Watch out for displays of specials or new foods that are, for the most part, bargains. These presentations are in your face deliberately, and organizations pay truckloads of money to be in your face!

- When it goes to those powerful specials in tempting displays or in food coupons—ask yourself, "Is it a deal if I don't have it on my list and it's not part of my program?"

- Know the areas where you are easily attracted to food. Write in your Journal and survey the segment on "Most loved foods that push me into excess weight gain," and audit your systems for keeping away from those difficult foods.

- Pick who you go to the supermarket to shop with. A few people who go with you can undermine your best expectations: kids who need sugary treats, family members who have various thoughts regarding what you ought to and shouldn't eat, and good-natured companions who may have an effect on your shopping.

- Read names if you are picking bundled or handled foods. (See what you should search for in the following segment on perusing food names.) As a savvy, key customer, state to yourself, "I will...":

- Plan ahead for your weekly food needs and make a composed basic food item list.

- Shop after you have eaten.

- Shop the dividers to buy new foods however much as could be expected.

- Read the names when you have to buy bundled or prepared foods.

- Stick to your list.

- • Leave the kids at home, if possible, so there is less impulse to purchase outside of your list.

- Abstain from going shopping for food with somebody who could attack your arrangement.

- Purchase just those things on your list and abstain from utilizing coupons since you have them for different things, not on your list.

- Avoid spur of the moment purchases and promoting ploys to make such buys.

- Shop with a help individual, or if you should shop alone, be sure you adhere to your list.

CAREFULLY READ FOOD LABELS

When you read food labels, you are searching for a lot of sugars, fats, fiber, or sodium in the list of fixings. Essentially, you have to know a couple more things about reading food names to guarantee that you're getting the entire picture. The first ingredient recorded is the most important arranged by weight; the last fixing recorded has a minimal sum in an amount in the specific item. Additives and flavorings should likewise be recorded.

Sugars: Names for sugar are glucose, sorbitol, sucrose, dextrose, lactose, xylitol, etc. Different types of sugars include corn sugar, unadulterated sweetener, darker sugar, crude sugar, mannitol, corn sugar, corn syrups, sorghum, molasses, and nectar. There are various distinctive fake sugars available today. New fake sugars are springing up in food items all the time. The best way to remain careful is to eat everything with restraint.

Fats: Components in many of the foods we eat are soaked in fats, including oils, grease, suet, shortening, and spread. Soaked fats are additionally found in meats, for example, hamburger, and other creature items, for example, egg yolks, spread, cheddar, sharp cream, and all milk aside from skim. Palm and coconut oils are likewise soaked fats. Unsaturated or polyunsaturated fats are found in fish and plant foods, for example, avocados, nuts, seeds, olives, and oils, for example, sunflower, soy, nut, and canola oils. Mono-saturated fats are olive oil and rapeseed oil. Omega 3 unsaturated fats are found in sleek fish, for example, salmon and mackerel.

Trans-fats, which means fluid vegetable oils that have been transformed into strong fats by hydrogenation, are found in margarine, many nibble foods, heated products, and seared food. The words hydrogenated or halfway hydrogenated methods trans-fats are in the food—generally prepared food sources. Fats are frequently used to make mayonnaise sauces, flavors, and plate of mixed greens dressings. Different names for fat are mono-glycerides, diglycerides, triglycerides, lecithin, lipids, egg yolk, and mayonnaise.

Salt: A mineral fundamentally made out of sodium chloride, salt, is basic for most life. It is one of the fundamental tastes and is utilized as a significant additive. Salt is found in fixings records for ocean salt, kelp, heating powder, preparing pop, monosodium glutamate, sodium saccharin, sodium nitrate, sodium propionate, and anything with sodium in its name. Sauces, flavors, plate of mixed greens dressings, onion salt, garlic salt, celery salt, canned tomato items, ketchup, bean stew sauces, grill sauces, Worcestershire sauce, cooking wines, escapades, miso, hydrolyzed vegetable protein, yeast, arranged mustards, soya sauce, tamarin, pickles, corned meat, handled items and cheeses can be high in sodium. A general rule is to constrain your admission of foods that contain more than one mg — sodium per calorie. Foods guaranteeing "low-salt" or "no-salt" on their marks are best—however, read the name to ensure the case is valid. Fiber: Diets are improved with fiber. Dietary fiber originates from plants and isn't processed in the intestinal tract yet might be used in the lower gut.

Various plants have various types of fiber: gelatin and gum (which are water solvent), and adhesive, cellulose, hemicellulose, and lignin (which are water-insoluble). Wellsprings of dietary strands are discovered distinctly in plant foods—for instance: entire wheat, entire grains, oat wheat, multi-grain, rye, oats, dark colored rice, wild rice, entire grain pasta, crisp foods grown from the ground, plates of mixed greens, beans, lentils, split peas, nuts, seeds, and dried products of the soil considerably more. They aid absorption and guarantee that the stomach and digestion tracts function admirably. In marking, the fiber substance of food is recorded in weight just as a level of the day by day admission esteem. Also, here's the last word on shopping for food: If you need somebody to buy staple goods for you since you feel that you are excessively occupied or accept that being in a market is unreasonably enticing for you at the present time—proceed.

Keep in mind this is about YOUR success, and success implies loving and taking care of yourself. When you are more certain about your capacity to the basic food item shop, return to your list of strategies that you feel are significant for you to pursue and go complete it.

FAMILY MEALS

Our general public is portrayed by busy people from every walk of life. We are occupied individuals in our business and in our private lives. Family life can be as entangled as it is occupied, as we attempt to be all over and everything for the remainder of our relatives. Our youngsters are the ones who will endure the most if they never realize what it feels like to have sound, formal dinners with discussion and family. Family suppers ought to be solid in sustenance—for the soul and mind just as the body. You can serve scrumptious dinners that are brisk, nutritious, and engaging for the whole family.

There are numerous sources to assist you with structuring and planning healthy family dinners: cookbooks, magazines, the web, and unique media programs. From these sources, you will find food organization and cooking methods that are lower in fat, sugar, and sodium. While there are great deals of pre-arranged sound foods at the supermarket that can be served rapidly for your benefit, there are many inexpensive food dinners you can make at home utilizing whole foods. For instance, look at certain plans in cookbooks for diabetics, low-fat cookbooks, or heart-savvy cookbooks for solid supper plans. Explore them all and most of all: plan, plan, plan!.

If being too occupied is your major challenge, there are a few procedures that can help conquer time-challenging weeks. For instance, be imaginative and amass freezer suppers on Sunday before the week begins. Have an assortment of dinners prepared for whatever state of mind strikes you and your family. Everybody could have something other than what's expected if they like. You can make cooler dinners that are sound and fun, as well. For all suppers, however, particularly family dinners, it is ideal to take a seat at the table to eat as opposed to eating in your vehicle or before the TV. The standard here is to slow down!

Set aside some effort to visit with the family, talk about the day, and put your fork or knife down if food is in your mouth. Bite your food as opposed to breathing in it! Appreciate each nibble and taste the food! If the family demands foods that you know are unmistakably not in your eating plan and you have a test with them, you may settle on a decision to remain in charge by eating your principle supper previously or after the family eats. While they eat, you can have a plate of mixed greens.

Along these lines, you are not enticed by their decisions are as yet at the table for discussion and participating in the family gathering. You realize what will work for you. Make an arrangement early. If you don't feel great getting ready family dinners, request support from your family for some assistance. You may be astounded what they think of it. The perfect, obviously, is to plan foods you would appreciate that are nutritious and good for your entire family. One father told me that he was not very good at arranging dinners and continued putting it off. He additionally said that his teenage girl was always delighted in preparing meals, so I proposed that he let his little girl plan the suppers for the week, and he could double-check them for taste and satisfaction. His food organizing challenge was understood.

Food preparation can be one of the absolute most noteworthy factors in making healthy meals. Be aware of food preparation descriptions, for example, deep-frying, coated or adding of fat/oil to cook. These techniques include a bigger number of calories and fat than is vital. Better strategies for planning healthy meals include grilling, baking, steaming, boiling, broiling, microwaving, barbecuing, roasting, poaching, braising, and stir-frying.

Here are a couple of tips to reduce the fat, sodium, and sugar in your cooking:

- Drain off the fat that collects during cooking.

- Refrigerate sauces, soups or stews, and flavors before serving so as to skim off the hardened fat that has ascended to the top. Warm them.

- In planning meats, cut back on excess as much at conceivable and expel the skin from poultry before cooking.

- When you pan sear, utilize a low-sodium stock instead of oil to cook meats and vegetables. To thicken sauces, use cornstarch or rice flour.

- In preparing, supplant fats with fruit purée or no-fat yogurt fitting for the formula.

- Reduce the measure of sugar or salt in a recipe.

- Reduce the measure of cheddar in the recipe (low-fat obviously).

- Avoid cooking your vegetable dishes with fat and salt or including fat and salt at the table.

- Use garlic, onions, peppers, or new herbs in your dishes.

- Add a dash of flavor to your dish; decrease the sugar and include vanilla or almond concentrates or cinnamon powder for the season.

Snacks are a significant piece of family dinners, whether they are eaten at home or while away. Organized and laid out in your kitchen, custom made snacks and tidbits have a few benefits.

When taken to class or work, they frequently free us from the stress of what we will have for lunch and questions regarding how to remain on our eating plan. Other than being savvy, pre-made snacks fend off us from enticing and normally less nutritious cheap food and eatery suppers. We know precisely what is in our pre-made snacks and can incorporate the best possible adjustments for ideal sustenance and good dieting. Assortment in lunch and snacks isn't an issue since we can bundle and convey hot and cold food sources. Scraps frequently make amazing snacks. Utilize a canteen for hot or cold foods; warm sacks and little cooler packs can guarantee freshness. Making snacks and bites at home takes effective planning.

Plan ahead for seven days of snacks and lunch that will cater to the entire family. Set a suitable time for collecting snacks sacks ahead of time—for certain families, the prior night functions work well, and for other people, the morning appears to be less difficult. I plan my lunch and snacks for my days off as well; then, when I'm getting things done, I realize I can adhere to my eating plan.

Put variety and nutrient-filled ingredients in every snack, keeping desserts, carbonated beverages, sodium, and fats to the base or disposing of them all together. If you need recommendations, ask your family, different guardians, or search for data on lunch proposals on the web. If you are enticed to nibble on the fixings as you set up the lunch meals, request that other relatives assist you with making them. If you are eating at home, pursue similar standards for all family dinners: sit together, take part in the discussion, put down your utensils between bites, chew completely, and turn off telephones, radios, and TV interruptions. Make the most of your time together over lunch!

CHAPTER NINE
HOW TO BURN FAT AUTOMATICALLY AND FEEL FULLER ON LESS

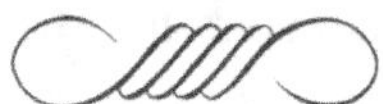

In this chapter, you're going to figure out how to reduce your size, become healthier, and feel full even when you're eating less food. Utilizing the simple and straightforward nutrition rules stated in this section, you'll effectively accomplish your ideal weight, and it won't appear as though you're on an eating regimen. In fact, you don't need to starve yourself or surrender your preferred foods. You'll likewise have no issue keeping up your new body shape since you're not going to do anything strange or extraordinary to achieve it.

Losing fat doesn't rely on fat grams, sugar grams, feast timing, food blends, macronutrient proportions, singular micronutrients, or any of a hundred other extraordinary diet program subjects. None of those things matters if you're eating excessively. At last, almost every weight reduction system returns full-cycle to whether it encourages you to keep up a calorie deficit. Remaining in a calorie shortage reliably, be that as it may, is a challenge on the grounds that many factors impact the amount you eat and number of calories you consume.

Energy balance is dynamic, which implies the measure of calories you require can change. Alongside thinking little of food utilization, neglecting to alter your calorie consumption when your vitality needs change is the most widely recognized reason for weight reduction levels. The central issue is, "What is the most effortless, proficient, and most beneficial approach to keep up that imperative caloric shortfall?" For my cash, I'll wager on what I call "high-low" food, a way to deal with food determination dependent on three significant standards:

1. Energy density, otherwise called calorie density, is the number of calories in a portion of food for every serving.

2. Nutrient density is the dietary benefit per serving (nutrients, minerals, phytonutrients, and fiber).

3. Satiety is defined by how full a portion of food or dinner makes you feel and how that influences the amount you eat. To boost fat loss while enhancing your wellbeing, you will likely pick foods that contain the most noteworthy supplement density, the highest satiety level, and the least calorie density.

Is a calorie, "Just a Calorie?" You might be thinking, "There's significantly more to nutrition than just calories, and a calorie isn't only a calorie!" That is the general purpose of eating nutrient-dense, normal foods. Clearly, 200 calories from pretzels and soft drinks won't give the equivalent dietary benefit or satiety as 200 calories of broccoli and salmon. Various foods can significantly influence your wellbeing, your hormones, and even your disposition, sharpness, and mental work.

Various kinds of foods can likewise have marginally various consequences for body structure at a similar gross caloric consumption. This can be clarified by the thermic impact of food, calories in stringy foods that aren't totally assimilated, and the impact of food on hormones and consequent craving. In any case, this doesn't negate the calorie law; it checks it. Representing every one of these components, when you take a look at the net outcome, you're left with precisely what the math directs: weight changes depend on calories in versus calories out. From a vitality balance perspective, a metabolizable calorie is only a calorie.

There's a major distinction between "don't count calories" and "calories don't count." Some diet regimen programs discourage calorie counting; they basically show you what to eat and what not to eat. The exceptional food blends or remarkable topic of the diet regimen is generally credited for the weight reduction. What they don't let you know is that their eating rules cause you to eat less consequently.

A DIFFERENT DEFINITION OF COUNTING CALORIES

At this point, you might be thinking, "God help us, not another calorie-counting program!" If so, take a deep breath. You won't need to check calories.

Truth be told, in case you're determined about not including anything, I won't demand it. I'll essentially request that you complete three things:

1. Recognize the calories-in versus calories-out equation.

2. Know about your bite sizes.

3. Increase or reduce your portions in light of your week by week results.

My definition of checking calories may not be what you think. Checking calories doesn't need to mean strolling around with a scratch pad or electronic gadget, recording each piece you eat consistently. Rather, you make a day by day menu plan as your eating objective for the afternoon. Utilizing this strategy, you possibly need to tally calories once when you make your menu.

This technique is proactive, not responsive. You record what you intend to eat first, then eat it, as opposed to eating first and afterward recording what you just ate. Consider it menu arranging as opposed to calorie checking. To counteract weariness and get a dietary variety, you can make various menus or make food substitutions from a similar class with comparable caloric qualities. Making your very own menus is simpler than you might suspect. Basically, pursue the ten Body Fat Solution food rules, and your menus will nearly make themselves.

CALORIES 101: ASCERTAIN YOUR DAILY MAINTENANCE CALORIES

One size doesn't fit all with regards to calories. It's senseless to endorse a similar measure of calories for everybody, particularly if it bumps people or dynamic and inactive individuals together. For instance, 1,500 calories daily may be ideal for most ladies to reduce fat; however, it could be semi-starvation for a gigantic and active man. The greater and increasingly dynamic you are, the more calories you have to have to keep up your weight. Keep in mind these focuses and that both can change. Likewise, remember that ladies are commonly littler than men, so ladies, for the most part, need around 600 to 800 fewer calories every day. Calorie needs likewise decline as you get more established. As indicated by exercise physiologists Victor Katch and Frank McArdle, the normal female between the ages of twenty-three and fifty has a calorie maintenance level of around 2,000 to 2,100 calories for each day and the normal male around 2,700 to 2,900 calories.

CALORIES 102: MAKE THE ALL-SIGNIFICANT CALORIE DEFICIT

To shed fat, you should make a caloric deficit. A caloric deficit, otherwise called negative energy balance, implies that the quantity of calories you devour is not exactly the number of calories you consume. You can make a shortage by diminishing your food admission, expanding your movement level, or both. If you require 2,800 calories for each day to keep up your weight and you eat 3,300 calories every day, you're in positive energy balance by 500 calories, and you'll put on weight.

If you eat 2,300 calories every day, you're in negative energy balance, and you'll get thinner. A caloric shortfall is a basic subtraction. To figure your optimal caloric admission for diminishing muscle to fat ratio, subtract 20–30 percent from your support level. 20% is viewed as a preservationist shortage, 30 percent a forceful shortfall. In case you're a normal male, and your support level is 2,800 calories for each day, then a 20 percent shortage is a 560-calorie decrease, which gives you an objective of 2,240 calories for every day. In case you're a normal female, and your upkeep level is 2,100 calories for each day, then a 20 percent shortage is 1,680 calories for each day.

It's commonly best to keep your calorie decrease preservationist from the outset. In case you're not getting the pace of fat loss you need, you can make a progressively forceful shortfall later by diminishing your calories a little further or expanding your movement. Overall, most ladies will decrease muscle to fat ratio adequately and securely on 1,400 to 1,800 calories for every day. Most men will accomplish healthy, safe, and effective fat reduction around 2,100 to 2,500 calories each day. Keep in mind that these are midpoints. If your body is huge and you're dynamic, utilize the upper end of these ranges. If your body is small in size or if you're inert, utilize the lower end of these ranges.

CALORIES 103: MODIFY YOUR CALORIE INTAKE OR EXERCISE OUTPUT ON THE BASIS OF YOUR RESULTS

There are numerous equations you can use to ascertain your calorie needs with accurate precision. In any case, don't be excessively worried about calorie calculations, since you'll need to modify your calories dependent on your week after week results in any case. All you need is a decent pattern. At last, it's progressively significant that you comprehend the 10,000-foot view of energy balance. Despite the number of calories you believe you're eating at the present time, if your body weight isn't changing, then you don't have a calorie shortfall. This implies one of three things:

4. You thought little of what number of calories you are eating.

5. You overestimated what number of calories you are consuming.

6. Both of the above-mentioned. Whatever the explanation, you have to make or restore a shortage by eating less or exercising more.

THE SELECTIVE REDUCTION OF CALORIES

There are two different ways to make a shortfall: increment your vitality use or decrease your food utilization. On the food decrease side, the following inquiry is, "Which food sources do you cut?" Do you basically eat somewhat less of everything? That would work, because any caloric deficiency will cause weight reduction. In any case, there's a superior way.

At that point, when a reduction in calories is called for, you specifically decrease the calorie-density basic sugars, dull carbs, and grains. That leaves the fundamental proteins, fats, and micronutrients from products of the soil. If the calories fall too low to even think about satisfying your vitality needs, you essentially include caloric counterbalance by somewhat expanding your lean protein and solid fats. In case you're an insightful reader, you may be thinking, "Hello, hold up a moment, aren't you making another low-carb diet in a mask?" Well, yes and no. Truly, on the grounds that we're expanding your caloric shortfall by diminishing certain carbs. No, because there are some significant contrasts in my methodology contrasted with "conventional" low-carb diets:

To start with, this diet plan isn't an outrageous low-carb diet. It's a moderate-carb sustenance program. Second, the measure of carbs you decrease isn't fixed; it's a variable dependent on your needs and inclinations. Third, the sort of carbs you wipe out directly from the beginning are the prepared carbs, refined sugars, and man-made carbs.

As a result, you additionally lessen normal starches and grains, which are calorie thick. There's no motivation to evacuate high-nutrient density foods like leafy foods. Fourth, the essential center isn't around carbs, yet where it ought to be — on the calories. Conventional low-carb slimming down mindset can sometimes lead to the misconception and judgment of alive and well and nutritious foods and makes carbs resemble the reason for heftiness. The reason for weight isn't carbs; it's an overabundance of calories, an abatement in physical activity, and every one of the components that lead to this vitality irregularity.

The Macronutrients:

Protein, Carbohydrates, and Fat Like calories, the correct admission of the three macronutrients—proteins, solid carbs, and fundamental fats—is basic. Be that as it may, if you essentially pursue the ten Body Fat Solution food runs, your macronutrient needs will be met, and you'll naturally be in the ballpark with every one of your numbers. What's most significant is to get the fundamentals first and locate a restorative macronutrient balance that keeps away from the boundaries. From that point, you can alter the arrangement to address your issues. Before we proceed onward to the ten principles, how about we quickly review the three macronutrients. The Power of "protein" originates from the Greek word proteos, which signifies "of first significance." This is fitting since, when you set up a feast, I need you to consider lean protein first.

Consider protein building material for the body on the grounds that the amino acids in protein are utilized as development material for almost every cell and tissue, including muscle. Protein is found in numerous foods, even vegetables, beans, vegetables, and grains. While this is significant for veggie lovers to know, when we allude to "lean proteins" in this program, we're alluding fundamentally to the lean wellsprings of complete proteins, ones that contain all the basic amino acids. Complete proteins incorporate chicken breast, turkey breast, lean red meat, fish, shellfish, egg whites, and low-or nonfat dairy items. Protein assumes some significant jobs in weight control. Slender protein encourages you to keep up your fit weight when your calories are confined. It additionally smothers your craving. Eating lean protein expands your digestion because of the thermic impact of food, which is how a lot of vitality you consume to process the food. Protein has a thermic impact of 30 percent. This implies, if you eat a lean protein food that has 100 calories, 30 of those calories are utilized to process the food, leaving just 70 calories of net vitality accessible. Sugars have a thermic impact of 10–15 percent, while dietary fat has the least thermic impact of just 3 percent.

CHAPTER TEN
PLANNING, ORGANIZING, AND IMPLEMENTING

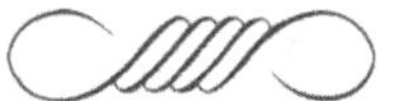

If we gave your fitness and health habits an unexpected assessment today, what might be the prognosis? Be sincere. Would your eating routine be a critical condition, in critical need of crisis treatment? Would your training program need a bit of fixing up to a great extent? Do you, at any point, have an organized training program? What about your lifestyle? Is your body enduring the impacts generally late nights, liquor use, or significant levels of stress?

Notwithstanding your current physical condition, the absolute quickest method to improve your outcomes is by planning and prioritizing. Your central goal is to recognize which regions throughout your life need prompt consideration and afterward sort out the entirety of your exercises around those needs.

By following the recipe, you'll learn in this chapter how you could go from a total stop to pedal to the metal and really show signs of improvement brings about less time. 80-20: The Magic Formula for Achieving More by Doing Less There's presumably no better method to set needs and increase your energy than observing the 80-20 rule.

It was first discovered in 1897 by Vilfredo Pareto, an Italian business analyst who saw a striking lopsidedness in the circulation of riches. He found that 20 percent of the populace had 80 percent of the cash and resources. In wellness, the 80-20 guideline is nonsensical. You may expect that all aspects of your preparation and food would have similar importance. Subsequently, you, as a rule, treat every viewpoint similarly. Be that as it may, the 80-20 principle applied to fitness and wellness says that 20 percent of your food, planning, and habits will create 80 percent of the adjustments in your body.

Understanding this guideline can be unpleasant from the outset since you'll understand that the vast majority of what you were doing each day created almost no outcomes. You may wind up feeling like the proverbial gerbil on the wheel—lots of action, yet going nowhere fast. Then again, it's a significant disclosure since it implies that it's completely conceivable to get more results because of doing less. When you see how to utilize this to further your potential benefit by actualizing the standard, it's a groundbreaking change in perspective. You understand that you don't need to perspire the little stuff, so in that sense, it's freeing. Your frame of mind turns out to be progressively loose, and the entire undertaking is less upsetting because you quit stressing over each modest detail.

Applying the 80-20 guideline is a procedure of recognizing needs and concentrating more on those and less on everything else. It's not time; it's action. It's the embodiment of working savvy. There are two different ways to apply the 80-20 standard:

1. Invest additional time and vitality on the imperative few (the 20 percent).

2. Invest less time and vitality on the unimportant many (the 80 percent). The million-dollar question is, how would you know the contrast between the significant needs and the paltry subtleties? What are the 20 percent of exercises that are creating most of your outcomes?

Finding and Eliminating Bottlenecks: Think of the way to your ideal weight and perfect body as a gigantic multilane expressway. Then envision there's something blocking at least one of the paths. As autos must converge to the other side to press through a restricted passageway, a gag point is made, making traffic back up for miles, hindering your movement time or, in any event, carrying you to a stand-still. Any individual who has ever been trapped in rush hour gridlock in Los Angeles or Chicago can identify with this since turnpike bottlenecks in those urban areas cause 25 to 27 million hours of delay each year. Unnecessary delays likewise happen in your fitness venture since at least one significant path of progress is blocked. Coaches regularly whine about their customers demolishing all their difficult work in the exercise center because, even that can't be expected to make up for a lousy eating routine. One change in your regular lifestyle routine, for example, lack of sleep, poor decisions in cafés, or end of the week gorging can demolish a whole seven day stretch of smart dieting.

A solitary restricting conviction, negative frame of mind, or enthusiastic issue can attack all that you do. Other basic limitations incorporate poor travel propensities, skipping breakfast, passionate eating, hitting the bottle hard, poor practice structure, wasteful practice projects, and irregularity in any part of your sustenance or preparing. Requirements can either be heavily influenced by you (inside) or out of your control (outer). For the most part, you'll find that the greatest requirements are interior. As Pogo stated, "We have met the enemy, and he is us." If you're not gaining ground toward your objective, there's quite often one significant requirement obstructing your way, and you quite often have authority over it. When you separate and get rid of it, your advancement begins to move through again at the most extreme conceivable speed. Your body's shape and size will begin changing so quickly it's practically alarming. A basic question or two can help flush with excursion the significant restricting imperative: What one snag is keeping down your advancement in each other territory? What one deadly defect has been keeping you from arriving at your objective? When you've bound the limitation, your need is to pour most of your vitality into settling that one major issue.

THE HIERARCHY OF NUTRITION

One of the ideal approaches to organizing is by utilizing the chain of command approach. Abraham Maslow's progressive system of necessities, a mental hypothesis of inspiration, was one of the most celebrated chains of command. Shown as a pyramid, basic physiological needs, for example, food, water, and rest framed the biggest part at the base, and regard or self-realization needs, for example, accomplishment and imagination, were the littler pieces stacked on top. As indicated by Maslow's chain of command, if the most fundamental life needs aren't satisfied, then they should become quick needs. Just when the basic endurance needs have been met can the higher needs be sought after. This pecking order idea is amazingly useful when you apply it to your preparation and sustenance. More than forty supplements are fundamental for your wellbeing, to give vitality, fabricate or fix body tissues, and perform different substantial capacities.

A caloric deficiency is a fundamental prerequisite for fat loss; however, outrageous and delayed starvation eats fewer carbs to reduce your metabolic rate. Caloric hardship additionally makes it hard to get the various basics. Food is fuel, and you need to top off the gas tank each day if you need to go anyplace. It is safe to say that you are getting enough fuel, basic amino acids. Protein is seemingly the most significant macronutrient when you're concentrating on fat loss. Protein causes you to clutch lean tissue while you're in a caloric deficiency, and it even smothers your hunger. Basic amino acids, which are the structure squares of protein, can't be made by your body, so you should get them from your food. Is it safe to say that you are eating a lean protein with every supper and meeting your day by day protein necessities? Fundamental unsaturated fats. Fundamental unsaturated fats are imperatively significant for cardiovascular wellbeing and various body capacities, including consuming fat. Like basic amino, the fundamental unsaturated fats can't be integrated into your body and should be gotten from your food. Is it true that you include solid fat sources, for example, salmon consistently? Fundamental nutrients and minerals. Nutrients and minerals are natural or inorganic mixes vital for the legitimate working of your body. They're basic because your body can't make them or can't make them in sufficient amounts, so you should get them from your food. Foods grown from the ground are among the most extravagant wellsprings of these micronutrients. Is it safe to say that you are eating them consistently? Water. Your body is, for the most part, water. Water is fundamental to the point that, without it, you'd pass on in merely days. Indeed, even mellow parchedness diminishes physical execution. Satisfactory water admission is likewise important to consume fat, ideally. Is it accurate to say that you are drinking enough water? These are the fundamentals that must frame the establishment of your pyramid. There are numerous minor subtleties that can take your sustenance to a more elevated level. In any case, if you understand you're inadequate in any of the basic pieces, that is the place your needs should go. Allude back to Chapter Six and the ten food rules to be certain your fundamental needs are met, to the exclusion of everything else. The Hierarchy of Training: The primary fundamental is that you are preparing. Any preparation is superior to no preparation. Numerous individuals go through a long time examining preparing methods, yet never begin. Numerous individuals, particularly ladies, are reluctant to lift loads. Yet, weight preparing is a higher priority than vigorous preparing. Weight preparing can give cardiovascular medical advantages, yet heart stimulating exercise can't give quality or solid advancement benefits. Your selection of activities ought to likewise be organized, utilizing a chain of command of significance. All activities are not made equivalent. Continuously make the compound free-weight activities, for example, squats, thrusts, deadlifts, lines, and presses your first need.

The workouts, for example, twists, triceps augmentations, and calf raises, are useful yet less significant, and accordingly, put rearward in the exercise. If you're at any point in a hurry and need to abbreviate your exercises, drop these detail practices first and consistently keep the significant developments. Most machines, except for certain workouts, take lower need than freeloads. If your lower body exercise comprises leg expansions, leg twists, inward thigh machine, and butt blaster machine, you have to take care of your needs. Start hunching down and deadlifting. You'll get progressively out of those two free weight practices than every one of the four of the machines joined. Cardio is lower on the activity chain of importance than weight preparing, yet significant in any case. The perfect program contains weight preparing and cardio preparing.

Cardio gives its very own one of a kind wellbeing and wellness advantages and expands your all-out calories consumed. Similarly, as with weight training, the kind of cardio ought to likewise be organized. Try not to pass judgment on a cardio exercise dependent on time alone. A twenty-to thirty-minute cardio exercise could consume the same number of calories as an hour-long exercise. The thing that matters is force. If you're healthy, fit, and have no orthopedic or therapeutic issues, then extraordinary cardio goes higher on the chain of importance, particularly if time proficiency is essential to you.

TRY NOT TO WASTE TIME

If 20 percent of your activities produce most of your outcomes, then by definition, 80 percent of your activities produce the minority of your outcomes and are generally insignificant. Worrying over details is the deadly problem in a large number of individuals' fat loss goals. For instance, we have Mike the Macronutrient Micromanager, who sweats over spreadsheets for a considerable length of time attempting to change the proportions of protein, carbs, and fat to the tenth of a rating point. Is it worth the issue? All things considered, take a look at it along these lines: If you're on a hunger diet that leaves you insufficient in protein, do you think it makes a difference whether your negligible calorie admission is adjusted impeccably to a 40-30-30 balance or whatever enchanted proportion you're attempting to hit? Then we have Annie, who is forty pounds overweight and needs to know whether she ought to eat natural products of the soil to assist her with getting thinner. Before I even begin to clarify any potential natural advantages, for example, dodging pesticides or getting more elevated levels of micronutrients, I ask her what number of foods grown from the ground she's eating now. I can't resist the urge to laugh when she reveals to me she isn't eating any vegetables whatsoever and just an incidental natural product. Yet, she has an issue kicking the day by day treat propensity. Wouldn't it bode well to cut the sugar and eat more foods grown from the ground before agonizing over natural versus conventional, or crisp versus solidified, or any of twelve different subtleties that don't make a difference if you're not eating any veggies? At long last, we have Pete the Pill Popper, who needs to recognize what fat killers to take—the whopper of every question and answer. If you become tied up with the cases in many promotions for diet pills, you'd leave away accepting you'd found the Holy Grail of weight reduction. Unexpectedly, in well-planned clinical research preliminaries, at any rate, 80 percent of enhancements publicized for weight reduction have never been demonstrated to work for people. Of the staying 20 percent, 80 percent of those items don't do what the ads guarantee they'll do. One broadly publicized fat-eliminator pill guaranteed that it would fix stomach fat and soften away 20 percent of your muscle to fat ratio in a quarter of a year. The examination recounted to an alternate story. A large portion of the investigations said it didn't work by any means. The other half said it worked; however, the outcomes were scarcely huge. One twofold blind, placebo-controlled clinical preliminary demonstrated just a single kilogram of weight reduction in a half year. A huge number of individuals surrender $240 for a six-month supply of an enhancement that delivered paltry advantages, which effectively may have been ascribed to something different, even the misleading impact.

Don't the Details Make a difference Too? A few people misconstrue the 80-20 principle to imply that nearly all that they're doing is useless. While that is not a long way from reality now and again, it's not so much exact. The 80 percent essentially speaks to bring down worth exercises. In case you're an aggressive competitor, propelled student, or refined calorie counter who has just aced every one of the basics and fundamentals, the subtleties matter. A great deal. Another significant achievement guideline is known as the triumphant edge hypothesis, which expresses that everything aides or damages; nothing is nonpartisan. This is particularly significant in sports, business, or aggressive undertakings, where the smallest edge tallies. Do subtleties make a difference? Approach an Olympic swimmer for whom the distinction between a gold and a silver award was one-hundredth of a second. Ask the sprinter who set forth and missed the decorations by a tenth of a second. If you're an expert competitor, then apparently unimportant subtleties, arranging, and execution are the distinction between leaving a mark on the world and being a spectator. Everything matters. Everything tallies. A little 100-calorie-per-day awkwardness in vitality—that is around four chocolate chips from the sweet snack at work—could make you fat if you kept it up for a long enough timeframe and everything else stayed equivalent. The 80-20 standard doesn't infer that subtleties don't make a difference. It says you don't stress over the subtleties until you've aced the fundamentals. As Goethe stated, "The things that issue the most should never be helpless before things that issue the least." Always Have a Plan—Never Wing It. Imagine strolling by a building site and soliciting one of the laborers, "Hello, what are you all building?" A specialist answers, "I have no clue." I wager you've never heard a wonder such as this, since beginning to manufacture something without an arrangement would be senseless. In any case, did you ever think it's just as senseless to go to a rec center, go shopping for food, or even take a seat during supper without an objective and composed outline for your sustenance and preparing? I once heard a statement from persuasive orator Jim Rohn that changed my reasoning for eternity. He stated, "Never start your day until you finish it." From the start, it seemed like a puzzle. How are you expected to complete your day before you start it? Then the light went on, and I understood that he was talking about arranging before acting. The sensible augmentations are, never start your week until you've completed it, never start your month until you've completed it, and never start your year until you've completed it. Activity without arranging is perhaps the greatest reason for disappointment. Arranging requires genuine ideas and exertion. It requires a peaceful, centered time with a pen and paper or PC, frequently with a mentor or accomplice. Proficiency specialists state that consistent time spent in arranging will spare you ten minutes in execution. When you apply this basic arranging idea to your sustenance, preparing, and way of life, the outcomes will stun you. Better results and increasingly productive utilization of time aren't the main benefits. Feeling ill-equipped or capricious makes tension and stress. That makes arranging and arrangement an amazing pressure reducer and certainty developer. Arranging and organizing around priorities start each day, week, month, and year on paper. Continuously work from a rundown, plan, or timetable. Compose a list of objectives, a list of day by day activity steps, an everyday plan, a week by week plan, a composed supper plan, a composed shopping list, and a composed preparing plan. Make need records, not plans for the day. Need records center around the imperative few. The plan for the day is generally jumbled with the minor many. The arranging procedure starts with an objective setting, since every one of your exercises must be sorted out around your high-need objectives and wanted a new way of life propensities. When your objectives are recorded as a hard copy, apply 80-20 reasoning. What is the one wellbeing, wellness, or body-weight objective that would have the greatest effect in your life? If you accomplished it in the following twelve weeks? Organize that objective by composing it on a card, conveying it with you wherever you go and perusing it regularly. Take a look at every one of the five Body Fat Solution standards—mental training, cardio training, quality training, food, and social help. In every one of these classes, what is the one most elevated need objective or activity step that will have the greatest effect in your life? Make your week after week calendar and everyday activity plan around these needs. Every day and Weekly Scheduling: Do you make meetings with your primary care physician? What about your dental specialist? Your bookkeeper? Your beautician? What about your life partner or noteworthy other—do you plan a period and a day for dates? (Neighborly tip: If you don't, leave visas are impending.) If you make arrangements for everything else in your life, for what reason would you leave your preparation for whatever pieces of time happen to be leftover every day? Prepare to have your mind blown. There never is whenever left finished. Strangely, your schedule will consistently top off each day except if you set needs and calendar squares of time for what's generally critical to you. You can begin the arranging procedure with only a pen and a clean sheet of paper. I prescribe putting resources into an arrangement book or time organizer. Planning every week ahead of time is simple since you, as of now, might suspect and arrange your life on a week by week premise. You'll additionally be setting body-weight and body composition objectives and outlining your advancement on a week after week premise, making seven days the ideal square of time for arranging your preparation and food. I propose composing your week after week preparing plan into your time organizer each Sunday evening for the up and coming week. Then each night before hitting the hay, survey your timetable and set everyday objectives and needs for the following day. Along these lines, your oblivious personality can assimilate and coordinate the data while you're dozing. You'll get down to business in the first part of the day with the center and course. At any rate, one of your day by day arrangements will be exercise. Record the specific time you'll be preparing, the activities or body parts you'll be working, and your objectives for the session. Be explicit. There's an enormous distinction between saying, "I'm getting down to business tomorrow," and saying, "Tomorrow at seven a.m. sharp at Gold's Gym, I'm preparing hip-predominant lower body, even push, level force, and lower abs, and I mean to break my own deadlift record."

THE COUNTDOWN METHOD

Another incredible arranging procedure is the "commencement schedule." I began utilizing this technique preceding my first weight training rivalry. It worked so well for me, I've utilized it from that point forward and have prescribed it to a large number of my customers who have additionally utilized it with colossal achievement. Utilizing a commencement, you'll get increasingly engaged and progressively persuaded as time passes as you see the cutoff time drawing nearer and closer. If you don't have looming cutoff times to give you a twinge in your stomach that shouts, "Make a move now or disaster will be imminent!" then you'll see it simpler to state to yourself, "I have a lot of time, so one cheat dinner or skipped exercise doesn't make a difference."

Then, when you understand you don't have time, all things considered, you freeze and participate in a last-minute scrambling practice or resort to outrageous strategies and risky solutions. Here's the means by which it works: get a divider or work area schedule—the sort that shows every week extending on a level plane over the page with an open square of room for every day—or make your very own eighty-four-day (twelve-week) graph on a PC in a word processor or spreadsheet. Circle the objective cutoff time or rivalry date on the schedule and imprint that as day zero. In each of the crates, start checking in reverse from the present day: T minus eighty-four days; T minus eighty-three days; T minus eighty-two days. This will program your oblivious personality to acquire you for an ideal arrival on your cutoff time date, similar to an F-14 on a plane carrying warship. Menu Planning: A composed menu might be the absolute most significant piece of your arrangement. The upside of working off a menu is that it's a proactive arranging system. Numerous individuals keep food journals or diaries, and I don't debilitate that at all since diaries are a fabulous device for training and responsibility. Nonetheless, journaling isn't a similar thing as working off a menu. With food diaries, you eat something and afterward record it. That is responsive. If you make a menu plan and then tail it, that is proactive. A menu plan is your eating objective for the afternoon. Beginning your day without a menu plan is an encouragement to a stray course at the smallest allurement or interruption. Working off a menu additionally implies that you don't need to include your calories consistently progressively. You possibly need to check your calories once when you make your menus. Then you essentially pursue the menu by gauging and estimating your food partitions. The perfect menu is one you make yourself utilizing a format and general standards of feast development, for example, the ten sustenance rules you learned in Chapter Six. You can make menus on a clear sheet of paper and include the calories by hand with a mini-computer, or you can utilize any of the business programming programs accessible available today. Spreadsheets, for example, Microsoft Excel, likewise work consummately for menu arranging and come previously introduced on numerous PCs. Sorting out Your Kitchen: Your following stage is to make a key arrangement for setting up your dinners, including how you will eat at home, at work, in eateries, and when voyaging. The best spot to begin is in your very own kitchen. I've seen coolers loaded up with so much garbage you'd need a GPS to explore your way through them. Kitchen pantries run a nearby second as the most jumbled spot in the home. There's most likely a great deal of stuff in your kitchen that isn't good for your new wellbeing and wellness objectives. Let it be known. Then start Operation Kitchen Clean Sweep. The greatest reason I hear is, "I would prefer not to squander anything." We put that one to rest in Chapter Four, so don't consider it. Toss it hard and fast. Because there's a large portion of a pack of potato chips in the pantry doesn't mean you ought to eat them and afterward start your program after the sack is done. If you're not going to drink sugary, fatty soft drinks any longer, then toss that two-liter cola bottle. I couldn't care less if you just got it and haven't split the seal. Pour it down the sink. It probably won't go to squander all things considered—it will likely wipe some rust off your funnels. If you have food stored in the storm cellar, carport, or some mystery hideaway, get those spots out. Dispose of all the messiness, all over the place. If all else fails, toss it out. When your kitchen is spotless, keep it clean. If the garbage's not there, you can't eat it. Kitchen Essentials: Next, ensure you have all the fundamental kitchen apparatuses, utensils, cookware, and holders you'll require. Notwithstanding the standard things found in each kitchen, like an icebox, broiler, and stovetop, here are a portion of the fundamentals I have in my kitchen: Optional things incorporate a blender and a George Foreman flame broil or some electric barbecue that can accelerate your planning time by cooking chicken breasts and other lean meats rapidly and in amount.

A rice cooker that serves as a vegetable steamer is a gift from heaven. Machines that enable you to cook in mass are a superb help. Office Clean Sweep: Once your house is all together; it's an ideal opportunity to get out of your office. Experience every one of your drawers and dispose of sweets, pretzels, chips, and other low-supplement, fatty] snacks. You'll be carrying solid tidbits to work starting now and into the foreseeable future. While you're grinding away, set up your workplace with little suggestions to keep you concentrated on your objectives.

Post rousing statements and photographs. Show your composed objectives conspicuously where you'll see them throughout the day. Shouldn't something be said about that associate seductress who drops off the doughnuts each morning? Advise her, "No, thank you," and ask her not to leave them anyplace in your sight, or you'll toss them out. If she leaves them in any case, hurl them and ensure she sees you do it. Keep in mind; individuals hate to squander "splendidly great food." I ensure she won't bring you doughnuts any longer. It has exactly the intended effect without fail—particularly If you dump them in the trash can directly over the pencil shavings and espresso beans. Arranging your workday likewise incorporates choosing what you will have for lunch. Try not to venture out from home toward the beginning of the day without knowing where you'll have lunch and what you'll be having.

If you figure you won't have a wide enough scope of alternatives to make a solid, low-calorie decision, then put together your lunch. No reasons. The equivalent goes for your midmorning and mid-afternoon snacks.

CHAPTER ELEVEN
ARRANGING TRIPS TO THE SUPERMARKET

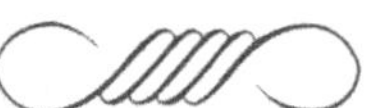

Dietitians gauge that 40 percent of store purchases are made on motivation. Now and then, you'll need to examine food marks at the store to settle on the better decision between two things, yet the entirety of your significant purchasing choices ought to be made ahead of time. Follow my shopping tips below, and you'll turn out each time with low-calorie, high food that draws you nearer to your objectives. Ensure you shop from a list.

Shopping records are anything but difficult to make by utilizing everyday menu designs and including the provisions required for seven days of menus. When you have your list, stay with it. As indicated by New York University sustenance teacher Marion Nestle, 70 percent of customers carry records into the grocery store; however, just around 10 percent stick to them.

- Try not to shop when hungry. I'm certain you've heard this counsel previously, yet do you heed to it?

- Never shop on an unfilled stomach.

- Be aware of your physical and emotional state, also.

- In case you're worn out or upset, you're bound to snatch low quality food on motivation.

- Shop rapidly. Did you realize that general stores play downtempo music to impact you to shop all the more gradually? It's valid. If you wait longer, you purchase more. Rather, with a list close by, perceive how quick you can hurdle through the store. It helps if you shop during off-top hours when there are no groups and shorter lines.

- Do the greater part of your shopping in the aisles of the store. 80% of the foods you'll need to eat all the time can be found on the outskirts of the store: natural products, vegetables, servings of mixed greens, potatoes, yams, lean meats, fish, fish, dairy items, and eggs. Be careful with food item promoting. In each square inch of the store, you're being advertised to always. Food organizations pay for prime areas on the racks.

- Watch out for craving animating colors, for example, red, orange, and yellow are utilized to cause you to notice foods. Adhere to your arrangement and don't be taken in by promoting, including wellbeing and weight reduction claims. Eat generally foods with one fixing and no name. 80% of the foods you eat every day will come without a mark (think products of the soil).

- If they have a mark, they'll normally have just a single fixing, as on account of lean meats, fish, eggs, or antiquated cereal.

- Become a specialist at checking the names.

- Prior to eating anything in a crate, can, or bundle, read the mark cautiously.

- Reduce the quantity of white flour or any refined sugars; for example, sucrose or high-fructose corn syrup, are high on the list.

- Do likewise if the fixings incorporate trans-unsaturated fats or synthetic substances with names you can't articulate. Additionally, observe the calories, serving size, and fiber sum. Watch for name escape clauses. As indicated by food naming laws, if there's not exactly a large portion of a gram of fat, the mark can say "fat-free." If there are less than five calories for every serving, the name can say "zero calories." Food organizations exploit these escape clauses by contracting their serving sizes. For instance, a run of the mill nonstick cooking shower will say "calorie-free" on the name, yet cooking splash is 100 percent oil. How would they pull off it? The serving size is a 33% of-a-second shower. Oppose drive buys at the register. Indeed, even as you're looking, regardless, you're being showcased too. Pretty much every checkout path has treats and soft drink inside arm's lengths.

- Shop for food supplies on the web. A study distributed in the International Journal of Behavioral Nutrition and Physical Activity found that individuals on fat loss programs who requested their staple goods utilizing on the web conveyance administrations bought 28 percent less calorie-thick foods than individuals who shopped in the grocery store.

ANTICIPATING RESTAURANT EATING

If there's one huge error that is bound to disrupt your program, it's making awful decisions at cafés. In many investigations, eating every now and again in eateries corresponds to the higher muscle to fat ratio. Everything bodes well when you take a look at how things have changed in the previous few years. In 1955, Americans burned through 19 percent of their food spending plan on dinners arranged outside the home. Today that number has dramatically increased to 41 percent.

The quantity of individuals now overweight has dramatically

increased with it. Stoutness has significantly increased. As indicated by the U.S. Branch of Agriculture, $222 billion is gone through consistently at cafés and $118 billion of that at drive-thru eateries. The huge issue: unhealthy dinners, to a limited extent, because of expanding segment sizes. Numerous ordinary café suppers contain 1,000 calories or more in principle course alone. If you incorporate a tidbit and treat, that could include at least 1,000. One cut of cheesecake can have 700 calories. Cheddar nachos or seared mozzarella sticks have around 800 calories, the "ordinary" servings that is. As indicated by a report in Men's Health magazine, the most noticeably awful nachos checked in at 2,740 calories. A run of the mill steakhouse prime rib or porterhouse could without much of a stretch fall in the 1,200-to 1,500-calorie extend. Suppose you had hors d'oeuvres, fries, sweet, and beverages with that. The National Restaurant Association reports that the normal individual eats out 4.2 times each week. With that recurrence, if you picked any of these "calorie bombs" each time you ate out, it would totally undermine each nutritious handcrafted supper you ate and all that you did in the rec center throughout the entire week.

Obviously, I understand that telling individuals they can't eat in cafés won't make me extremely well known, so my progressively moderate idea is essentially to downplay eatery eating. One of the qualities I've found in most of the lean individuals is that they like to keep tighter command over their wholesome admission by making their very own large portion suppers. If the national normal is four café dinners for every week and you don't need a normal individual's body, then don't do what normal individuals do. Do what lean individuals do. Keep eating at the cafe a few times each week and settle on the correct decisions when you're there. Notwithstanding how regularly you feast out, you need to instruct yourself about the healthy benefit of eatery food and have an arrangement in advance.

- Start with low-calorie plates of mixed greens rather than fatty hors d'oeuvres.

- Stay away from broiled foods, for example, French fries, onion rings, and calamari.

- Inquire if you don't know how something is readied, particularly about additional sauces, oil, spread, or other shrouded calories.

- Look into menus and calorie data on the web and settle on a sound decision ahead of time.

- If you don't have the foggiest idea of what number of calories are in a dish, don't eat it.

- Pick broiled chicken or fish for lean protein. Pick lean sirloins or filets and get nine-to twelve-ounce cuts or littler.

- Request steamed vegetables as side dishes.

- Request dry heated potatoes, sweet potatoes, or darker rice as sides or part of the primary course.

- Request crisp natural product for dessert.

- Split a customary sweet with a friend.

- Try not to clean your plate—take a doggie pack home with you.

- Eat until you are 80 percent full.

- Never stuff yourself.

- Try not to eat at buffets.

ARRANGING YOUR WEEKENDS

Unless your Saturdays and Sundays follow a similar schedule to what you pursue on weekdays, it's imperative to design your ends of the week ahead of time, particularly your dinners. A study led at Washington University and distributed in the diary Obesity found that adjustments in timetable, dinners, and way of life practices on ends of the week were sufficient to cause weight increase or hinder weight reduction for the whole week. Numerous individuals can't understand why they're not getting results when it appears as though they invest a lot of exertion throughout the entire week.

The appropriate response is that two days of extravagance can fix five days of work. Making arrangements for Holidays, Birthdays, and Special Occasions Planning is likewise instrumental for exploring your way through occasions, birthday events, parties, and other unique events. I accept that these are events where it's superbly suitable to unwind and appreciate the food, family, and fun that are a piece of these unique occasions. Be that as it may, this doesn't mean overeating or tossing all alert to the breeze. Stay away from all-or-none reasoning. You don't need to pick between getting a charge out of the special seasons or remaining lean and solid—you can pick both.

Occasions and other get-togethers can undoubtedly be worked into your 10 percent consistency rule. Be that as it may, when you focus on 90 percent consistency, respect your guarantee to yourself. A typical example, particularly every November and December, is the "I'll start when" mentality. For reasons unknown, three occasions—Thanksgiving, Christmas, and New Year's—some way or another convert into about a month and a half of relentless dietary destruction. It's imperative to place this in a legitimate viewpoint. It's extremely just three days you need to manage.

Truth be told, it's just a couple of suppers. Appreciate the occasion food with some restraint. The remainder of the period it's preparation and nutritious eating, not surprisingly. If you discover yourself saying, "I'll start when I move beyond the special seasons," be cautious, since that sort of reasoning typically reaches out a long ways past January 1, and you'll generally be hoping to begin when conditions are perfect. They never are. Making arrangements for Vacations and Travel: Because you're voyaging doesn't mean you can't pursue your ordinary food and preparing routine. You invest a lot of energy arranging the flight, the vehicle rental, the lodging, and different subtleties of your excursion; why not prepare and food?

Here's the absolute most dominant method I've utilized for health and wellness: each time I travel, I set an objective to return home as fit as when I left. Here are the means by which to do it:

- Get lodging with a kitchen. Numerous inn networks offer rooms with a full kitchen. Or attempt transient loft or condominium rentals. Search the Internet, and you might be amazed at the sort of cabin accessible and now and then at preferable costs over inns.

- Go food shopping following checking in. Subsequent to checking in, make a straight shot to the neighborhood supermarket, shopping list close by. Any place you are on the planet, if you have a kitchen and a well-loaded icebox, your supper arranging and food readiness is very little, not quite the same as when you're home.

- Check the neighborhood eatery menus ahead of time. When you travel, almost certainly, you'll have more café suppers than expected. Utilize all the eatery arranging techniques you adapted before and consistently ponder what you'll eat each time you eat out.

- Prepare various types of foods and pack healthy snacks for drives, flights, and day trips. For long flights and drives, nothing beats convenient dinners and tidbits that you can take with you. You can figure out how to make a variety of compact foods, including various kinds of cereal flapjacks, solid burgers, and sound sandwiches. Traveling, flying, or driving is never a reason for poor eating.

- Work out your exercise plan in advance. Continue utilizing your time organizer or timetable book when you're away from home. Continuously work from a composed arrangement.

- Pick your training area ahead of time. You can do bodyweight practices directly in your lodging. If you like, utilize the Internet to find a rec center before your outing. Bring ahead of time and inquire as to whether there is day by day or week after week rates. Inquire as to whether your inn has an exercise center or an alliance with a nearby fitness center.

If you use an exercise center in your neighborhood, check whether they are associated with different clubs around the nation. Make physical diversion part of your sightseeing plans. On one ongoing excursion, I spent a whole day climbing on the slopes of a wonderful national park. On another, I leased a bicycle and rode for miles along a beach. I've additionally seen other individuals, a significant number of them unfit, tooling around outside on those high-quality bikes. Which would you pick?

THE SUREFIRE WAY TO IMPLEMENT NEW HABITS AND LIFESTYLE CHANGES

There's no chance to get around it—to handle an issue like a muscle to fat ratio, which has such a large number of causes, you should make changes in each aspect of your life. You need to eat better, train reliably, deal with your feelings, change your reasoning, get the help you need, and set up everything together into a solid way of life. In any case, there's extraordinary power in organizing and focusing on the absolute most significant errand at some random time.

Numerous individuals attempt to do excessively, too early. The amazingly roused sorts may pull it off, yet the vast majority who make a plunge and roll out clearing improvements at the same time only dissipate their center, diffuse their endeavors, and end up with a lower achievement rate over the long haul. Another propensity, as a rule, takes around twenty-one sequential days to shape. If you center on each essential objective or conduct change in turn, while keeping everything else in a holding design, you can shape seventeen new propensities in a year.

With this methodology, one year from now, you will be such a changed individual, you'll need a telescope to think back to where you began. Locate your greatest restricting imperative, adhere to the 80-20 principle, and utilize the progressive system to deal with picking the most sensible spots to begin. Every individual has one of a kind qualities and shortcomings, so you'll need to painstakingly pick which territories you need to organize and concentrate on first. Here's one case of how the initial six habit changes may play out.

7. Hit the sack at ten to eleven p.m. sharp, so you get seven to eight hours of value rest.

8. Take up yoga, contemplation, or unwinding activities to help lessen pressure.

9. Start having breakfast each day, which you may have skipped regularly. Attempt regular oats, blueberries, and an egg-white scramble with one entire omega-3 egg.

10. Exchange the leg "conditioning" practices you were accomplishing for weight squats and deadlifts.

11. Quit drinking liquor or lessen to one to two beverages a few times per week.

12. Quit drinking pop and change to water or unsweetened green tea as your essential refreshments.

CHAPTER TWELVE
EATING OUT: STRATEGIES FOR DEALING WITH EMOTIONAL EATING OUTSIDE YOUR HOME

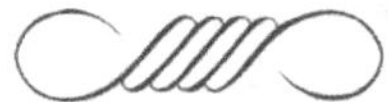

With our fast-paced ways of life, I think individuals now and then eat out more than they eat at home. Eatery and inexpensive food eateries, buffet meals, get-togethers, occasion meals, huge family social occasions, and excursion dinners can become uncommon difficulties for the greater part of us. Why? There are numerous reasons. When we eat out, we see that since we are not responsible for fixings, arrangement, or in small sizes, "feasting out" signifies "getting out" or deserting our food plan. We may get confounded or feel vanquished by the number of decisions we should make when we eat away from home. Lastly, we may make presumptions about what is fitting conduct when we're eating out or even give ourselves authorization to binge.

A few people have not many challenges with eating out, yet they may battle with eating plans at home. Still, other individuals find that they are in charge when they eat at home, yet a gathering or eating out can be shocking for their eating plans.

Regularly, we don't recollect every one of the things that work for us in a period of tumult, when feelings are running high or when our quick paced world stretches us as far as possible. Know about one's self-talk at that time. What are you letting yourself know? Is it accurate to say that you are looking into effective techniques or feeling despair on account of negative considerations? Decide to compose what works in the diary, utilize the diary, and keep mindful and change your self-talk. Work on that self-talk and alter territories of concern. Take 20 seconds to allude to the fitting segment—particularly this segment on eating out—and be set up for all outcomes with the goal that you can stay in charge and be fruitful.

Have an arrangement all set in your mind before you break the flow from your home meal plan. More than once, we have said, "To hell with the arrangement, I'll simply begin once again on Monday." It isn't an alternative—and it is anything but a sensible methodology. You can deal with every one of your difficulties through mindfulness and arranging! In North America, the cafe experience is frequently appraised on the measure of food in singular servings. The pattern has been that the normal client will gripe whenever served a sensible portion, by all accounts dependent on the nature of the food, but on the amount of food on individual plates. You have to prepare when you eat out in eateries. When placing an order, request a smaller part or a half-portion. Lots of eateries will readily do this. If the eatery doesn't agree, request a "take out" compartment to accompany your dinner.

This gives you the chance of passing judgment on your own part size and putting what you won't eat in the holder to bring home. Do this before you dive into the supper, and you will find that you most likely have enough in your holder for another dinner!

The reward: You won't be enticed to binge. A few eateries will guarantee that they don't have littler divides as a choice. However, they will furnish a plate with less food on it—in spite of the fact that they will charge you the maximum. This is really a sensible choice. If you eat the bigger feast, what is the genuine cost you are paying regarding feelings, blame, fault, or disgrace? Is it justified, despite all the trouble to forfeit smart dieting, trouble with your association with food, and to endanger your associations with the ones you love?

Here is a list of systems I have discovered supportive when advising individuals about eating out concerns and difficulties:

- Call the café early and have the menu faxed to you with the goal that you can choose what to arrange early that accommodates your eating plan.

- Pre-order your food to guarantee achievement if you are truly not certain about your capacity to arrange astutely before other individuals.

- Ask your host if it is OK to arrange first, so you are not enticed by what others are requesting.

- When you request, ask how things are readied. Inquire as to whether your request can be broiled or poached rather than fried.

- Order broiled veggies with your supper rather than pasta or pureed potatoes with sauce.

- Be cognizant with regards to requesting food with flavors, cream sauces, or sauces when all is said and done. Request them as an afterthought, so you can control the sum you expend. Simply dunk your fork into the sauce for enhancing as you take a nibble of food.

- Be mindful of requesting food that accompanies serving of mixed greens dressings, nuts, high sodium meats, cheeses, bread 3D squares, nacho platters, olives, and guacamole. Request serving of mixed greens dressings as an afterthought—

dunk your fork in them for enhancing as opposed to pouring them on your plate of mixed greens.

- Offer to part a supper with a friend if it is suitable. Approach your server to bring another side plate with the goal that you can partition the dinner into two segments. Cafés are frequently glad.

- Ask the server beforehand to carry your plate when you are finished.

- When you are finished eating, place your knife and fork on your plate. Treat your plate like a clock: place the knife and fork together with handles at 5 o'clock, indicating 10 o'clock. Push the plate only a couple of inches from you with your thumbs on the edge of the plate to flag you are finished. If you have been utilizing a paper napkin, place it over your plate. (Legitimate behavior implies that you would not do this with fabric napkins; they ought to just be set on the table close to your plate.) These are signals to your server that you are done with your supper.

- • If you decide not to eat the full segments you have been served, inquire as to whether you can have the rest of it to go.

FAST FOOD

Normally, fast-food eateries serve foods that are high in fat, sugar, sodium, and starches. Late drifts in good dieting have incited some fast-food chains to make some solid decisions. Anyway, those things are not as well known, in some cases, sit on the rack for broadened timeframes, some of the time turn sour, and very regularly are immediately supplanted in the menu. Fast food ordinarily keeps to things that are prevalent and sell reliably, for example, high-fat substance burgers, fries, and carbonated refreshments stacked with sugar.

Fast food eateries have additionally experienced esteem in the amount of their food. "Super-sized" suppers can be twofold or even triple the segments of fat, sugar, and sodium that we regularly devour in a whole day! If you decide to go to a fast-food eatery, plan to go to one where you will use sound judgment. One methodology is to arrange a children's feast to exploit the littler size; give the toy to the children. Look on the web and become more acquainted with a few fast food menus, so you know the rates and dietary benefits of their things and can make sense of what will work best for you early — that way, you are set up with a strategy.

Think about all the squandered vitality related to decision making and the squandered vitality if you don't settle on informed choices. The outcomes in your self-talk could be: blame, thrashing on yourself, disgrace, and emotions of loss of control. These emotions could ruin the entire occasion, in addition to influencing your determination to keep up your good dieting arrangement. Relax! Eating fast food is unavoidable—so why not make it pleasant and keen! Settle on shrewd decisions. Select fast food suppers that will fit into your day by day eating plan and keep to your objectives.

This might be simpler than it sounds if you recall thoughts regarding balance. For instance, envision that you enable yourself to have one little request of fries with a broiled chicken burger, mayo as an afterthought, with juice or water to drink. Gradually eat each fry in turn, tasting each nibble, appreciating the supper. Understand that you don't need to complete the fries, realizing you are content with just having 6–8 pieces. Settle on a choice that the remainder of the fries are not worth going short on different foods later in the day. Acknowledge that, although a couple are delicious, they are oily and too salty to even think about eating the whole bit. You realize that eating every one of them may give you an annoyed stomach, and you choose it's not justified, despite any potential benefits to eating them all. Poise implies you decide to be content as you pursue your arrangement and feel glad for yourself. You've put your breathing device on first: you are dealing with yourself and breathing simpler about your association with food.

Well-Being: "It will be awful! I don't have the foggiest idea of what to request to keep on my arrangement!" That is the way it will be. That is the thing that you have let yourself know, in this way you will make it so. Instead, you may state, "I will set myself up early, find out about my decisions, and settle on the best choice for my well-being." That is the thing that you will probably do.

BUFFETS

The scandalous buffet is regularly charged as "Everything YOU CAN EAT!" as though this were the objective of buffet feasting. Some dread the buffet table; some adore it! Regardless of which side you are on, the visual effect of the buffet spread is sometimes overwhelming. The primary thought that strikes a chord concerning decisions was— what decisions are to be made, yet what are the best worth choices. A few people need to get their cash's value. Typically, the last decision to be made is, "Is the thing that on this buffet table solid and does it fit into my eating plan?" Buffets sensibly connect with us in a great deal of self-talk because there is such a significant number of decisions to be made about such a large number of enticing dishes.

Self-talk may be very surprising for every individual, except it regularly comes as a test to our feeling of decency. It doesn't need to be. If you are vexed about the value contrasted with the amount of food you intend to devour, who truly pays? It is safe to say that you are practical or sharp? Examine what is happening in your mind. Be progressively mindful of what you are informing yourself regarding food. Again and again, we have negative self-talk! Consider this. I did when I directed individuals. I would believe that it has cost a few people—in one year alone—3300 dollars to shed 45 pounds. I needed to inquire as to whether they were going to pass up being affected by their negative discussion about their association with food.

They had a decision to make. Is it safe to say they would get every piece of significant worth from an eatery or buffet supper by devouring as much as they could, or would they say they would connect an incentive to the nature of their feasting out? I would regularly transcend their protests and legitimizations by soliciting, "Shouldn't something be said about the cost of your well-being?" If buffets alarm you, don't go to one until you are alright with picking the correct foods and eating as indicated by your eating plan. Cost is extra; accept that you are paying for the experience, not the amount you can eat.

Here are a few methodologies for eating out at a buffet:

- If it is a cooperative choice to go to a buffet, and you are awkward with that decision, inquire as to whether anybody minds heading someplace else. If you feel bolstered, disclose that to the individuals in your gathering.

- Ask if you could meet them at the eatery after they eat. Or state that you are tied up to that point, and you will seek an espresso after.

- If you wind up heading off to the smorgasbord café, request a menu as opposed to picking the smorgasbord alternative. Feel certain of this great decision and maintain a strategic distance from the buffet table.

- Ask to be situated far away from the smorgasbord. If the smorgasbord is in somebody's home, sit far away from the smorgasbord table.

- If you decide to participate in the smorgasbord, study the spread for savvy decisions and furthermore for thoughts that will advance your prosperity. Adhere to your arrangement.

- Tell yourself that the foods on a smorgasbord table consistently look obviously superior to the taste. In reality, this is likely obvious because the foods are set up in enormous amounts and kept warm or cold for quite a long time as opposed to being readied new for singular plates.

- Choose a littler plate if you can. If a littler plate isn't accessible, then remain inside the inward ring of the supper plate and don't put any food past that edge.

- Have a little soup to begin or an enormous serving of mixed greens.

- Have only a spot of what you might want to attempt. When you place the food on your plate, orchestrate it with the goal that foods don't contact one another.

- Take your time. Plunk down and make the most of your food. Taste each bite; appreciate the organization.

- Have an organic product for dessert.

- Share a sugary pastry. If you should, however, have only a couple of nibbles. Appreciate them. Enjoy the flavors. Enable yourself to have the taste without overindulging.

- When you are finished eating, place your knife and fork on the plate and cover your plate with your paper napkin. Move the plate away from you two or three inches. This flags you are done eating and a server can expel your plate.

- Resist the compulsion to return to the table for quite a long time.

Be straightforward with yourself about your eating design and be in charge. Relax!

GET-TOGETHERS

In many societies, numerous get-togethers are associated with foods. In your home, at work, and around your companions, you may feel responsible for your food. However, get-togethers may show an entire diverse arrangement of difficulties for you. Weddings, organization feasts, mixed drink parties, potlucks, retirement festivities, leaving parties, political meetings, craftsmanship opening gatherings, and church picnics are only a couple of instances of get-togethers that frequently serve food. The greatest test is that the food is generally free! My most exceedingly terrible time is "free" food at a gathering, meeting, or at another person's home.

As I examine the food table, I consider new plans, new food thoughts, food sources I don't typically have close by or don't ordinarily eat because they are on my "dangerous foods" list. Like such a significant number of individuals, when I'm in this circumstance, my first thought is that I should top off with free food. I am mindful that, in my school years, this demeanor helped me to increase 15 additional pounds. This is such a notable marvel in new undergrads in Canada and the States that it is regularly alluded to as the "Green bean Fifteen"! I presently realize that "getting my fill" appeared in my midriff! Presently, as a grown-up, I am mindful that at a get-together, I can decide to have one taste of a food and be fulfilled. I have figured out how to move my spotlight and rather focus on the event, the individuals, and the social parts of the occasion as opposed to the food.

Here are some more methodologies that can assist you with concentrating on the occasion and not the food:

- Plan your day when you realize you will go out later. Pack your lunch and snacks prior in the day. Else you will be eager to such an extent that you will try too hard when you get to the occasion.

- Compensate for an event that you realize will be focused on food: plan additional activity and equal out your everyday food admission.

- Ask what will be served, so you realize how to prepare it in time.

- Plan to eat with some restraint and alter your bits as need be. Pick solid foods.

- If you should have a sweet pastry, select one that is your least favorite, so you do not eat a lot of it.

- Ask your host or leader if you may carry a dish to the occasion—make it something that you can fit into your eating plan.

- Do you have a helpful individual with you? Tell that individual early about any food or eating difficulties you hope to experience. Discussion the help you need.

- Show up to the occasion later to maintain a strategic distance from the tidbits. Eat before you go.

- Pre-divide your plate with foods that fit your arrangement and just eat what is on your plate to abstain from picking.

- Focus on the non-food themes and on different visitors.

- Keep a solid beverage in your grasp consistently; make it a full or half-full glass to guarantee nobody inquires as to whether you need a beverage.

- Keep a handbag, or a plate, cutlery, and a napkin in the other hand to shield you from snacking at the food or topping off your plate.

- Keep the discussion going as you avoid the table or the treats.

- Help the hosts by taking empty plates or cups the kitchen to abstain from being enticed to snack at the food contributions.

Here are some close to home instances of procedures I use. As you probably are aware, I love chocolate brownies. However, if they have nuts in them, I am less inclined to eat them and enjoy them. Along these lines, if I have brownies on my very own occasion, I purchase ones with nuts in them. At Halloween, I get the chocolate bars that simply don't taste great to me, so I avoid them. A choice is to plan the get-together to occur at your home. Have a lot of sound options on the menu. Maybe you could get ready just what you know you need to remain on track as opposed to having enticing foods on the menu that are not a piece of your arrangement. Plan to serve a few foods that you enable yourself to eat, so you don't feel denied.

If planning an occasion at your home is excessively unpleasant or is an over the top allurement with food planning, propose that another person have the occasion. Thoroughly consider it—what will be better for you? If you do have the occasion at your home, do you trust you can control things better? Make sense of this. Have an arrangement in any case. Here are some self-disclosure journaling questions that may assist you with seeing progressively about your association with food at get-togethers.

HOLIDAYS AND FAMILY FESTIVITIES

Holidays can be a challenge for us all. There is one holiday for each month in America—and maybe more if we incorporate strict and ethnic occasions. For some families, occasions, for example, weddings, commemorations, birthday events, and reunions are events celebrated with food. Thus, with regards to eating out, at any rate once per month, we have the chance to be tested in the good dieting division. Where do we start? You have to tune in to your positive self-talk, know, prepare, have techniques set up and inhale each day—or you could be in a tough situation. Possibly you sense that you are now in a tough situation. It's OK—take it each day in turn, and you can deal with these events. Your packed food schedule didn't occur without any forethought. Be caring to yourself and work through this diary; keep it with you and use it! Take the entirety of your systems for eating out and apply them to holiday and family festivities too.

Plan ahead and choose what you will do together, not to try too hard. On the event, ensure you have a sample of everything if you wish. Simply don't surpass your everyday food consumption plan. Maybe you have a most loved occasion or family food. Appreciate it, however, balance it inside your day or choose to practice more to redress. Discover some help, focus on partition size, tune in to your self-talk, and change it if essential. Hold returning to mindfulness and your systems. Remind yourself about your objectives, why you need to be sound.

GET-AWAYS

Being away from home resembles eating out three times each day, so survey your techniques in this part, "Why You Eat." When you are on an excursion, utilize a meal plan that ensures you remain a similar weight or keep up your weight. Be savvy, healthy, be sound, and be effective! How and what would you be able to design? Here are some explicit get-away techniques to increase the ones we have just secured:

- Plan ahead and find out about the foods that are in your movement region.

- Be safe with foods! Counsel your nearby trip specialist and your well-being facility about risky foods in underdeveloped nations.

- On the street, bring a cooler and fill it with healthy food and snacks–organic product, squeeze, and hacked up veggies.

- When in an inn or motel, approach early for a kitchenette; inquire as to whether your room has a microwave and cooler.

- At your goal, go to prescribed nearby food markets for sound tidbits and feast fixings.

- Ask if the kitchen in your inn, motel, or resort highlights solid menu options.

- Eat with some restraint

EMOTIONALLY SUPPORTIVE NETWORKS: GETTING ENOUGH AIR

Having individuals who bolster you is significant with regard to your weight, the executives, and dealing with yourself. This emotionally supportive network gives positive consolation while simultaneously keeping you responsible. Here are a couple of general thoughts regarding how emotionally supportive networks work. Individuals in your care group ask how they can best help you in the challenges you face with eating and food. Bolster individuals don't chasten you or treat you gravely when you have had an awful food experience; rather, they tune in, offer proposals, and ask how they can help you later.

At different occasions, you may require your care partners to be firmer with you than on different occasions. Be clear with them ahead of time that you depend on them to help you in specific manners and not in others—speak with them and reveal to them what you need. Together, you and your care partners can have any kind of effect. Try not to control your helpful individuals. They are there for you. I realize it can happen because I have done it—I've controlled somebody who was attempting to help me so as to get what I needed temporarily. Luckily, it didn't work since I could have endangered my objectives to practice good eating habits.

Monitor what works for you. Every individual has an alternate approach, and every individual has various needs. Some like help to be conveyed delicately, however solidly; others acknowledge productive encounters, inspirational talk, and fervor. Still, others favor severe support. You choose what you need right now and be adaptable enough to transform it as your needs change.

SUPPORT FROM HOME

Specifically, our home support depends on the individuals who live with us and are generally acquainted with our needs and difficulties. If your emotionally supportive network is comprised of relatives or individuals who live with you and are not exactly alluring, it is imperative to chat with these individuals. Tell them how glad it would make you if you had somebody on your side to help you. If you have individuals who need to be on your help group, but are really are out to attack your prosperity, you might need to constrain your time with those individuals until you feel less enticed to bargain your arrangement and increasingly enabled to stay with it.

Maybe you live without anyone else. Who else could give home help? A few thoughts for help individuals who don't live with you but who know about your home life may be a nearby family member, a companion or colleague, a parent or kin, your neighbor, a rec center accomplice, your fitness coach or weight reduction advocate, or your chiropractor or specialist.

Here are a couple of ways your home emotionally supportive network can work successfully:

- When you are enticed to have foods that are not part of your program, food sources that you have distinguished as being hazardous, or if you figure you may start to gorge on food, your help people will be aware of those perils and inquire as to whether they can do or say whatever would assist you with moving beyond this scene. For instance, they may help with an interruption system to assist you with forgetting about food.

- When you feel enticed by foods, converse with your helpful individual immediately and request that the person help you. Try not to anticipate that that individual should think about what you are thinking or police everything you might do.

- Ask your help individuals to move high-hazard foods to a zone you are ignorant of or that is difficult for you to reach.

- Suggest that your care partners do not eat high-calorie foods before you, or if nothing else inquire as to whether it OK to eat before you.

- Support individuals ought to be urged to inquire as to whether you need some rousing consolation to deal with your eating program. Maybe they could help you to remember your objective to eat good food, deal with your weight, and not feel caught or worried about your food decisions.

SUPPORT AT WORK

Do you have an emotionally supportive network at work? If you invest a great deal of energy at work, you will require support there similarly as you need at home. If you feel great doing as such, request that individuals at work assist in bolstering your good dieting objectives. Work can be a hazardous situation if there are colleagues or individuals in your work environment who are not on a similar wavelength as you in attempting to practice good eating habits.

Some colleagues or companions will need you to eat as they do with the goal that they don't feel so terrible about what food and well-being decisions they are making. If so, enroll some collaborators to help you. Likely, they will perceive these as difficulties for themselves, and you may find that you will shape a common bolster group. With mindfulness, eagerness, procedures, positive self-talk, and a decent, emotionally supportive network, this could be your key to progress!

At work, your help individual or group is there for you. Like your help individuals at home, these supporters don't chasten you or hate you when you have had a terrible involvement in food. Rather they ask how they can support you. They get you persuaded, keep you propelled, and cheer you on if that is the thing that you need. They remind you how significant your objectives are.

When you are going to eat something that isn't in the arrangement and is unfortunate, speaks with your help individuals: request that they help you, don't simply accept it's their accountability to comprehend what is happening in your mind. Your help individual would then be able to assist you with maintaining a strategic distance from the circumstance. Maybe they will help with one of your interruptions to get you away from food. Perhaps they will help by moving high-chance foods to a territory out of your sight and reach. Your work bolsters individual or group will be delicate to eating high-hazard foods before you. They can investigate with you a few inspirations to keep to your arrangement and objectives to be successful.

If your emotionally supportive network at work is not exactly alluring, maybe it is essential to converse with them. Tell them how glad it would make you if you had somebody on your side to help you. If you have an emotionally supportive network that is out to attack the entirety of your prosperity, you might need to constrain your time with those individuals until you feel progressively good about being around them in circumstances where enticing foods are being served. Keep occupied with work and ventures until you feel increasingly sure about this.

If there are no genuine help applicants in your work environment, attempt other people who could bolster you where you work. Is there somebody that you believe works near your office? Is there somebody that you constantly see during noon? When you do discover some help in your workplace, monitor what works for you. Every individual has an alternate approach, and every individual has various needs. You choose what you need and change it to fit.

Here are a few methodologies that you and your work environment support group can do together to help one another:

- Keep occupied with your work. It is imperative to keep centered and abstain from pondering food.

- Plan your snacks with your breaks; bring solid snacks and snacks from home.

- Always eat from your work area.

- Drink water during the day and have your water bottle full.

- Resist the impulse to keep desserts and snacks on or in your work area.

- Get up and stroll around if you are situated throughout the day!

- Challenge the workplace to choose progressively nutritious tidbits and suppers.

- Switch to more advantageous choices for office birthday, move, or retirement festivities—for instance, attempt a natural product flan as opposed to a chunk cake with thick icing.

- Ask if the sound tidbits can be placed in one organizer and less nutritious bites sorted out in another cabinet that you won't go into.

- Get the workplace roused to begin strolling at noon.

- Encourage others to pursue your propensity for taking the stairs as opposed to the lift.

If your working environment doesn't present specific difficulties—that is incredible—however, imagine a scenario in which you move to a new position in an alternate office or even to an alternate organization. You could wind up in an alternate working environment dynamic later. I suggest that, regardless, you answer the inquiries beneath in this diary, move a portion of those plans to your Journal, and afterward occasionally, particularly if your work environment changes, survey what is essential to you and what works. You may decide to impart a portion of these plans to your work environment, or if you have framed a shared help group, you may jump at the chance to examine a portion of these thoughts together.

If they feel that it is sheltered to do as such, a few people will converse with the individual who is persistently pushing food and clarify that this conduct might be hazardous for others attempting to control their food consumption. To evade that individual, you can eat in an alternate zone, make outside lunch arrangements, or get things done outside the workplace. If an experience is unavoidable, consistently be lovely to the food pusher. For instance, when I wound up in an office with an individual who was continually pushing food on others, I kept my plate loaded with solid food sources and pleasantly stated, "Not this time—I have something as of now."

Much the same as the systems you use at home, interruption strategies can be essential to assist you with enticing or testing foods and food circumstances at work. Contingent upon your particular work, you may have the option to fit a portion of these interruptions into your workday. Here are five classifications that may support you:

6. Things that should be possible rapidly during work:

   - Take a restroom break. Enjoy your reprieve early and appreciate the nibble you arranged.

   - If you are responsible for reusing and need to clear the little containers, do it now.

   - If you have to go to verify the mail or drop something in another office, do it now.

7. Busy exercises during work—things that will absolutely remove your psyche from food or occupy a ton of time:

   - Engage in any venture that requires close scrupulousness.

   - Set a motivation for your next gathering or review the minutes from the last gathering.

   - Work on your yearly report.

   - Contact customers.

8. Things you can do on breaks at work:

- • Go for a walk.

- • Walk the stairs.

-

- • Run a task.

- • Balance your checkbook.

9. Things that are unwinding during breaks:

- • Take a breather outside.

- • Go into the meeting room if it's empty and unwind.

- • File your nails.

- • Go to your vehicle for a rest and have somebody call you in a short time after your break is finished.

10. Things you can do with others or with others around you:

- • Plan the workplace softball match-up.

- • Plan the staff BBQ.

- • Organize the following office philanthropy occasion.

- • Start an office book club, sports lottery, or class arrangement.

When you have a challenge with food and eating at work, choose which classification will fit into your work routine. Select one of the exercises to finish, and if you need more interruption, then proceed with choosing another action. You may find that you can consider just a couple of interruption classifications in view of the sort of work that you do. Maybe your classifications are, for the most part, fit to exercises that you can do during snacks or breaks. That is fine—simply record pragmatic interruption techniques that fit you and your work environment. If you telecommute, you will have some extraordinary interruption thoughts from those you would have in an increasingly traditional office circumstance. Whatever your work environment, if food and food circumstances are a test, be set up to plan your very own interruption classifications. This strategy works! You will occupy yourself from considering food so you can continue ahead with your work—and conceivably proceed onward to greater and better things.

COMPANIONS AND SUPPORT

Companions can be an extraordinary help—or they can be an issue. A few companions can be exceptionally strong, while different companions can need you to remain unfortunate, so they have somebody to be undesirable with. Try not to confuse support with compassion. Try not to believe that, by sharing food, you are getting support; you could wind up becoming involved with another person's pity party. That isn't the target. If you get great help from companions and are a decent help to other people, you would be shocked how well you will do. I comprehend there will be days that you won't give or get impeccable help; however, quiet yourself at the time and consider your self-talk. Gain power by utilizing your Distraction Techniques. Remind yourself why it is imperative to be solid. Get support from companions and, thus, be a mentor and an incredible model! If your emotionally supportive network is not exactly attractive, maybe it is significant in any event to converse with your companions and let them realize how glad it would make you if you had somebody on your side to help you in arriving at your objectives. If you feel that your companions may unknowingly or incidentally damage the entirety of your endeavors to control your food admission, you might need to constrain your time with them until you feel progressively great around circumstances where you might be enticed to surrender your program. Try not to control companions' help. They are there for you. More than family or work connections, companions might be the most powerless to our controls on the grounds that, out of kinship, they need to satisfy us and not feel they have over-ventured the limits of good kinship. There are uncommon difficulties in requesting that companions bolster you—be delicate and know about them! Yet, additionally, know about the endowment of a companion's help; it might be the most valuable blessing you claim or can give. Do you and companions consistently assemble around food? When you are with companions, keep occupied with exercises and activities that don't include food until you feel progressively sure of remaining in charge. Plan getting together after supper or for espresso. Make the most of your kinships, yet additionally, recall the agony related to eating undesirably as opposed to breathing simpler about your association with food. Keep your fellowships invigorating and steady!

IN CONCLUSION

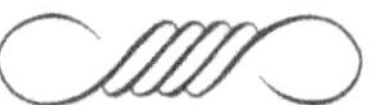

Here are a couple of definite instances of techniques and indications to support you on your voyage to a healthy wellbeing while successfully managing emotional eating:

- Unless you have a lot of weight to lose and you can't traverse with the dress you have, hold on to purchase smaller attire until you arrive at your objective.

- Alter some exemplary pieces you effectively possess until you accomplish your objective weight, or relying upon how a lot of weight you intend to lose, purchase just a couple of outfits to endure this progress time until you arrive at your objective.

- Get free of your bigger apparel. Give the garments or put them in a recycled shop or transfer store. Get a portion of your garments there too—you may locate some awesome outfits there while you change to your objective weight!

- For inspiration, experience your wardrobe and compose your garments from the biggest size to the littlest size. Mess around with your storeroom as you progress through the sizes from enormous to little. Make certain vestments small objectives.

- Hang outfits that you are practically prepared to fit into before your room entryway, so you physically need to stroll past them in the first part of the day and night. These "objective outfits" will help you to remember what you are doing.

- Write notes containing positive self-talk and certifiable articulations. Stick them everywhere throughout the house to remind yourself about your objectives. Compose your objectives on the notes too.

- Wear marginally more tightly fitting garments to remind you all the time that you have to eat better to quit being awkward. Indeed, even go to the extraordinary of putting on a somewhat tight swimming outfit under your apparel for the day to keep you propelled. When you get too agreeable is the point at which you are bound to eat inaccurately. This is works, however!

- Picture yourself 5 or 10 pounds lighter—or 20 pounds lighter! Go to the supermarket and buy a 5, 10, or 20-pound pack of potatoes and put them in a knapsack. If your back will permit it, convey this potato-filled pack around for a day. Feel the help by the day's end when you remove that rucksack. See what shedding those pounds can feel like? Pounds not lost distinctly to be found once more—you've freed yourself of those pounds for good!

- Visualize yourself in your ideal weight. What will your body feel like at that point? Your body will feel extraordinary. Indeed, even 10 pounds has an effect. Thus, eating great and doing activities will make you feel much improved. If you are keeping up your objective weight. Imagine your feeling of success as an individual who can smile at your relationship with food.

Motivation, amazing thoughts, positive energy, and a general feeling of well-being are the prizes of utilizing the Strategies and techniques delineated in this book. You just have to envision yourself at your objective weight and realize that you are the creator of your own success story. By what means will your apparel fit? What will it feel like to settle on healthy food choices? How empowering is it to feel that you are not just settling on savvy decisions with regards to food and eating, yet that these are your decisions! Don't give up! Don't relent! I will be cheering and rooting for you!